Dear Alyssa

It has been a pleasure to meet you
and work with you over the past three weeks.

Thank you for your participation and
contributions to our work and on behalf
of all of us at IEH, best wishes in
all that is ahead ... travel safe

Michael Ryan
17 March 2020

and the IEH team
University of Melbourne

TRACHOMA

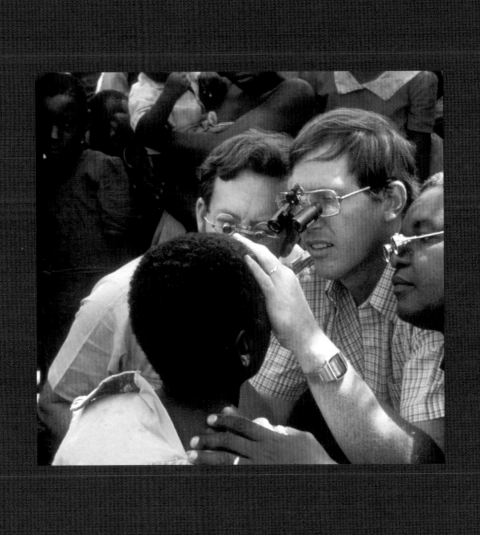

TRACHOMA

A BLINDING SCOURGE
FROM THE BRONZE AGE TO
THE TWENTY-FIRST CENTURY

Hugh R Taylor

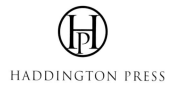

HADDINGTON PRESS

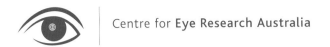
Centre for **Eye Research Australia**

First published in 2008 by Centre for Eye Research Australia
32 Gisborne Street, East Melbourne, Victoria 3002, Australia
Phone: (61 3) 9929 8360
Fax: (61 3) 9662 3859
Email: cera-info@unimelb.edu.au
Website: www.cera.org.au

Produced by Haddington Press Pty Ltd
Box 3182, Domain Road P.O., South Yarra, Victoria 3141, Australia
Phone: (61 3) 9866 2758
Fax: (61 3) 9866 2751
Email: haddingtonpress@bigpond.com
Website: www.haddingtonpress.com.au

The National Library of Australia Cataloguing-in-Publication entry:

Author:	Taylor, Hugh R.
Title:	Trachoma : a blinding scourge from the Bronze Age to the twenty-first century / author, Hugh R Taylor
Publisher:	East Melbourne, Vic. : Centre for Eye Research Australia, 2008.
ISBN:	9780975769591 (hbk.)
Notes:	Includes index.
Subjects:	Trachoma Trachoma–History Eye–Diseases. Blindness–Prevention Eye–Care and hygiene.
Dewey Number:	617.7

Text and cover design by Andrew Cunningham – Studio Pazzo
Printed by Everbest in China

10 9 8 7 6 5 4 3 2 1

Trachoma painting on front cover: courtesy, Jennifer Summerfield and the Nganampa Health Art Collection, permanent display in the Umuwa office of Nganampa Health, via Alice Springs, Northern Territory, Australia; photograph of painting courtesy, Cyndi Cole. The painting is by Jennifer Summerfield, an assistant health educator of Nganampa Health Council, South Australia and is used as a health promotion instrument. The pupil of the eye represents the instructor, while the iris represents Umuwa, the administrative and training centre. The eyelashes represent the Aboriginal Health Workers learning about trachoma and general eye health. The footprints represent the health workers returning to their communities symbolised by a flower shape in each corner. The flower petals represent members of the community surrounding the health workers who are discussing trachoma and its prevention in their communities. The smaller eyes represent blind and painful eyes and the white dots signify trachoma follicles. The elongated thin "worm-like" structures represent the varying degrees of scarring tissue in the tarsal conjunctiva. Somewhat hidden toward the corners are acronyms used for different stages of the disease.

Photograph on page 16: reprinted from Survey of Ophthalmology, 47, Allen SK, Semba RD, The Trachoma "Menace" in the United States, 1897 to 1960, 500–9 © 2002, with permission from Elsevier.

Photograph on page 88: courtesy, Michael Ward.

DEDICATION

To Liz

Trachoma, and the efforts to control it, make a terrific tale. Dr. Hugh Taylor is just the person to tell it. Dr. Taylor is probably the most influential expert in the field, and certainly the most tireless advocate for the WHO's elimination program. The book is a comprehensive *tour de force*—the story spans centuries from the pharaohs to 2020, and from the laboratory to rural villages. What's more, it reads well ...

TOM LIETMAN
F.I. PROCTOR FOUNDATION, UNIVERSITY OF CALIFORNIA, SAN FRANCISCO

Trachoma is a neglected, often blinding disease, of antiquity, common in neglected people. Hugh Taylor relates very poignantly the story, full of pathos, of the long battle to eliminate blindness from this scourge, from the face of the earth. He shows us that there is light at the end of the tunnel, with victory in sight.

R PARARAJASEGARAM
FORMER PRESIDENT, INTERNATIONAL AGENCY FOR THE PREVENTION OF BLINDNESS
CONSULTANT, WORLD HEALTH ORGANIZATION

This is a unique book, which gives a very comprehensive and detailed insight into trachoma and its control. The history, impact and pathogenesis of trachoma, along with the clinical and epidemiological aspects of the disease, are covered in an excellent way, with numerous valuable references; the same goes for the overview of the evolution of trachoma classification systems, and a very didactic section on modern diagnostic techniques. The author also discusses many scientific and programmatic matters, often based on his vast field experience. A very valuable reference book for all those who want to learn much more about trachoma and its control.

BJORN THYLEFORS
FORMER DIRECTOR, PROGRAMME FOR THE PREVENTION OF BLINDNESS, WORLD HEALTH ORGANIZATION

I am delighted to stress the importance of this book that adopts a comprehensive approach to stress the very special nature of trachoma, a disease that shifted from a global threat to a marker of poverty.

SERGE RESNIKOFF
COORDINATOR, CHRONIC DISEASES PREVENTION & MANAGEMENT
WORLD HEALTH ORGANIZATION

This book on trachoma is a great work. I believe it is an important milestone in the study of trachoma. In recent years many people speak about trachoma but often know very little about the disease. I do hope this book will become an important reference for all.

K KONYAMA
DEPARTMENT OF OPHTHALMOLOGY
JUNTENDO UNIVERSITY SCHOOL OF MEDICINE, TOKYO

This book, by a leading ophthalmologist who has devoted more than 30 years to research on trachoma, is the first monograph on trachoma—the leading infectious cause of blindness—to have been published since the 1960's. It includes a fascinating account of the history of this ancient disease, detailed descriptions of its clinical features, pathogenesis and treatment, and a critical review of strategies for its control. It looks forward to the prospects for its elimination as a cause of blindness by the year 2020, as proposed by a Global Alliance convened by the World Health Organization. It will be of interest to ophthalmologists, public health and infectious diseases specialists, and all those interested in the history of medicine and the control of infectious diseases.

DAVID MABEY
LONDON SCHOOL OF HYGIENE & TROPICAL MEDICINE.

Among the infectious causes of blindness, trachoma continues to be the leading contributor globally and there is no single source of information on this important subject that is current. This monograph by Hugh Taylor fills this void and should immediately find a niche for itself. The author's background and wide experience in trachoma makes him uniquely qualified to undertake this onerous task, which he has completed most efficiently and elegantly. This is a "must" for all ophthalmology and public health libraries as well as for all professionals involved in the fight against trachoma globally. This book will remain a magnum opus on trachoma for many years to come.

GN RAO
PRESIDENT, INTERNATIONAL AGENCY FOR THE PREVENTION OF BLINDNESS
CHAIRMAN, VISION 2020

This book sheds light on the past, present and future of trachoma control. Professor Taylor has been involved in the front line of trachoma control, and represents a perfect blend of basic researcher and public health officer, ideally placed to successfully deliver the fascinating story of trachoma across decades and countries.

SILVIO P MARIOTTI
COORDINATOR, GLOBAL ALLIANCE AGAINST TRACHOMA,
WORLD HEALTH ORGANIZATION

This book is the most comprehensive review of trachoma, a disease that has afflicted mankind for centuries and which continues to cause disabling blindness throughout many countries of the world. Dr. Hugh Taylor captures the history of this disease and the advances that have been made over the years in diagnosis, treatment, and control. The book objectively reviews what is known about the epidemiology and pathogenesis of trachoma and how we can utilize effective interventions including advancements in diagnosis and treatment to limit its spread. This book will become a classic for all scientists and clinicians in helping achieve WHO's plans for trachoma elimination by 2020.

THOMAS QUINN
DIRECTOR, JOHNS HOPKINS CENTER FOR GLOBAL HEALTH

About the author

HUGH RINGLAND TAYLOR, AC, was born in Melbourne and trained in ophthalmology. After first working on trachoma with the late Fred Hollows, he became a faculty member of the Johns Hopkins University where he conducted pioneering studies on trachoma and other causes of blindness over 13 years. In 1990, he became the Ringland Anderson Professor of Ophthalmology at the University of Melbourne, and later the founding director of the Centre for Eye Research Australia (CERA). In 2008, he became the Harold Mitchell Professor of Indigenous Eye Health at the University of Melbourne. He has studied trachoma in five continents for over 30 years, advised the World Health Organization and served the International Agency for the Prevention of Blindness, Vision 2020 and the International Council of Ophthalmology. He is Australia's most published ophthalmologist with more than 650 scientific papers, 16 books and over 60 book chapters. He was appointed a Companion of the Order of Australia (AC) in 2001. He and his wife Elizabeth have four children and three grandchildren.

Foreword

TRACHOMA IS AN ancient disease and has long been a major cause of ocular discomfort and visual disability and blindness. It was once prevalent around the globe. Indeed, the right of passage most feared by would-be immigrants to the United States at the turn of the 20th century was their eye examination on Ellis Island—evidence of active trachoma precluded their entry.

Happily, trachoma has receded from most wealthy countries, presumably with improvements in living standards, particularly better hygiene practices. But it remains prevalent among the economically "bottom billion". As Professor Taylor points out, trachoma still remains a significant problem in many Aboriginal communities in the Australian outback.

Research during the past four decades has shed important new insights into the reasons trachoma persists among the poor—and given the world a proven intervention, SAFE ("Surgery for trichiasis, Antibiotics, Facial cleanliness and Environmental improvement") that properly applied allows populations to leap-frog the poverty trap and control, if not entirely eradicate trachoma as a blinding entity.

Professor Hugh Taylor has spent much of his remarkable career at the center of the trachoma research revolution and played a major role in the development and application of all four components of the SAFE strategy. This authoritative and richly illustrated text, the first full explication on trachoma's origins, consequences and control in decades, is destined to be a classic in the field.

Alfred Sommer MD, MHS
Dean Emeritus and Professor of Ophthalmology,
Epidemiology and International Health
The Johns Hopkins University

Contents

List of figures

List of tables

Acknowledgements

NOWADAYS, IT IS rather bold to write a single-authored book. However, I wanted to cover the field from a single and hopefully, consistent perspective. I am well aware that no one can be fully up-to-date across a field as diverse as trachoma, and that some of my views and opinions are not universally held. To ensure I had not overlooked significant bodies of work or made egregious errors of commission or omission, friends and colleagues have kindly reviewed each chapter to make sure they can be understood, are comprehensive and accurate. I very much want to thank them for their time and thoughts. I greatly valued this input, which in some cases was considerable when I had strayed. In alphabetical order, I want to thank Robin Bailey, Matthew Burton, Gerry Byrne, Ian Clarke, Chan Dawson, Charlotte Gaydos, Tom Grayston, Tom Lietman, Silvio Mariotti, Ramachandra Pararajasegaram, Tom Quinn, Serge Resnikoff, Julius Schachter and Sheila West. I also want to acknowledge the great debt I owe to those colleagues and mentors who have taught me so much over the years including Fred Hollows, Barrie Jones, Bob Prendergast, Art Silverstein, Bjorn Thylefors and Judy Whittum-Hudson. In addition, I want to thank Gabriel Coscas, Chan Dawson, Wallace Foulds, Hu Ailian, Tom Lietman, Claude Michel, Michael Ward, Sheila West and Heathcote Wright who provided photographs and other information. Otherwise the photographs in this book have come from a lifetime collection. I have acknowledged the contribution of others wherever I have known that the photograph was originally given to me by someone else. If I have inadvertently overlooked an acknowledgement, I apologise in advance to my colleague. Similarly, written consent was not obtained from each individual photographed, although verbal consent to take and use the photograph was always obtained.

The bulk of this book was written during a three-month sabbatical at Cambridge University. I want to specifically thank Keith Martin who made that sabbatical possible, Peter and Anne Watson for their wonderful pastoral care and friendship, Monica Mauer and Caroline Ondracek for help with references, Christian Gaetani for help with the figures and, in particular, Judy Carrigan whose unfailing commitment and whose extraordinary and untiring assistance has helped in so many ways from start to finish. I thank and recognise the financial support for the preparation and publication of this book from the University of Melbourne, Christian Blind Mission International, Pfizer Inc. and particularly Noel and Sylvia Alpins. I must also thank and recognise the contribution made by Diane Brown, my editor, Andrew Cunningham, my designer, and Paul McSweeney of Haddington Press. Finally, I must thank my writing companion from the attic who shared so many cups of coffee and walks along the Cam while I was working on the project, and who put up with me and my absences during the previous 30 years while I was off doing trachoma work—my wife Elizabeth.

Hugh R Taylor
Melbourne, December 2007

Summary

THIS BOOK IS a comprehensive review of trachoma, from antiquity through to the present, with predictions about the future elimination of this ancient blinding scourge. Known since Pharaonic times, this infectious cause of blindness has been targeted by the World Health Organizaton (WHO) for elimination by 2020. Currently 84 million children in 56 countries are affected and 1.5 million adults are blinded by trachoma.

Trachoma: A Blinding Scourge from the Bronze Age to the Twenty-first Century reviews the historical evolution of our understanding of trachoma, its clinical appearance, its epidemiology, the disease processes involved and the four-pronged SAFE Strategy used to combat the disease.

Introduction

To know trachoma well one must have examined,
treated and followed up thousands of cases
Karl Lindner, 1949

THE YEAR 2007 marks a number of milestones for trachoma. *Chlamydia trachomatis*, the bacterium that causes trachoma, was first identified in 1907 and first cultured in 1957. The World Health Organization (WHO) launched the Global Initiative to Eliminate Blindness from Trachoma (GET 2020) as a public health problem in 1997. Data from 2002 show the number of people who are blind from trachoma is decreasing.

One hundred years ago trachoma was a major problem worldwide. Before then, it had been a major political problem in European countries as a significant cause of infection and disability in troops, and also among the urban poor in slums created by the Industrial Revolution. Trachoma has now been eliminated from most developed regions, but the disease still affects some 84 million people in 56 developing countries.

Although great progress has been made, there is still much work to do to eliminate trachoma as a major blinding disease. Those areas in which trachoma persists are the most difficult to address. Trachoma has been named as one of the major diseases in the new WHO initiative on Neglected Tropical Diseases and its control is closely linked with a number of the Millennium Development Goals. The distribution of azithromycin by Pfizer is a model for successful public–private partnerships, a key strategy for poverty alleviation and disease control promoted by the United Nations (UN) Global Fund.

I am not sure if I live up to Lindner's standards, but in this book I reflect on what I have learnt about trachoma from my experiences, both in the field and the laboratory. I wanted to review findings over the last 30 years and indicate how they have helped us combat the disease. I explore what old information has been rediscovered and what new information has changed the way we understand or deal with trachoma. Were there lessons from the past that we had overlooked? I have also tried to assess whether we were actually making the best use of new knowledge at our disposal.

This approach brings together a diverse range of information about trachoma, from cellular and molecular biology to public health policy, and places this information in a historical context. This is not a simple textbook, nor a technical book on the microbiology or molecular genetics of chlamydia. I have tried to convey an understanding of trachoma that would be useful for those working in the field, and for those responsible for designing, supervising or funding trachoma control activities. By introducing a somewhat broader social and historical context, I hope this book will be of interest to a wider audience working in public health and social development. In addition, it should constitute an important summary of the subject and therefore find a place in the libraries of ophthalmologists and medical schools.

Currently there are no books devoted to trachoma, although chapters on the subject appear regularly in textbooks. The last major book on trachoma published in English is MacCallan's in 1936. Bietti also published a book in English in 1967 that detailed his work on trachoma vaccine development. The WHO has published a series of very useful and important manuals that deal with specific technical or practical aspects of trachoma control, and the quadrennial series of reports presented at international chlamydial meetings is an outstanding source of information.

This book tells the story of trachoma. It starts with the ancient writings and understanding of trachoma. It outlines the explosion of trachoma in Europe associated with the Napoleonic Wars and the Industrial Revolution, and the social impact that trachoma had including the development of specialisation within medicine. The second chapter reviews trachoma in the 20th century, with the development of control programs and the elimination of trachoma from the developed world. The next three chapters review the clinical recognition and grading of trachoma, the laboratory methods for diagnosis and the biology of chlamydia. Chapter six reviews the epidemiology and individual risk factors which highlight facial cleanliness in children as the final common pathway. The next chapter examines the pathology and the importance of cellular immune response and repeated episodes of reinfection. Fifty years of work on trachoma vaccines is then explored in chapter eight, followed by a review of the integrated approach to trachoma control, the SAFE Strategy, including the use of azithromycin. The concluding chapter evaluates the current status of trachoma and its gradual decrease in a number of areas over time. I have tried to complete the circle between specific and targeted interventions and general socioeconomic development. In this final chapter, I also address some of the issues around the persistence of trachoma in Australian Aboriginal communities.

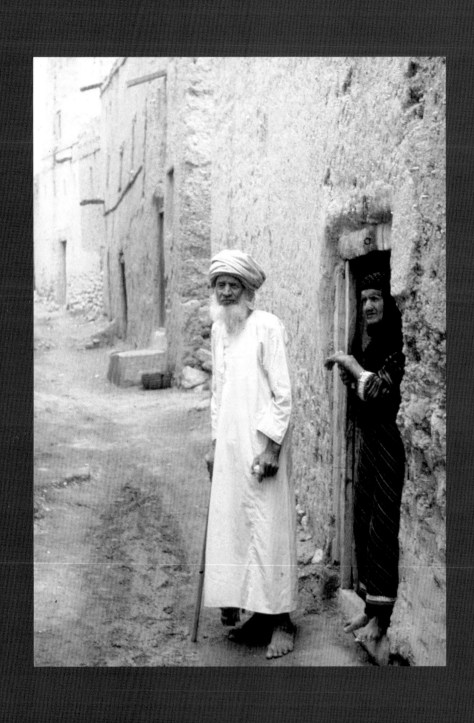

CHAPTER ONE

Trachoma is an ancient disease and a weapon of mass destruction

We have to try hard and to practise,
so that we can describe the past, recognize
the present and predict the future
HIPPOCRATES, 420 BC

HOW MANY TIMES have we read a paper that starts something like this?

Trachoma is a disease that has come with us from antiquity. It is discussed in ancient Egyptian texts, written on papyrus and even in early writings from ancient China. Chronic infection with the organism, *Chlamydia trachomatis*, can lead to blindness. The disease came to prominence in Europe during the Napoleonic Wars when tens of thousands of British and French troops returned with trachoma after fighting in Egypt. It spread rapidly through the armies of Europe where the troops lived in crowded and insanitary barracks (1).

Other papers may start with:

One quarter of all blindness in the world is due either directly or indirectly to trachoma. At present, it affects some 300 to 500 million people, with some seven to 10 million people who are blinded by this disease. Although once common worldwide, over the last century trachoma as a blinding disease has disappeared from most cities and towns of developed countries and today is most commonly found in the poorest arid rural areas of underdeveloped countries. These are the areas where hygiene is the most inadequate (2).

More recent papers may quote figures from the 2002 estimate by the World Health Organization (WHO) of 84 million people with active trachoma and 7.6 million with trichiasis (3).

However, the history and evolution of our understanding of trachoma is more complex and much more interesting. Furthermore, it is important to have an understanding of the evolution of our knowledge of trachoma, as it contains many clues that are relevant to today's efforts to finally eliminate this ancient blinding disease so well described by Hippocrates in 420 BC.

The early history of trachoma

Some have asserted that trachoma first arose in the peoples in Central Asia and then spread eastwards into Asia and westwards into the Middle East and the Mediterranean (4). It seems more likely that trachoma as such was first seen in the early

settlements in Mesopotamia, the so-called "Fertile Crescent". The ocular strains of chlamydia first diverged from the genital strains some two million to five million years ago, about the same time as *Homo habilis* and *Homo erectus* evolved (5) (see Figure 1.1).

The strains of chlamydia that affect other species separated even earlier. The variation within the trachoma biovar of *Chlamydia trachomatis* developed about a million years ago. This shows the very early association of chlamydial ocular infection and human evolution. Human ocular chlamydial infection must have been sufficiently common to allow chlamydia themselves to survive over time and must date back some millions of years. *Homo sapiens* did not evolve until about 120,000 years ago and did not aggregate into large communities until the end of the last Ice Age about 10,000 BC. People aggregated in the earliest settlements and towns that were formed in Mesopotamia. The increased crowding and poor

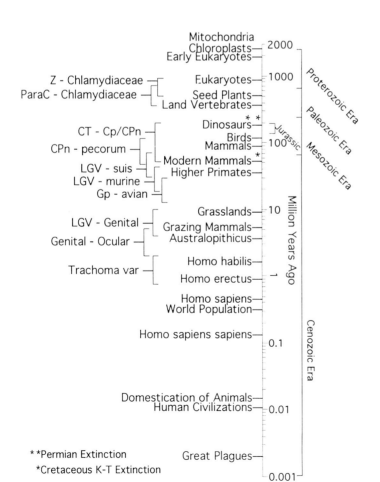

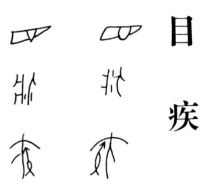

LEFT **Figure 1.1** The evolutionary history of *Chlamydiales* (Stephens 2002 (5); courtesy, Richard Stephens).

ABOVE **Figure 1.2** Transcription of Chang Dynasty (16th to 11th century BC) from Chinese writing on bones. The words "disease" and "eye" have been reproduced by Eugene Chan (Chen Yaozhen) 1981 (8) (© Chinese Medical Journal, reproduced with permission).

hygiene in these early settlements would have been key determinants for the development of what we recognise as trachoma—the endemic blinding disease. Blinding trachoma is seen to be different from occasional episodes of chlamydial inclusion conjunctivitis that still continue to occur around the world, even in the most developed countries.

This early settlement and the historical trade routes that developed westward along the north and south coasts of the Mediterranean and eastward into Asia give plausible means for the "spread" of trachoma that accompanied human agriculture and settlement and the building of houses and villages. Centuries before Christ, trachoma was probably well known and widespread in the four great river valleys that sheltered the development of early civilisations; those of the Yangtze and Hwang Ho in China, the Indus and Ganges in South Asia, the Euphrates and Tigris in the Middle East and the Nile in Egypt (6).

References to trachoma in China date back to the 27th century BC when Emperor Huang Ti Nei Ching had surgery for trichiasis (8). Inscribed animal bones and tortoise shells dating from the 16th to 11th centuries BC include references to a range of eye disorders (8) (see Figure 1.2). However, the earliest specific references to trachoma that could be found by Eugene Chan (Chen Yaozhen 1899–1986), both a great ophthalmologist and a great Chinese scholar, date back to the Northern and Southern Dynasties (420–581 AD). He noted the traditional Chinese terms for trachoma included "pepper-seed-like lesions" and "millet-like granules". Pannus and trichiasis were well known. The use of copper compounds and the rubbing of the lids with octopus bone and garlic were traditional Chinese treatments of great antiquity. Trachoma is also believed to have existed in Sumeria in the Bronze Age and epilation forceps, dating from around 2600 BC, were found in Ur (9) (see Figure 1.3).

Writings attributed to the Indian surgeon Susruta (between 1000 and 500 BC), describe the roughening and thickening of the inner surface of the eyelids as well as the development of trichiasis and entropion (10). Treatment involved scarification followed by a variety of topical medications including ginger, rock salt, honey, sulpharsenic acid and ferrous sulphate. Trichiasis

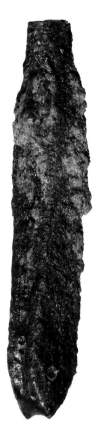

Figure 1.3 Bronze Age epilation forceps from Ur (2600 BC) (© the Trustees of the British Museum).

was treated with either surgical incision of the lid, with everting sutures made of human hair, or cauterisation of the lash follicles.

Julius Hirschberg (1843–1925) wrote an amazing 11 volume history of ophthalmology between 1889 and 1905. Hirschberg was a practising ophthalmologist who lived in Berlin but also travelled widely. He read ancient and modern Greek, Latin, English, French, Italian and Arabic. Frederic Blodi did ophthalmology an enormous service by translating this opus into English (11). This work has provided an enormously rich source of information on the evolution and development of ophthalmology from the earliest records available at the time. It benefits greatly from Hirschberg's ability to read the original documents. He pays particular attention to the two major eye diseases—trachoma and cataract.

Trachoma was common and well recognised in ancient Egypt. The Ebers' papyrus was discovered in Thebes in 1872 by George Ebers. It is the oldest

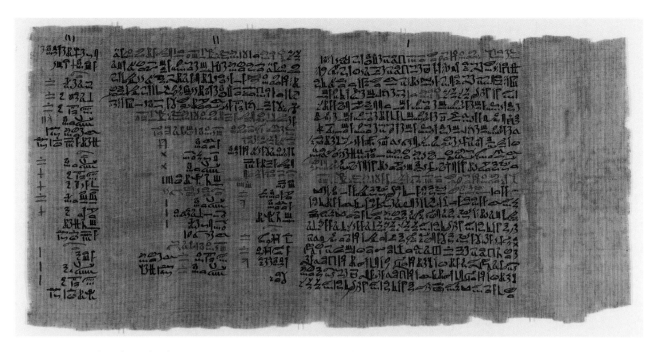

Figure 1.4 A sheet from the Ebers' papyrus (1553–1550 BC) (Papyrus Ebers, Kol. I-III, Universitätsbibliothek Leipzig).

known "book" on medicine and was written in the 18th Dynasty between 1553 and 1550 BC (see Figure 1.4). The papyrus basically contains a collection of prescriptions and only in passing does it mention various diseases by name. It is thought that there were companion volumes on diagnosis and surgery that have not survived. One-tenth of the 700 or so prescriptions in the Ebers' papyrus were to treat eye disease. Much Egyptian medicine was based on topical treatment, a variety of biological products including onions, myrrh and gazelle excrement. These were to be applied to the eye with the feather of a vulture. Blood from lizards or bats was to be applied to the eyelid after epilation, the only surgical procedure mentioned in the papyrus that has survived. Mineral components such as lead sulphate, lead acetate and kohl (made out of soot or finely ground antimony powder) were also applied to the eye. It is interesting to note that many of these remedies are still in traditional use in Egypt today (12).

Epilation forceps have been found in tombs of the New Empire Kingdom (1570–1070 BC) as well as pots containing copper and zinc oxide, and lead and antimony sulphates (4). These pigments are used to make "kohl", a mascara-like substance commonly used to outline the eyes, as well as to treat conjunctivitis. MacCallan also refers to the funeral stele belonging to the earliest known ophthalmologist, Pepi-Ankh Iri, who served the court of the Sixth Dynasty in about 2500 BC.

Although there are many biblical references to eye disease and blindness, trachoma is not specifically mentioned in the bible. However, when St Tobias used fish bile to cure his father Tobit of blindness, he was probably treating trachoma (13,14) (see Figure 1.5). Fish bile and bile from animals was an accepted treatment for trachoma. Goat bile was later used by the Romans to treat trachoma and eel and ox bile were widely advocated to treat eye disease in 16th and 17th century Europe. Sterile isotonic solutions are difficult to make and store and have only become available in the last century. Before then, people used naturally available solutions: blood, urine, breast milk or bile. Their use was widely recommended and practised, although the concepts of sterility and isotonicity were unknown.

Ophthalmia was well known to the Greeks and is referred to in several of the plays written by the Athenian playwright Aristophanes (466–388 BC), including Plutus (388 BC) and the Frogs (405 BC), and in the writings of Plato (427–347 BC). Trachoma became particularly troublesome during the long siege of Athens during the Peloponnesian War (431–414 BC) (15). This was a major war between the two leading states of Greece, Athens and Sparta. It marked the zenith of the power of Athens, the losers. The siege caused the prolonged over-crowding of people within the Athenian city walls.

In the play of the same name, Plutous, the god of wealth, had been blinded by Zeus so he could distribute wealth without prejudice, and not according to merit. Aristophanes' play relates that Asclepius, the god of healing, had tried to restore the vision of Neoclides with an ointment of fig tree sap, garlic, lentisk and vinegar. This ointment was applied to the everted eyelids but it caused considerable pain. Plutous opted for an alternate cure for his blindness and with the help of the daughter of Asclepius, Panaceia, he covered his head with a purple cloth and two snakes emerged from the temple and licked his eyelids and restored his vision.

Plato wrote at length about healthy lifestyles and gave advice as to where one should live to reduce the likelihood of developing ophthalmia. Plato suggested ophthalmia was contagious and Aristotle (384–322 BC) went further and concluded that one could catch trachoma just by looking at someone who was infected. This controversy about the "infectivity" of trachoma flared again in the early 1800s (16) and was not really settled until Pasteur's work in the 1880s led to the identification of bacteria and the establishment of germ theory.

Ophthalmia or trachoma was an important cause of morbidity and vision loss in ancient times. As Hirschberg points out, almost every medical writing that has survived from ancient times included at least some reference to trachoma, its diagnosis or treatment (10).

Hippocrates (460–380 BC) is the earliest of the Greek physicians whose writings are known. There are some 70 books attributed to him and these include descriptions of trachoma, which he termed "ophthalmia" and "lippitudo" (bleary or dripping eye). He recognised the fig-like appearance of the everted upper lid and "trichosis", the term he used for inturned lashes. In *About the Air*, he gave advice to avoid the cold winds from the north which caused severe ophthalmia, as well as the warm south winds which would cause a wet and mild ophthalmia. In one of his famous aphorisms (Aphorism VI 31), he stated that ocular disease can be cured by drinking wine, by bathing, purging, bloodletting, or by a cleansing medication.

Hippocrates describes four eye operations only; three were for trachoma (*About Vision*). The first was for the scarification of the granular

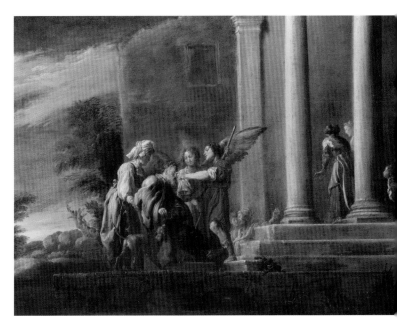

Figure 1.5 Painting by Fetti of St Tobias curing his father's blindness (Fetti, Domenico. Healing of Tobit. The State Hermitage Museum, St Petersburg © The State Hermitage Museum).

conjunctiva, ophthalmoxysis. This procedure used a dense, clean piece of wool wrapped around a wooden stick to scarify the everted tarsal conjunctiva. The abraided surface was then treated with "copper bloom" to form an eschar or scab. Second, if the lids were markedly thickened, Hippocrates recommended the surgical excision of as much of the fleshy granular tissue as possible. This was followed by cauterisation with a heated iron and copper bloom treatment. The third operation Hippocrates described was a suturing method to correct entropion and trichiasis. Two hair sutures were passed through the lid and tied tightly to evert the lid. The sutures would eventually slough out. His last eye operation was an anterior chamber paracentesis to drain a hypopyon. He also advocated local bloodletting by incising the scalp in the parietal area (*Common Diseases*). This led to two millennia of almost tortuous incisions, bloodletting, cupping and leaches variously applied to the temple, scalp and neck.

Aurelius Cornelius Celsus (25 BC to 50 AD), a Greco-Roman physician who lived in Provence, is best known for describing the four cardinal signs of inflammation. He wrote an encyclopaedia of medicine that included descriptions of cataract and trachoma (17). He used the Latin term "aspritudo" for "rough" to describe trachoma and he reiterated the subsequent development of trichiasis:

> This roughness is usually a sequelae of an inflammation. Occasionally it is more advanced, occasionally less developed. Sometimes the roughness results in severe tearing which in itself may increase the roughness. In some patients it lasts only a short time, in others a long time or never disappears at all. In this chronic form some physicians scarify the thickened and hard lids (on the inner surface) with a fig leaf or a rough probe or a knife. The lid should be daily rubbed with medication. This should only be performed in cases of chronic or severe roughness and should not be frequently repeated. The same objective can be better achieved by diet and by appropriate medication. We therefore recommend gymnastics, baths, frequent heating of the eye with warm compresses, the food should be spicy and diluted. As a medication we recommend the imperial collyrium (an ointment made of copper, iron, zinc and antimony) (10).

If an ointment was not available the bile of a goat or very fine honey could be used. The treatment preferred by Celsus for trichiasis was cautery of the lashes with a hot iron needle—ancient "electrolysis". He also recommended several other surgical methods for treating trichiasis including lid surgery using women's hair for sutures.

Pedanius Dioscorides (40–90 AD), a Greek physician originally from Asia Minor but who practised in Rome, was the first to use the Greek word "trachoma" to describe the roughness of everted eyelids. Dioscorides wrote the first pharmacopoeia and describes some 600 medicinal plants. The pharmacopoeia included a wide range of animal, vegetable and mineral products to treat trachoma including copper sulphate fashioned in pencils and the use of a fig leaf to scarify the lid. Treatments ranged from egg white to the ear of a mouse, mother's milk to frogs' blood.

Claudius Galenus (Galen) of Pergamun in Turkey (129–200 AD), a practising physician who also couched for cataracts, built on and extended the work of Hippocrates and provided a comprehensive summary of Greek medical knowledge. His writings were translated into Arabic and ultimately provided the foundation for renaissance medicine in western Europe. His collected works total some 22 volumes, but this also includes material attributed to him and almost certainly written by others (10). In his work on the eye, "De Oculis", the term "trichiasis" is used for the first time and four stages of trachoma are described: psorophthalmia, choma (trachoma), sycosis, tylosis (roughly translated as itch, rough, scarred and trichiasis). These four stages were more fully described by Aetius of Amida (502–575 AD). This staging foreshadows MacCallan's Classification nearly 2000 years later.

With the fall of the Roman Empire, the centre for medical knowledge, and in fact all western learning, moved to Alexandria and its fabled library. Paulus of Aegina (625–690 AD) was a Greek physician who worked in Alexandria at the peak of the Byzantine era. His *Medical Compendium in Seven Books* became the standard Byzantine medical text. He described trachoma as a disease of the inner surface of the lids with four stages, rough (trachoma), fig disease, scarred and trichiasis. Wine and red iron ore were used topically followed by ointment. Cuttlefish bone or a raspatory (lid scraper) were used to smooth out the roughness (18). Trichiasis was treated by the removal of an ellipse of skin by pressure necrosis of a fold of lid skin held tightly between two tied sticks. MacCallan found this method was still commonly used by the Fellahin in Egypt in the 1900s (4) and it is still in use in Oman in the 1980s. Boldt concludes:

> Trachoma even in ancient times was a common and familiar disease, not only in Hellas Proper, and the coasts of Asia Minor, Sicily and Lower Italy, but also in the Hellenic Empire of the Roman Emperors, which embraced the countries bordering on the Mediterranean Sea (15).

The development and spread of Islam from the eighth century led to a flowering of Arabic knowledge and discovery. Arab authors used the term "jarab" (or scabies) to describe trachoma. Between 800 and 1300 AD some 60 textbooks on ophthalmology were written in Arabic (18). Arabic scholars were centred in Baghdad, Cairo and Damascus where specialist eye clinics existed. Other centres included Jerusalem, and Cordoba and Seville in Spain. The authors included

Christians and Jews as well as Muslims.

Honian ibn Is'hag (808–873 AD) (also known as Johannitius), a Christian physician in Baghdad, wrote "The ten treatises of the eye". He was the first to write in detail about pannus or "sabal". The corneal vascularisation in trachoma had not been described by the Greeks or Romans. Arab ophthalmologists such as Al Razi (850–924 AD) (also known as Rhazes) and Ammar ibn Ali Al-mawsili (996–1020) described several different surgical methods to remove pannus. Al Razi remonstrates "in eye inflammation remember to evert the lids and you will find trachoma". He also gave a description of snow blindness and described how the reflection of the sun's rays contributed to this condition (19).

The classic Arabic textbook on ophthalmology was written by Isa ibn Ali (d. 1010 AD, also called Al-Kahhāl, the ophthalmologist). He lived in Baghdad and wrote an encyclopaedic textbook of ophthalmology that survived intact. It was largely based on the extensive Greek writings and was the first systematic textbook of ophthalmology in which the chapters followed an anatomic sequence: each chapter was arranged systematically in which more important and frequent diseases such as trachoma, cataract and conjunctivitis received more attention (18). Probably the most famous of the Arabic writers was the Persian physician and philosopher Ibn Sina (Avicenna) (980–1037) who wrote 450 books, although his description of trachoma is quite cursive (18).

Arabic texts emphasise the important distinction between acute ophthalmia and chronic, blinding trachoma. The "oculists" of the 19th century had forgotten this distinction and this became a point of intensive debate and disagreement (18). Even the First World Health Organization Expert Committee on Trachoma in 1952 argued whether trachoma always had to start with an episode of acute purulent conjunctivitis, or whether it could start insidiously (20). Eventually the Arabic learning and leadership started to wane in the 14th century. At the same time, the Renaissance was gaining strength in southern Europe.

Interesting insights into the management of trachoma come from documentary fragments found in the genzia or storeroom of the Ben Ezra Synagogue in Cairo. These documents were left by ninth to 14th century Jewish doctors and

pharmacists (21). They defined Ramad (trachoma) as having four stages, with the description of sago grains or a cut fig for active trachoma. To treat trichiasis they recommended either epilation or surgery to remove lid skin. There were specialists who only treated eye diseases and who charged three dirhems a week for treatment, although the poor were treated for free.

It had been suggested that St Francis of Assisi (1182–1226) acquired trachoma during the Crusades and became blind as a result (22). St Francis visited Palestine on at least two occasions between 1218 and 1221. By 1223 he was described as having severe trachoma and trichiasis (see Figure 1.6). He was blind when he died in 1226. Many returning crusaders and pilgrims to the Holy Lands may have returned with trachoma which they introduced to Italy and elsewhere in Europe in the 13th century (22).

During and after the Renaissance not much attention was paid to trachoma in Europe:

The clear anatomical definition of granular conjunctivitis used by the ancient Greeks was obscured by the Arabs who used rather unclear descriptions and called the disease also scabies or herpes; only after Napoleon's campaign in Egypt was the Egyptian eye disease again the centre of medical attention. However, due to the epidemics caused by Napoleon's campaign, surgical treatment of trachoma was re-introduced during the first third of the 19th century and dominated the treatment during the last one-third of that century (18).

The first European text on ophthalmology, *Practica Oculorum*, was by Benvenutus Grassus of Jerusalem who worked in a monastery in Salerno, Italy in the late 13th century. Salerno was the first medical school in Christian Europe (7). He

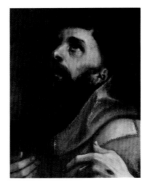

Figure 1.6 St Francis of Assisi (Annibale Carracci c. 1587) (© Ministero per i Beni e le Attività Culturali Soprintendenza Speciale per il Polo Museale Napoletano).

classifies the acute stage of ophthalmia as a sanguine disorder to be treated with herbal remedies. Granular (follicular) trachoma and trichiasis were phlegmatic disorders; the first to be treated with excision of granules followed by the instillation of egg whites and trichiasis by epilation or double armed compression lid sutures (23). Peter the Spaniard (1210–76) also worked in Salerno. He was a Portuguese physician, later Pope John XXI, who wrote *Liber de Oculu*, a reiteration of the works of Galen, translated by Honian ibn Is'hag (7).

European references to trachoma continued to appear in the 14th to 16th centuries including Guy de Chauliac (Avignon 1300–68), Fabricus (Padua 1537–1619) and Ambroise Pare (Paris 1510–90), although in Hirschberg's opinion, they added nothing of value and reiterated previous work, often incorrectly (18). Writings of trachoma also originated from France, Germany, Holland, Spain, Portugal and England (15,24). It is hard to tell which reports actually deal with blinding trachoma and its sequelae as we know it, and which describe the effects of episodes or epidemics of acute or chronic untreated bacterial or viral conjunctivitis.

A number of Europeans who had visited Egypt over the years commented on the presence of ophthalmia. In 1598 Baron Harant of Poljitz, Bohemia commented that the masses of flies on children's eyes were the cause of their frequent eye infections (4). In 1683, the Venetian consul in Cairo, Prospero Alpino, noticed the seasonal epidemics of conjunctivitis that occurred in summer (25). The Frenchman Tourtechot de Grenger labelled Egypt the "land of the blind" after a visit in 1745 (25).

The Egyptian or military ophthalmia

Egypt and eye disease were branded into European consciousness during the Napoleonic Wars (1798–1815), starting with the Battle of the Nile and the Egyptian Campaign (1798–1802). Probably the best review of the devastating epidemics of ocular infections that first occurred amongst European troops in Egypt in the 1800s is given by Max Meyerhof in a presentation to the Royal Society of Medicine in 1931 (26). He recounts how on 1 July 1798 Napoleon Bonaparte landed near Alexandria

with 40,000 French troops and marched to Cairo which he reached on 9 July (see Figure 1.7). During the march through the Egyptian desert in the middle of summer, the troops suffered from delirium and thirst (probable heat stroke), dysentery and night blindness. Without proper protection one must wonder whether there was some component of photokeratitis, "snow blindness" associated with this "night" blindness. Certainly at this early stage in the campaign xerophthalmia is unlikely. After winning the Battle of the Pyramids on 21 July and occupying Cairo, a military hospital had to be established at Giza to accommodate the wounded, those with dysentery, and those with ophthalmia.

By 17 August that year, the soldiers, particularly those on guard duty, were advised to take precautions and protect their eyes during the cooler moist nights, because the humidity was thought to lead to "inflammations of the eyes which without being dangerous, are very troublesome and painful." These initial epidemics of ophthalmia were probably due to infection with the Koch-Weeks bacillus (*Haemophilus aegyptius*) (26).

However, the epidemic of ophthalmia spread rapidly and became more severe by late September. In one battalion, 125 of 350 men had ophthalmia, now complicated by marked lid swelling, chemosis and purulent discharge that together effectively blinded the affected soldiers. Despite their loss of vision, they still had to man the trenches and "their muskets were pointed at the enemy by their comrades whose sight had not been affected." Although self-limited in many cases, other cases persisted for months (26).

An expedition to upper Egypt had to be aborted in October 1798 when 1400 developed ophthalmia from a force of 3000 men. On evacuation "there were more blind men than there were healthy. Every soldier who was able to see or who had only one eye attacked served as a guide for several comrades who had, however, to carry their arms and baggage." Although initially most infections resolved without corneal involvement, by the end of the year many cases became "complicated" with corneal lesions including "specks and staphylomas hypopions and other diseases" (Assalini quoted by Meyerhof (26)). The intense sunlight was thought to be the principal cause of these changes.

On 25 November 1798 Napoleon evacuated 150

amputated or blind soldiers who were forced to land in Sicily, where all were captured or killed. A second convoy of 200 blind soldiers was sent back to France in February 1799. They reached France safely, where some with dense corneal opacities had optical iridectomies that partly restored vision. In Egypt, the ophthalmia subsided during the winter of 1798 to 1799 and was less severe in the following year, when it was overshadowed by epidemics of plague amongst the troops.

The French physicians and military surgeons firmly believed that the ophthalmia was related to the damp, cool evening air in the delta regions—the noxious night vapours—but they also blamed the hot winds blowing from the south. The French rejected the notion that ophthalmia could be contagious. In contradistinction, the English rapidly formed the impression that ophthalmia was transmissible. The argument about whether trachoma was contagious raged until Pasteur's demonstration of the existence of bacteria and the

proof for infectious agents contained in Koch's postulates.

In Egypt, further outbreaks of acute ophthalmia were also experienced by the Turkish Army that initially fought alongside the British, but later fought against them. However, it was the British Army who seemed to suffer most from the Egyptian ophthalmia, and for whom copious documentation exists. After winning the Battle of the Nile, the British Navy blockaded the Egyptian coast from August 1798 to September 1801. The British forces were not affected by ophthalmia until their troops landed outside Alexandria in March 1801; the "sun-glare, dust of the desert and humidity" caused the rapid development of ophthalmia. Even though it was believed that the ophthalmia may initially have been acquired from the "myasm", once established, cases were quickly recognised by British surgeons as being contagious. Edmonston published a comprehensive account of his experience with troops returning from Egypt (27).

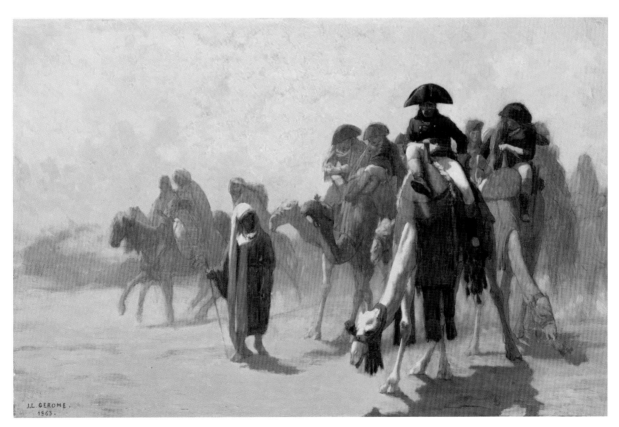

Figure 1.7 Napoleon leading his troops in the desert (Gerome, Jean-Leon 1863. Napoleon in Egypt. The State Hermitage Museum, St Petersburg © The State Hermitage Museum).

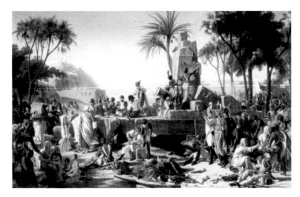

LEFT **Figure 1.8** British troops around an oasis during the Egyptian Campaign (1801–1802).

BELOW **Figure 1.9** Australian troops encamped at Giza in 1915. On the left of Artillery Road are the lines of the first Australian Divisional Artillery and on the right those of the third Infantry Brigade and the divisional engineers behind them (Australian War Memorial, negative number CO1880).

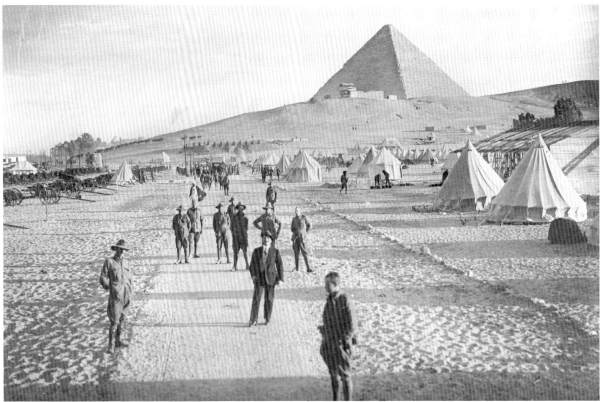

A division of 8000 men from India, half of whom were British and half Indian, had 1600 soldiers develop ophthalmia in September and October 1801 and 158 became blind (26) (see Figure 1.8).

The descriptions of acute purulent conjunctivitis with corneal ulceration and perforation are entirely consistent with seasonal epidemics of gonococcal conjunctivitis more common in Egypt in the latter part of the year. Differences were noted in the relative infrequency with which officers were infected and the need for frequent and careful washing of hands and eyes. Edmonston particularly noted how infection was passed from one soldier to another, especially when they were confined in barracks or in ships quarters when returning to England. Men sleeping in the same bed or even the same room would be infected within 24 hours. It was common practice to have two or even four men share one bunk. However, Edmonston like Aristotle, suggested infection could be contracted just by looking at a case, a view rejected by Vetch (16).

An outbreak of acute conjunctivitis, "Ophthalmia Gibraltariensis", occurred in Gibraltar which was identical to that seen in Egypt. It occurred as troops returned from Egypt and a similar outbreak also occurred in Malta. In both islands ophthalmia rapidly spread to the civilian population. The same thing also occurred in Britain:

> After the peace in May 1802, the regiments were disbanded in England and the soldiers carried the infection with them to the civil population, the lower classes of which did not at the time have such notion of cleanliness ... Ophthalmia appeared at the same time in the most distant parts of Great Britain and that particular modification of it, denominated Egyptian ophthalmia is now (1806!) familiar to almost every medical practitioner ... (Edmonston quoted by Meyerhof (26)).

The Egyptian ophthalmia continued to rage through military institutions. John Vetch (1783–1835) gave a compelling and celebrated description of the incapacitating effect it had in the second battalion of the 52nd Regiment of Foot, where between August 1805 and August 1806, 606 of 700 soldiers developed ophthalmia, 50 became bilaterally blind and a further 40 unilaterally blind (16). He redescribed the granulations under the upper lid and the use of silver nitrate and copper sulphate. He was firm in his conviction of the infectious nature of the disease, which he demonstrated with a number of experiments by transferring infection with infected secretions. Vetch enforced strict hygiene measures that reduced transmission (28). In particular, he warned of the danger of the common use of towels and hand basins by soldiers and the need to isolate infected soldiers.

In 1804 Sir Patrick Macgregor reported on the outbreak of ophthalmia in the Royal Military Asylum, a boarding school for the children of soldiers who were serving overseas (29). The infection was apparently introduced by two Irish brothers and over six months or so, nearly 400 children were affected with ophthalmia with six becoming bilaterally blind and 12 losing one eye. Three of the nurses at the asylum were also affected, again confirming the contagious nature of ophthalmia.

British troops returned to Egypt in 1807 in an attempt to remove the Turks, who had taken control after the British had defeated the French and then retired. During this ill-fated and under-resourced expedition the British Army was affected by further outbreaks of ophthalmia, as did the British garrison in Sicily when the troops returned to England (26).

By 1811, 2317 British soldiers were bilaterally blind (30). Macgregor wrote that the ophthalmia has "crippled many of our best regular regiments to such a degree as for a time to render them unfit for service" (30). The British Army implemented several changes to curb ophthalmia. First, it recognised that ophthalmia was communicable and therefore all troops needed to be inspected and any cases were to be isolated. Second, it recognised the importance of cleanliness and prohibited soldiers from using the same tub or water for washing. Faces had to be washed under running water and each soldier was to be issued with his own towel. Third, bedding was seen to be an important method of transmitting infection. Pillow cases were introduced and sheets and pillow cases had to be washed regularly. These measures did much to curb the ophthalmia, although trachoma continued to be a problem throughout the British Army, particularly in centres where many troops passed through, such as Malta, Gibraltar and Cape Town. In the Crimean War (1861–67), 4% of all disability in the army was due to ophthalmia and 5% of the total discharges were because of blindness, although these rates were approximately half what they had been in the 1830s (30).

In the 1882 expedition to Egypt, British troops were issued with blue veils and a pair of goggles. Their eyes were to be freely bathed in clean pure water. Again no two men should ever use the same water and every man had to have his own towel, which was to be washed daily. This regime worked well until the troops went into battle. Subsequently 9% developed ophthalmia (30) and this has been attributed to infection with the Koch-Weeks bacillus (4).

Hundreds of thousands of British and other colonial soldiers, including those from Australia, passed through Egypt during the First World War (1914–18) (see Figure 1.9). Although trachoma was still widespread in the civilian population, few cases of conjunctivitis occurred in these soldiers (26,31). This is a testament to the improvement in standards of British military hygiene from 1801 to 1915. However, in this war many Turkish prisoners of war did have trachoma (4). Although at the time the Egyptian ophthalmia was regarded as a single entity, there clearly was a problem of not being able to differentiate between multiple causes of conjunctivitis. With little in the way of therapy and no diagnostic resources other than signs and symptoms, these Georgian military surgeons were operating in an uncharted area. Many infections must have been mixed infections with chlamydia being concurrently passed with other bacteria, especially the seasonal epidemics of Koch-Weeks conjunctivitis (*Haemophilus aegypticus*) and gonococcal conjunctivitis (either *Moraxella catarrhalis* or *Neisseria gonorrhoea*) (32). Meyerhof also mentions another outbreak of relatively mild ophthalmia that was both "very contagious and joined with a kind of influenza" (26), possibly an adenoviral keratoconjunctivitis.

Meyerhof subdivides Egyptian ophthalmia into four different diseases:

1. acute catarrhal conjunctivitis caused by Koch-Weeks bacillus that may become purulent and severe, but usually resolves without permanent sequelae (usually seen in the early summer when flies increase and before the weather became too hot).

2. acute purulent conjunctivitis due to gonococcus and occasionally with secondary infection from streptococcus or pneumococcus. Untreated, this frequently led to corneal ulceration and perforation or opacification (usually seen in late summer after the flies return as the high temperatures fall somewhat).

3. post-gonococcal conjunctivitis with residual papillary hypertrophy and occasionally ectropion of the lids. In the 1930s he advocated a strong solution of silver nitrate to treat this or ectropion surgery for the more severe cases. The clinical description of this is somewhat reminiscent of chronic staphylococcal conjunctivitis.

4. "genuine" trachoma with its four stages as classified by MacCallan.

Meyerhof recognises the easy confusion of an initial acute bacterial conjunctivitis that was then followed by the chronic blinding changes of trachoma. He makes the point strongly that trachoma can develop insidiously on its own without the need for an antecedent acute conjunctivitis. This was a particularly contentious point and as mentioned, even in the 1950s some

contended that trachoma always started as acute, purulent conjunctivitis (20,33).

The seasonal epidemics of flies in Egypt would have undoubtedly contributed to the rapid spread of infection. The fly population is also likely to have increased considerably around the soldiers and their camps. The accumulation of faeces and other rubbish around the hastily erected army camps would have provided excellent breeding sites for flies.

The Egyptian ophthalmia in Europe

In 1830 William Mackenzie (1791–1868) (see Figure 1.10) wrote *A Practical Treatise on the Diseases of the Eye* which became the definitive British textbook of ophthalmology for the next half century (29). Mackenzie differentiated three types of ophthalmia relevant to this discussion of trachoma. He borrowed heavily on the experience of Vetch and the other military surgeons.

The first ophthalmia was catarrhal ophthalmia or conjunctivitis *puro-mucosa atmospherica*. This acute conjunctivitis was the ophthalmia that "attacked the British and French armies in Egypt (and) was an atmospheric puro-mucous conjunctivitis, but that it afterwards degenerated into a contagious, perhaps infectious, disease". However, it was thought that catarrhal ophthalmia was usually acquired because of atmospheric changes, especially exposure to cold and wet conditions or to the night air (34). Wet feet were also an important cause. It usually presented as a mild conjunctivitis, but in severe cases chemosis may develop when bloodletting and purging were required. In some cases the cornea also was involved and could perforate.

The second condition characterised by Mackenzie was contagious ophthalmia or purulent ophthalmia, also known as the Egyptian ophthalmia. The severity of this purulent condition was thought to vary with climate, the time of year and the constitution or general state of health of those when they become affected. It was less severe in women than

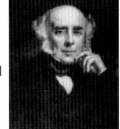

Figure 1.10 William Mackenzie (Lebensohn JE. An Anthology of Ophthalmic Classics. Baltimore: The Williams & Wilkins Company, 1969).

men and the right eye was more frequently affected. Unlike catarrhal conjunctivitis that often started with a foreign body sensation, the first symptoms of contagious ophthalmia were a marked discharge and lid changes. Chemosis could be marked and coupled with marked swelling of the lids. The purulent discharge usually decreased after 12 to 14 days and with time, granular (follicular) changes could be seen in the conjunctiva (see Figure 1.11). The inflammation often extended into the cornea, causing ulceration and perforation. Pain was a prominent feature, particularly with corneal involvement. The granular prominences were thought to be enlarged acini of the Meibomian glands. Much attention was directed to identifying and classifying the different types of pain and defining specific therapies for each type of pain (see Table 1.1).

Mackenzie goes on to stress that "in every case in which this ophthalmia has spread through a regiment, a school or a family, there has been a suspicion of actual contact by means either of fingers of the patients or of towels or other utensils which they were in the habit of using in common". Mackenzie sets out recommendations to prevent the spread of trachoma amongst soldiers (see Table 1.2) and quotes Dr Vetch: "Each company has a separate room in which the intercourse among the men is necessarily great. Many things are used in common ... washing their faces in the same water ... and having recourse to the same towel". Vetch subsequently demonstrated the contagious nature of the purulent conjunctival mucous by applying it to the urethra and producing typical gonorrheae (16). Another surgeon of the times, Dr Guillie, also demonstrated the infectious nature by transferring pus from one eye to another (29). This interesting and confusing experimental differentiation of ophthalmia and gonorrhoea has been reviewed recently by Benedek (35).

Mackenzie recognised a third condition, ophthalmic granular conjunctiva, that also caused trachoma. It was characterised by the thickened, fleshy and rough membrane lining the lids, especially the upper lid. He explained at some length that this was not actual granulation tissue, but the granular appearance was due to changes in the Meibomian follicles. Without treatment, the great thickening and roughness of the tarsal

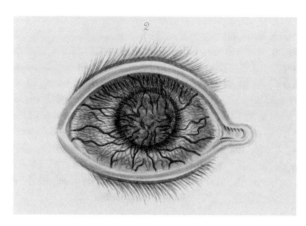

Figure 1.11 The effects of granular conjunctivitis "combined with a hazed condition of the cornea which is marked or streaked by numerous conjunctival vessels carrying red blood. The greater numbers are situated on the upper part of the globe, where the eyelid exerts most pressure. The term 'Pannus' has been given to this complaint" (Morgan J. Lectures on Diseases of the Eye. 2nd ed. London: Samuel Highley, 1848).

conjunctiva would lead to the total opacity of the cornea.

In cases of granular ophthalmia, a good prognosis could be expected if there were "sufficient clothing, proper diet, restriction from intemperance, good air and judicious medical treatment" (Hippocrates' aphorism restated). Treatment should include "scarification of the conjunctiva, the application of escharotics and the use of counter irritation". Several days after scarification or incision of the eyelids silver nitrate pencil was to be applied to the tarsal conjunctiva. This should be repeated every two to three days and then could be replaced with copper sulphate. The juice of the root *holcus avenaceus* and red precipitate salve could be used. It was considered of utmost importance to keep a blister open on the nape of the neck until the eye was healed.

Alternatively, a skilled surgeon can remove the roughened conjunctiva with a "small and very sharp lancet shaped knife ... (using) a steady motion". Although this operation causes "very considerable pain", one had to be careful not to remove too much conjunctiva as the consequent scarring would cause more damage to the cornea than the disease itself. All this was essentially the same treatment as first recommended by

Table 1.1: Treatment options for the ophthalmiae, Mackenzie,1830 (29)

1. Bloodletting – to depress the strength of the response; (i) venous, (ii) arterial, (iii) leeches, (iv) the use of incision of the conjunctiva. It is "the veriest of folly" to bleed very large quantities of blood for Egyptian ophthalmia because it does not work well; one would need to remove too much blood to have a good effect and there are other milder forms of treatment. However, for chemosis, 10 to 40 ounces of blood should be removed from the arm using a large orifice. The patient should sit or stand to ensure syncope. This should be repeated every 24 to 36 hours if the symptoms have not abated. Scarification of the conjunctiva should be repeated every second or third day.

   One to 20 leeches can be used over the temples and on the side of the nose. Consideration to be given to transection of the temporal artery, scarification or cupping at the temple.

   Consideration could also be given to cutting individual conjunctival blood vessels, 360 degree conjunctival resection or anterior chamber paracentesis.

2. Purgatives – depletory to remove excess fluids, especially calomel and jalap, for the sympathetic effect. Purgatives should be used in all cases of trachoma.

   Local treatment – irrigation of the eye with lemon juice has been advocated, as has irrigation with urine and salt water.

3. Emetics – to stop digestive organs causing irritation elsewhere in the body, to lower circulation and to relax the skin. Not useful in trachoma.

4. Diaphoretics – useful adjuvants to lower inflammation by increasing perspiration. Diaphoretics should be used as soon as the active inflammation has subdued.

5. Alteratives – to reduce inflammation and to remove effused coagulable lymph. These, particularly mercury, are essential for use in uveitis and internal ophthalmia. Alteratives are the most useful in severe cases linked with venesection.

6. Tonics such as cinchona were especially useful for scrofulous ophthalmiae. Sulphate and quinine were also used.

7. Narcotics – laudanum for pain, applied locally to the temple or forehead, as well as opium and calomel.

   In addition, belladonna or hyoscyamus can be used to dilate the pupil. They are delivered as an ointment smeared on the eyebrow and are particularly important for internal ophthalmia.

8. Refrigerants – cold water. Although tepid water can also be used; as it evaporates it will also cool by latent heat. Nitre is used as an internal refrigerant and as a diuretic.

9. Astringents including lead acetate and zinc sulphate give uniform bad results; instead, silver nitrate and murias hydrargyri are recommended.

10. Stimulants and escharotics – silver nitrate, but only in solution and never used as an ointment on its own. One could also use vinum opii.

11. Counter irritants – rubefacient liniments, blisters and "issues", particularly useful for chronic disease.

12. Dietetical – an improvement in the mode of life, including protection from glare, fresh air, rest, quietness, a good diet and regulated exercise.

Table 1.2: Recommendations for the prevention of trachoma, Mackenzie,1830 (29)

1. Prevent exposure to night air; soldiers on guard should cover their heads well and should avoid currents of air.
2. On the appearance of the first case of ophthalmia, the daily and minute inspection of every individual.
3. The instant separation of those affected.
4. Avoid excessive crowding.
5. Advise people of the contagious nature of ophthalmia and to avoid touching their eyes or using a shared towel.
6. Have soldiers carefully wash their faces and eyes with separate vessels of water under the supervision of the officer.

Table 1.3: Treatment for chronic entropion, Mackenzie,1830 (29)

(Note: chronic entropion develops after ophthalmia tarsi, a late condition of the Egyptian ophthalmia)

1. Simple, remove a transverse fold of skin and suture.
2. Cause an eschar with sulphuric acid applied to the skin on wool.
3. Complex cases, remove the tarsus:
   (i) Excise the lower half (Jaeger)
   (ii) Extirpation of the cartilage (tarsectomy) (Saunders)
   (iii) Two perpendicular vertical lid incisions (Ware)
   (iv) Combined incision of the lid plus skin excision (Crampton).

Hippocrates and passed on through Galen, the Arabic texts and subsequent Latin and European translations. Mackenzie also listed a number of operations that could be used to treat chronic entropion and trichiasis (see Table 1.3)

Dr Julius Boldt, a regimental surgeon in the Prussian infantry, published an outstanding book on trachoma. The English translation of this was prepared by Herbert Parsons (1868–1957) and published in 1904 (15). He gives an excellent summary of the early European experience of trachoma and many have subsequently used Boldt as a reference. Boldt traced the spread of ophthalmia through Europe. Following the landing of French troops at Sicily in 1801, Italian troops started to be affected. An epidemic raged for years through Italy and peaked in 1813, but continued intermittently until 1826. Italian troops stationed in Hungary in 1809 took the infection with them.

The Napoleonic Wars (1805–15) had Europe in upheaval with large armies hurriedly recruited, quartered in temporary barracks, marched across Europe and fighting with and against soldiers from many countries. The Prussian Army was mobilised in 1813 with universal conscription. The first affected Prussian troops had been stationed with French soldiers in the Baltic provinces. When these troops returned to their barracks after the Battle of Waterloo (1815), ophthalmia spread extensively and then waxed and waned. From 1813 to 1821, 25,000 Prussian troops were affected and 1100 were bilaterally blind. Similar outbreaks occurred in the Austrian Army after 1815 with epidemics continuing until 1851. The Russian Army was not affected until 1818, when ophthalmia first appeared in its garrison in Warsaw, and by 1839

nearly 80,000 Russian soldiers had been affected. Epidemics continued throughout the Crimean War (1854–6).

A major epidemic broke out amongst the Dutch and Belgian Armies in 1815, but a further severe epidemic occurred in Belgium in 1834. This left 4000 Belgian soldiers "totally blind" and another 10,000 partially blinded. To solve this problem, all the affected soldiers were discharged in 1834 and "by this brilliant but disastrous experiment the last trace of doubt as to the contagiousness of trachoma was dispelled" (15). This settled the controversy that had raged between the "Contagionists" and the "Anti-Contagionists" or "Compressionists":

> The latter would not hear of any other cause for the extraordinary epidemic of trachoma in Belgium than the glare of light reflected from the white tunics of the infantry, and the continuous compression of their necks by their cravats. Yet the epidemic was not in the least diminished by complete change of uniform (15).

This disaster in Belgium by and large partly led to the First International Congress of Ophthalmology convened in Brussels in 1857.

Outbreaks of ophthalmia are recounted in the Swedish, Danish and Portuguese Armies through to the 1860s. As with the British Army, the other European armies placed variable emphasis on the selection of recruits who were not infected, cleaning and disinfecting old barracks, separating patients with ophthalmia and following the lines of treatment already outlined.

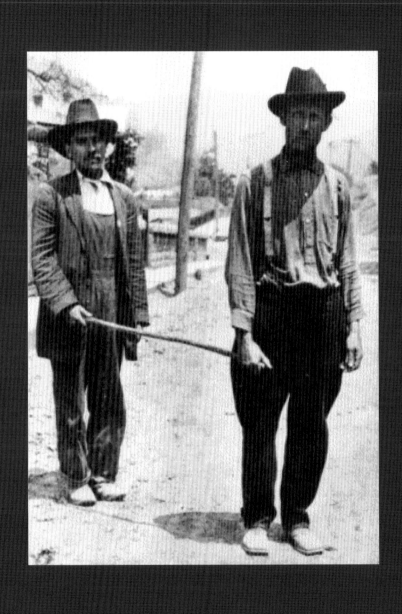

CHAPTER TWO

Trachoma development, institutions and the 20th century

Trachoma retreats as civilization advances

ANDRE CUENOD, 1901

THE NAME 'TRACHOMA' used to be almost synonymous with all eye disease and blindness. In a way somewhat reminiscent of Helen of Troy, trachoma was the disease that 'launched a thousand hospitals', and even more careers over the last two centuries. It was the reason that the famous ophthalmic hospitals were established around the world during the last century. These hospitals include Moorfields in London, the Massachusetts Eye and Ear Infirmary in Boston, and even the Royal Victorian Eye and Ear Hospital in Melbourne (36).

In this chapter, I will examine trachoma in more developed countries by reviewing the impact trachoma has had on the practice of medicine and the evolution of ophthalmology, and observing what was happening as trachoma disappeared from these countries.

Institutions formed in response to trachoma

Eye hospitals

In late 18th century Britain ophthalmology had one of the worst reputations for quackery in the medical profession, but it became the first and possibly the most successful medical specialty (37). Before 1800, most eye care was provided by travelling surgeons:

who palmed themselves upon the public under the name of oculists, operated at fairs and markets and in public places, upon raised platforms, something after the manner of itinerant showmen of the present day, and whose arrival in any town or village was announced by blast of horn (38).

The most famous of these was Chevalier John Taylor (1703–72), an English cataract surgeon who "travelled and stayed in the continent, in a carriage drawn by four horses, and its panels emblazoned all over with eyes, indicative of his calling" (38). He was appointed ocularist-in-ordinary to King George II (39).

The explosive appearance of the Egyptian ophthalmia forced a reconsideration by established medicine about the role and importance of eye disease. The Egyptian ophthalmia was so unexpected, so widespread, so incomprehensible and so horrid that every medical practitioner had to know something about it (16). An immediate response in the army was to form separate eye hospitals to take care of soldiers with ophthalmia. This was replicated in civilian life and hospitals, such as the Royal Infirmary for the Diseases of the Eye and the London Dispensary for Curing Diseases of the Eye and Ear, were both founded in 1805 in London (see Figure 2.1). The Dispensary became the London Eye Infirmary, the London Ophthalmic Hospital and ultimately Moorfields Eye Hospital. The military and political imperative to do something about trachoma helped raise the funds to establish these hospitals.

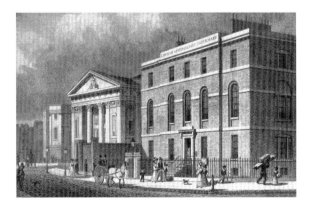

Figure 2.1 The London Ophthalmic Infirmary first erected at Moorfields in 1822 (Treacher Collins 1929 (39), engraving by R. Acon from a drawing by Tho. H. Shepherd).

The introduction of ophthalmia also occurred at a time of growing social and political concern about the adverse effects of the Industrial Revolution and the philosophic content of utilitarianism. Among other things, utilitarianism advocated that it was the responsibility of the community to enable the visually disabled and blind to undertake productive work (37). Equally, the philosophy of the Enlightenment viewed the progressive development of humans to a superior order of being. Those who were deprived of their sight were also deprived of the ability of reaching full comprehension and thereby enlightenment. This gave both a moral and philosophical impetus to address ophthalmia and its consequences.

Although the Royal Infirmary was established by Jonathan Wathen (later Sir Wathen Waller, 1769–1853) three months before John Saunders (1773–1810) established the London Dispensary, Saunders positioned himself as the father and originator of British ophthalmology (37). Saunders was a controversial figure, but his early death in 1810 was followed by years of controversy between his supporters and advocates and his detractors. The new eye hospitals were particularly valued and well attended. Following the lead of the hospitals in London, similar eye hospitals rapidly appeared throughout England, Europe and the New World. In Britain, 52 Eye or Eye and Ear Hospitals were established (40). In most instances these hospitals were initially set up to deal with ophthalmia or trachoma.

With new eye hospitals came the need for eye doctors to staff them and this led to further controversy. Prior to the early 1800s, physicians had shunned ophthalmology and left it to charlatan surgeons and travelling oculists. With the upsurge in the need to care for those with ophthalmia, physicians could no longer neglect eye disease and suddenly ophthalmology became a mainstream activity. There was ongoing controversy for over 50 years as to whether ophthalmologists should be separate specialists or whether they should be generalists, with an interest in ophthalmology. There were powerful advocates for both sides. William Wilde (1815–76), an ophthalmologist in Dublin, displayed the eloquence that his more famous son Oscar became renowned for and gave an impassioned justification for separate hospitals

Table 2.1: Announcement of the First International Congress of Ophthalmology to be held in Brussels in 1857 (41)

Without wanting to terminate any other program, we can say that the issue of military ophthalmia, a disease that for years has affected the many armies of the continent, and also daily claims new victims in the civilian population amongst whom unfortunately it is propagated, will take an important place in our deliberations. An exact statistical analysis of this disease in different countries; a study of the ways by which it is introduced; the examination of the proper measures to halt its progress; the results that could be obtained or expected following their application; and the discussion of the indications of cure and the most satisfactory treatment methods and ways to apply them will help to clarify the nature of the disease—imperfect though our knowledge is—and to exercise a beneficial influence on its prophylaxis and treatment.

and professionals (38). After the invention of the ophthalmoscope by von Helmholtz (1821–94) in 1850, physicians started to examine the eye in even greater detail and the ophthalmoscope became as much a tool of medicine as the stethoscope.

In addition to the establishment of eye hospitals and the creation of the specialty of ophthalmology, the number of people blinded from ophthalmia was also a spur to the ongoing development of specific homes and institutions for the blind. Another driver for this, of course, was the presence of children blinded by ophthalmia neonatorum. The high rates of trachoma in children in orphanages and other institutions led to special trachoma schools being established in and around London in the 1870s and 1880s and then elsewhere (30). Attention was given to housing the children in small groups, washing and bathing were performed frequently, and the children received regular treatment with copper sulphate or silver nitrate.

International organisations

One of the first international medical meetings was the International Congress of Ophthalmology held in Brussels in 1857. This meeting had two goals: to discuss military ophthalmia (see Table 2.1) and to discuss the ophthalmoscope that since 1850 had completely changed the scope and outlook of ophthalmology (41). At the end of the meeting Albrecht von Graefe (1828–70) gave the first presentation of his revolutionary cure for (angle closure) glaucoma—peripheral iridectomy.

As previously discussed, military ophthalmia was a major political concern and threatened national security across Europe. Its spread to the civilian population was of particular concern in Belgium. After the Napoleonic Wars, the Belgium Army had 4000 soldiers blind and 10,000 partially sighted (15):

in their desperation the authorities emptied the barracks of suffering and blinded soldiers, epidemics of unprecedented proportions spread amongst the civilian populations, transferring the political and military problem into a social calamity of the first magnitude (41).

Although much was discussed at the first International Congress, little could be done about trachoma. The International Congress reconvened four years later in Paris and with interruptions during the World Wars it has continued to meet regularly. The International Congress of Ophthalmology is the oldest international medical meeting, and in 1929 its organising body was formalised with the formation of the International Council of Ophthalmology. In that year, the International Council participated in the creation of two further organisations, the International Association for the Prevention of Blindness and the International Organization Against Trachoma (41).

Led by Charles Nicolle (1860–1936), Nobel Laureate for Medicine in 1928, and Victor Morax (1866–1935), Le Ligue Contre le Trachome was founded in Paris in 1923. With the International Council, the League helped found the International Organization Against Trachoma (IOAT) that first met in Geneva in 1930 (4). The IOAT continues to meet annually in association with either the International or the European Congresses of Ophthalmology and has provided an important and ongoing forum under the current leadership of Gabriel Coscas. The League continues to publish *Le Revue Internationale du Trachome*, a journal started in 1923 by Morax.

The International Association for the Prevention of Blindness first met in 1930 and held annual meetings until the 1950s with a break during the Second World War. The Association entered into an official relationship with the newly formed WHO in 1948. In 1975, the Association was recast as the International Agency for the Prevention of Blindness (IAPB) under the leadership of Sir John Wilson of the Royal Commonwealth Society of the Blind, with both the International Council of Ophthalmology and the World Blind Union as founding members. The IAPB has grown to be the major international organisation co-ordinating global activities for the prevention of blindness (42) and with the WHO, the co-founder of Vision 2020: The Right to Sight Initiative (43).

Although the League of Nations was established after the First World War, at that time there was no separate organisation comparable to the World Health Organization. The international functions relating to health were predominantly organised and co-ordinated by the League, either through its own health organisation or the International Red Cross. In 1929, the League of Nations Health Committee endorsed and reprinted the report on trachoma prepared by the ICO and recommended that "States members should lend [their] full moral support" (44).

In 1931 there was concern that trachoma was "the principal cause of blindness in certain Mediterranean districts and in hot countries." It had "considerable significance from an international standpoint, because of its worldwide distribution and because of the restrictive measures against immigration". An enquiry into "the legislative, public health and medical measures adopted in different countries for the prevention and cure" of trachoma was established (45). The International Council of Ophthalmology, the International Association for the Prevention of Blindness and the International Organization Against Trachoma advised both the League of Nations and the International Red Cross about vision issues and trachoma. The report on trachoma was published by the League of Nations in 1935 (46). The World Health Organization was established in 1947 and the Association also established an official relationship with the WHO in 1948.

At that time, the WHO and UNICEF established a number of vertical programs including trachoma. A study group in trachoma was established in 1948 (47). The First Expert Advisory Committee on Trachoma met in 1952 and was charged by a resolution of the Third World Health Assembly (48) to "study the problem of trachoma with a view to submitting practical recommendations" as to "the possibility of successfully eradicating it [trachoma] by the application of modern methods of control" because "in a great number of countries trachoma and a number of other related ophthalmias constitute an urgent health problem" (20). This Committee and the subsequent groups that met in 1956 (33), 1962 (49) and 1966 (50) consisted of a number of people heavily involved in trachoma research (see Figures 2.2, 2.3). Some have been quite critical that when charged to submit "practical recommendations" their reports contained a list of 28 problems for future research (51).

Working with UNICEF, the WHO initiated trachoma control programs in 11 countries including Morocco, Tunisia, Algeria, Taiwan, Burma, India, Oman, Vietnam, Brazil, Libya and Sudan, and by 1962 had treated 7.5 million people. Other programs were run in Argentina, Uruguay, Poland, Hungary, Yugoslavia, the USSR, Turkey, Palestine, Japan, China, Egypt and South Africa (52). The basic strategy was to use tetracycline ointment, provide trichiasis surgery and promote education programs addressing individual and community hygiene. Some of these programs were highly successful, but others ran into problems that often led to frustration and disappointment (53). After 1957 when it became possible to culture chlamydia, a vaccine seemed an attractive pathway for a quick solution. In the 1960s and 1970s as the WHO moved from vertical intervention programs to a more horizontal primary health care approach, specific disease programs, such as the trachoma programs, gradually fell away. In some countries such as Thailand this decrease in trachoma activity was linked to both the development of primary health care capacity and the decrease in trachoma (54).

The Alma-Ata Conference in 1978 clearly stated the principles of primary health care and summarised them in the catch call of "Health For All" (55). In 1978 this was associated with the recasting of the WHO vision-related activities from a trachoma program to a prevention of blindness program. This had been preceded by World Health Assembly Resolution in 1975 (WHA 28.54 (56)) and the selection of prevention of blindness as the

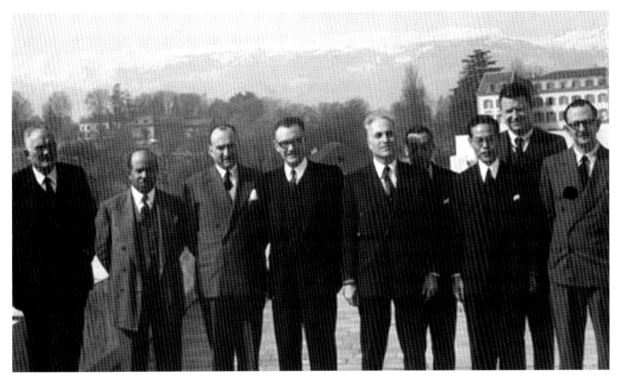

Figure 2.2 First Expert Advisory Committee on Trachoma outside The League of Nations building, Geneva, 1952; from left to right: Pages, El Tobgy Bey, Bietti, Larmande, Nataf, Moutinho, Mitsui, Thygeson, Maxwell-Lyons (courtesy, Chandler Dawson).

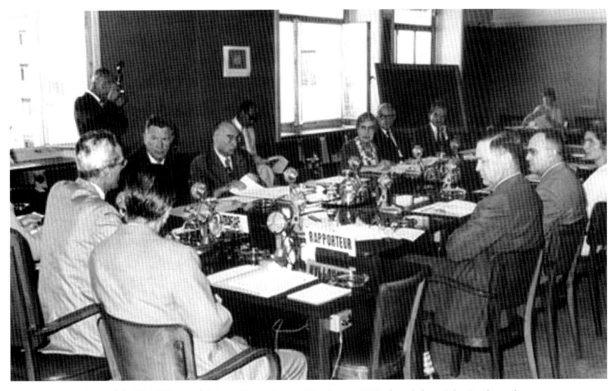

Figure 2.3 Members of the Third Expert Advisory Committee on Trachoma, 1962; from left to right: Snyder, unknown photographer, Larmande (foreground), Thygeson, Bietti, unknown, Mann, Carvalho, WHO staff, Scott (foreground), Kamal, WHO secretary (in background), Litricin (courtesy, Chandler Dawson).

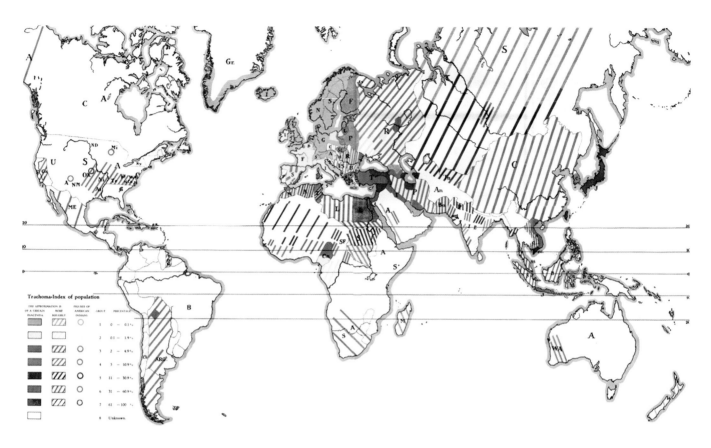

Figure 2.4 World map of trachoma prepared by the International
Council of Ophthalmology, 1929 (Wibaut 1929 (58) courtesy, ICO).

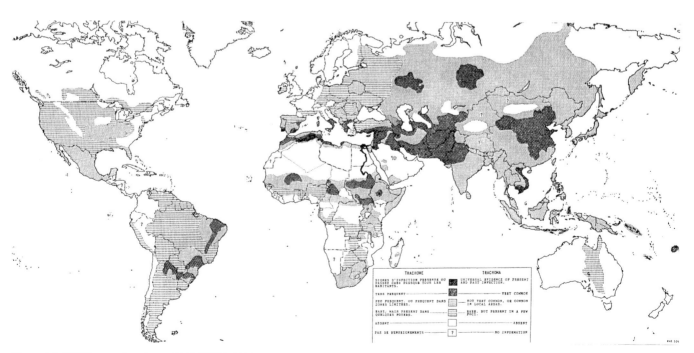

Figure 2.5 WHO map of trachoma 1949 (WHO 1949
(59). © 1949 WHO, reproduced with permission).

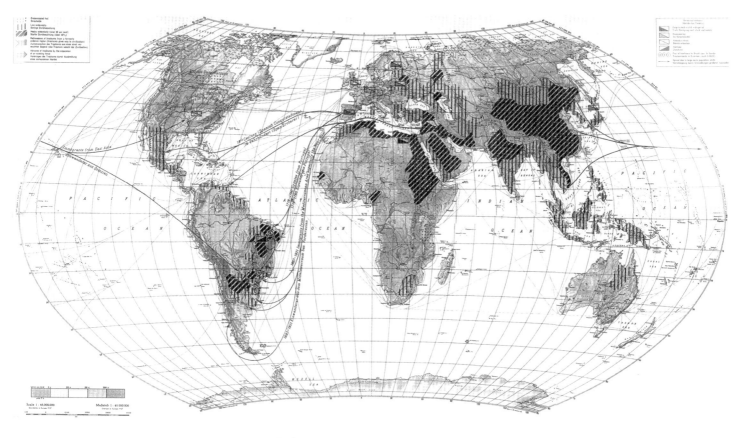

Figure 2.6 Global distribution of trachoma 1930–1955 (Siebeck 1961(9),
reproduced with permission of the Heidelberg Academy).

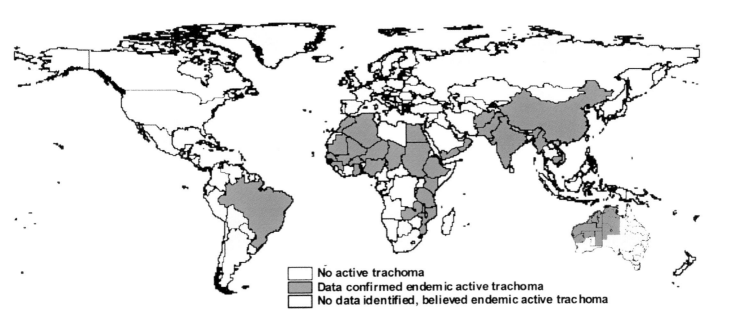

☐ No active trachoma
▨ Data confirmed endemic active trachoma
☐ No data identified, believed endemic active trachoma

Figure 2.7 Map of available active trachoma data in children by WHO region
(Polack et al 2005 (62), © 2005 WHO, reproduced with permission).

theme for World Health Day "Foresight" on 7 April 1976. The new WHO Prevention of Blindness Program (PBL) concentrated on cataract, xerophthalmia and onchocerciasis, in addition to trachoma. Subsequently, it was expanded to include deafness (PBD). Its mandate has continued to broaden with the launching of the Vision 2020 Initiative in 1999 to include childhood blindness, refractive error and low vision (57).

Trachoma in the 20th century

World maps

Although many had listed countries with trachoma, the first major effort to develop a systematic global picture of the distribution of trachoma appears to be the work of the International Council of Ophthalmology undertaken by F. Wibaut in Amsterdam. He spent two years working on an extensive survey during which he distributed a questionnaire to representatives of all the existing ophthalmic societies (58). This remarkable undertaking was presented at the International Congress in Amsterdam in 1929 (see Figure 2.4). Wibaut summarised the current knowledge of trachoma that indicated that no races seemed to be immune and women were affected more severely than men. Trachoma was a disease of the poor; it was contagious, secondary infections were important, its incubation period was four to 10 days, transmission took place in the family, children aged less than seven years had the highest prevalence and younger children were infected by older brothers and sisters. The control measures recommended were control of the national frontiers, compulsory notification, and the examination and treatment of schoolchildren and army recruits. More trained staff were needed in affected countries and free treatment was advocated for the poor. To eliminate trachoma, general hygiene measures and the improvement of the general welfare were needed, as were scientific investigation and international collaboration.

In 1949, the WHO undertook an initial mapping exercise of trachoma (59) (see Figure 2.5).

In 1961 a major world atlas of endemic diseases was published (60). Included amongst the comprehensive lists of diseases was trachoma. A world map was produced and more detailed maps

of several continents were included, with a narrative description of the presence and severity of trachoma and associated conditions (see Figure 2.6).

In Europe only Denmark, Norway, Sweden and Switzerland were free of trachoma, although probably at this time trachoma had disappeared from Glasgow leaving the United Kingdom also trachoma free. The trachoma clinic run by the Glasgow Royal Infirmary in the docks area of Glasgow ran until the 1960s (61). Trachoma was now recognised to be widespread both in North Africa and sub-Saharan Africa, and throughout Asia and the Pacific. Trachoma was also a problem in Brazil and the southern cone countries of Latin America, with occasional reports from other countries in South America; focal areas occurred in Canada, Mexico and the United States.

The most recent attempt by the WHO to map the global distribution of trachoma shows that trachoma has now disappeared from all the "easy" countries in Western Europe, North America and many countries in Asia and the Pacific that previously had a low prevalence (62). By and large, trachoma persists today in those "hard" countries in which it was a major problem 50 years ago (see Figure 2.7). Polack also prepared maps on the distribution of trichiasis.

Country examples

Now we will look at some developed countries in which blinding endemic trachoma disappeared over the 20th century. In these countries it is hard to tell whether the trachoma control activities played an important role in the elimination of trachoma. It seems quite likely that the isolation of children in trachoma schools and their improved hygiene were important, but health education in the absence of material improvement of the environment is unlikely to have made a great or lasting impact. The newly available antibiotics hastened the disappearance of trachoma in some areas. The only report of a specific attempt to eliminate trachoma by environmental change that I am aware of was the slum clearance of the ghetto areas in Amsterdam (63).

United Kingdom
In the first half of the 18th century, in addition to being a major military problem, there was an

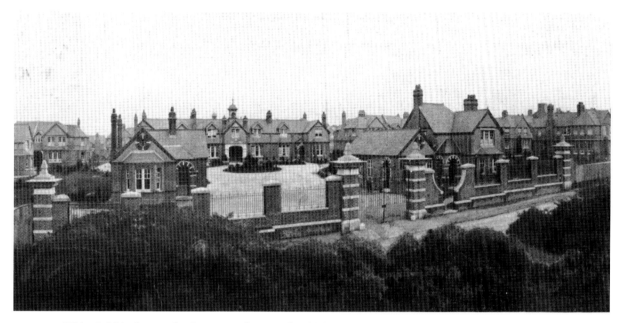

Figure 2.8 White Oak Trachoma School or Hospital in Kent for children with trachoma (late 19th century) (© Peter Higginbotham, <http://www.workhouses.org.uk>).

epidemic of ophthalmia in the civilian population. At the peak of the Industrial Revolution, people were flooding to the cities and living in appalling conditions in crowded tenements and the work houses of the urban slums, so well described by Hogarth and Dickens. In 1848 Poor Law schools were established for the poorest of the poor. Ophthalmia was noted to be a particular problem in children in these schools and often the conditions were quite terrible. In 1873, 400 children with ophthalmia were removed from one Poor Law school and treated successfully in a special "school" for a year (30). In 1875 Edward Nettleship (1845–1913) reported that active trachoma ranged from 17% to 66% in the Poor Law schools, and 9% of children had impaired vision due to corneal scarring and other trachoma schools were established across England (64). In 1888 the Central London District School established the "Hanwell Ophthalmic School". This school was replaced in 1903 by two new schools, White Oak in Swanlea (see Figure 2.8), Kent and High Wood in Brentwood, Essex. These schools had separate cottages for small groups of students, live-in nursing staff, spray taps in showers and numbered pegs for each child's towel. The number of children admitted progressively

decreased until in 1938 only 10 children had been admitted (64). The High Wood school had been closed in 1918 and the other, now also known as the London Country Council Hospital, finally closed in 1944 when there was no more trachoma reported (65). The advent and use of sulphonamides accelerated the treatment of remaining cases. Similar schools in other English cities were closed once trachoma had altogether disappeared (66).

In the UK, trachoma aggregated in the institutionalised groups; children living in the Poor Law schools and troops living in crowded and substandard barracks. Personal hygiene was compromised in both crowded settings. However, trachoma was also gradually disappearing from other areas of Britain, although the documentation is patchy. Trachoma was made a notifiable disease in Glasgow in 1914 and so better data are available for Glasgow than any other city in Britain (64,67). In Glasgow, a specific trachoma clinic was established, all notified patients were treated, and their contacts examined and treated, if needed. Until 1933 the number of new cases remained more or less constant at about 20 cases per year. This number had fallen to just seven new cases in 1937 (64). The rest of England followed a similar trend although it was less well documented.

However, the picture was very different in Ireland. In 1903 trachoma cases formed less than 1% of eye outpatients seen in seven major hospitals throughout Britain, but trachoma still accounted for 3% of patients seen in Dublin (30). Trachoma had been rife in the Irish workhouses established in 1841 with some 15% to 33% of people affected. Severe epidemics of eye disease were reported in 1849 and 1850 after the great famine (30). Wilde refers to an epidemic of ophthalmia in Ireland in 1701 although it seems unlikely that this was caused by trachoma (38). In 1937, two to three per 1000 schoolchildren in the Republic of Ireland still had trachoma (9) and the disease caused 9% of blindness (66). After the Second World War trachoma gradually petered out.

United States

It is unclear when trachoma first arrived in North America and there are no clear indications that trachoma had been a pre-existing problem in either North or South America before the arrival of Europeans. It has been supposed that trachoma was introduced by European migrants during colonial times (68). Others point to the waves of immigration from Ireland and Central Europe after 1848 until the early 1900s (30,51). Some proposed that trachoma was brought from Asia by migrating Indian peoples in prehistoric times (4,69). It may well be that ocular chlamydial infection had been longstanding and it was the changed living conditions that increased the transmission frequency that led to blinding trachoma.

The Massachusetts Eye and Ear Infirmary which opened in 1850 was modelled on Moorfields (37) and other similar specialist eye or eye and ear hospitals were set up across the then United States. The US Army was well aware of the problems of military ophthalmia. Dr J.S. Hildreth, Surgeon-in-Charge of the US Army Desmarres Eye and Ear Hospital in Chicago, presented a review of recent cases of gonorrhoeal and purulent ophthalmia at the inaugural meeting of the American Ophthalmological Society in 1865 (70). Parenthetically, he proposed using pressure dressings for patients with profusely purulent corneal ulcers, a suggestion some of his audience vehemently disagreed with.

Epidemics of purulent ophthalmia were observed in the USA from 1825, but whether these were related to trachoma or other causes of acute conjunctivitis is unknown (15). Boldt also quotes that 40% of the wards of a workhouse in New York had trachoma in the 1890s, although the prevalence of trachoma in Southern California was less than 1%.

In 1897 Surgeon General Walter Wyman (1848–1911) of the US Marine Hospital Service declared trachoma to be a "dangerous contagious disease" and instructed his medical officers to examine all immigrants (30). Would-be immigrants or aliens were also excluded if they were imbeciles, epileptics, insane, paupers, or if they had tuberculosis or other loathsome or dangerous contagious diseases that included trachoma, cholera, typhus, ringworm or other fungal infections (71). All those suspected to have red, watery or sore eyes were to be examined.

Trachoma came to be the central character "on the national stage of infectious disease and immigration" (72). Newly arrived immigrants personified the threat of trachoma to the community and local outbreaks of trachoma were blamed on immigrant children and their families. The aetiology and epidemiology of trachoma were poorly understood. However, it was clearly recognised by the public, professionals and politicians alike that trachoma was extremely contagious, and could be spread through touch and direct contact, and was particularly prevalent in areas where the weather and personal hygiene were poor. The presence of trachoma was used as a political weapon to stigmatise immigrant groups, especially eastern European Jews and migrants from the eastern Mediterranean and Asia (72). Trachoma surveillance of immigrants also became the major activity of the United States Public Health Service (USPHS). It "protected the nation against imported germs" and 80% of its resources were directed to the medical examination of immigrants (see Figure 2.9). Between 1897 and 1924, some 21,756,875 immigrants were examined and 33,847 (0.16%) were debarred because of trachoma (72). Trachoma was responsible for rejection of 44% of those with infectious disease and 9% for those debarred for all reasons (see Figure 2.10).

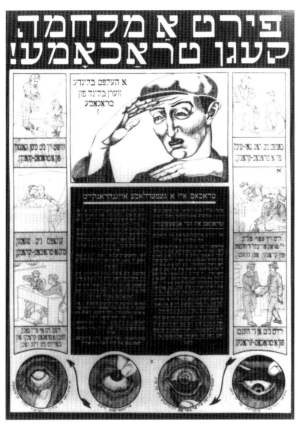

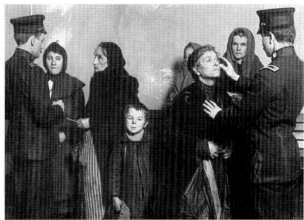

LEFT **Figure 2.9** Trachoma poster, fund for the relief of Jewish victims of the war in eastern Europe and the Federation of Ukrainian Jews, London, 1923 (Markel 2000 (72), from the Archives of the YIVO Institute for Jewish Research, New York).

BELOW **Figure 2.10** US public health officers examining immigrants for trachoma at Ellis Island, New York, 1911 (© Corbis).

All immigrants were examined with a painful double version of the upper lid, so the upper fornix could be examined as well as the tarsus. Often a button hook or forceps were used. Even President Theodore Roosevelt was concerned about the chance of cross contamination and after a visit to Ellis Island he commented that "the doctors made the examinations with dirty hands and with no pretence to clean their instruments" (72). Suspect immigrants had the letter T marked in blue chalk on their clothes and were sent to spend five days in the Contagious Disease Hospital to see if they recovered from acute conjunctivitis or whether they had trachoma (71).

Even though there was frequent argument about whether a particular person had trachoma or not, or whether a case of trachoma was infectious or cured, a final ruling was made and over 95% of those with trachoma were deported. To be deported was a crushing blow and often broke up families and the deportee returned to their homeland penniless. A USPHS officer in Baltimore stated "Deportation is unquestionably a hardship

… One had better have smallpox than severe trachoma" (71). After rigorous examination by a Board of Inquiry, a fortunate small percentage of those with trachoma were permitted to remain in the Hospital for treatment that took six months on average (72). The treatment consisted of resting in a dark room with cold compresses and irrigation of the eye three or four times daily with silver nitrate or argyrol solution. More severe cases would be treated with follicular expression and scarification followed by copper sulphate treatment. Grattage with rubbing of the tarsal conjunctiva with a steel brush dipped in bichloride of mercury was also used. Once "cured", immigrants were admitted to the USA.

In 1902 a fine of US$100 was imposed on the shipping companies for every case of trachoma they brought to the United States (30). This induced the shipping companies to set up their own screening centres in Europe to detect trachoma in their passengers before they embarked. Centres were set up at country borders and at the major ports of embarkation in England, Ireland, Germany and

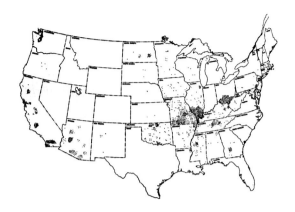

ABOVE **Figure 2.11** The "trachoma belt" in the United States in 1940 (Gradle HS. Incidence and Distribution of Trachoma in the United States. Sight Sav Rev.1940; 10:13–8, reproduced by Allen & Semba, 2002 (74). Reprinted from Survey of Ophthalmology, 47, Allen SK, Semba RD, The Trachoma "Menace" in the United States, 1897 to 1960, 500–9 © 2002, with permission from Elsevier).

RIGHT **Figure 2.12** The "blind leading the blind" as a result of trachoma (McMullen J. The government's work in the eradication of trachoma. Mod Hosp.1917; 9:163–5, reproduced by Allen & Semba, 2002 (74). Reprinted from Survey of Ophthalmology, 47, Allen SK, Semba RD, The Trachoma "Menace" in the United States, 1897 to 1960, 500–9 © 2002, with permission from Elsevier).

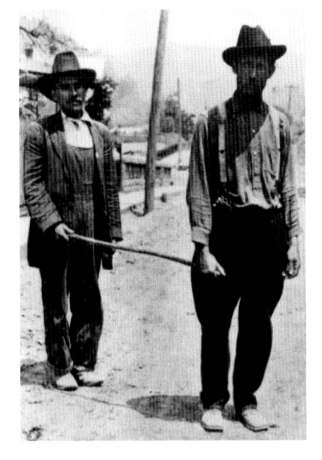

Italy. Some centres such as that in Naples was actually staffed by USPHS officers. One centre, Atlantic Park in Southampton, was still in operation in the 1930s (73). An increase in the number of people with trachoma was reported in London reflecting those who had been rejected by the shipping companies (30). It was common to have 2% to 5% of prospective immigrants rejected—85% because of trachoma (72). In 1901 a similar problem occurred in Montreal after the US authorities had started to examine all those entering the USA from Canada (30). In 1902 the Canadian Government enacted legislation to prohibit entry into Canada to those with trachoma.

By 1905 the US Congress had mandated that every single immigrant to the United States had to be examined for trachoma and US immigration service facilities, such as Ellis Island in New York, Locus Point in Baltimore, and in Boston,

Philadelphia and elsewhere became centres for screening (74). The examination on arrival might be more cursory for First and Second Class passengers, but it was rigorous for those Third and Fourth Class "Steerage" passengers (72). All passengers would have already been screened once or twice before they boarded the ship. From 1905, a million immigrants arrived in the USA each year until the First World War when the numbers halved. It is interesting to reflect on the amount of time, money and effort that was spent on these trachoma activities.

Little attention was given to endemic trachoma within the USA until 1911, when Dr J.A. Stucky of Lexington, Kentucky reported the frequent occurrence of trachoma in eastern Kentucky (75). The Committee on the Prevention of Blindness in the American Medical Association, pressed the US Public Health and Marine Hospital Service to assess the prevalence of trachoma, its mode of spread and measures for prevention (74). A number of surveys followed that defined the "trachoma belt" in the USA (68) (see Figure 2.11).

Trachoma was widespread, from the Allegheny Mountains and rural Appalachia through to Kansas and Oklahoma. The highest prevalence of trachoma reported amongst Americans (exclusive of Indians) was 13% in Kentucky, but the average rates of trachoma for Indian populations was 23%. Trachoma was a particular problem in the south west and mid west, and a prevalence of 92% was reported in Indian boarding school students in Oklahoma in 1912 (76). Trachoma also occurred on the east and west coasts. This was attributed to immigrants from Europe and Asia living in substandard and crowded housing after their arrival. In total, 35 of the 48 states in the USA reported cases of trachoma (68).

Many drew attention to the fact that Afro-Americans had much lower rates of trachoma than the Europeans amongst whom they lived and worked (30,68,69,71). At that time trachoma was also believed to be rare in sub-Saharan Africa, although this misconception was later corrected. It was noted that Africans in the West Indies had high rates of trachoma but this apparent conundrum remained unexplained at that time (30).

Allen and Semba have given a very good overview of the efforts to control trachoma in the USA (74). Their report includes a photograph of "the blind leading the blind" as a result of trachoma (see Figure 2.12) reminiscent of the photographs of onchocerciasis in Africa, and other photographs included in Stucky's paper (75). Briefly, the control measures aimed to treat every existing case and to prevent new cases from developing by means of health education. Education campaigns were used to teach people about the spread of disease and to encourage the improvement of personal hygiene. In 1913 the US Congress made a specific allocation of US$25,000 to combat trachoma (74).

The importance of family transmission was well recognised, as was the link to poor personal hygiene (75,76); the use of a common towel was "an almost certain invitation to disease" and "improvement in economic status with its concomitant improvement in sanitation and

housing" was seen as the key to elimination of disease (6). Living conditions were remarkably similar to those often reported from less developed areas of Africa today. People lived in "the rudest kind of hut … No windows, a lean-to chimney, a little stove in that room and in this room live the parents and anywhere from seven to 13 children … Everyone wiped on the one towel" (77). In Ohio, another area with a high prevalence of trachoma, most houses had outdoor privies, no running water and there was no garbage collection.

Boarding homes were considered to particularly facilitate the spread of trachoma, where people would often sleep two to a bed, with eight to 10 workers sharing a single room, sometimes sharing beds between night and day shifts (74). Trachoma was found to be a particular problem in New York, especially in the schools and in the Lower East side. This has been linked to migration especially from Ireland and later central Europe (30), although it seems likely that the appalling crowding and insanitary conditions in the tenements were also very important factors. A visit to the Tenement Museum in New York will confirm this view. Up to half the children in orphanages in New York had trachoma in the late 1800s (78). As in London, special trachoma schools were established in New York in 1912 and these also emphasised hygiene and daily washing.

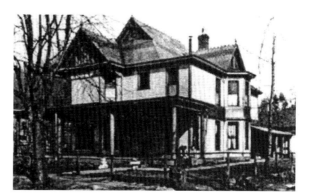

Figure 2.13 Irvinton House, the former US Public Health Service Trachoma Hospital in Pikesville, Kentucky (McMullen J. The government's work in the eradication of trachoma. Mod Hosp. 1917; 9:163–5, reproduced by Allen & Semba, 2002 (74). Reprinted from Survey of Ophthalmology, 47, Allen SK, Semba RD, The Trachoma "Menace" in the United States, 1897 to 1960, 500–9 © (2002), with permission from Elsevier).

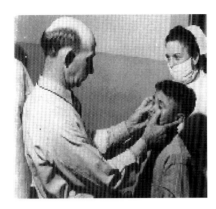

Figure 2.14 Dr WP Whitted examines eyes of trachoma patient, Trachoma School, Fort Defiance, Arizona 1941 (from collections of the National Archives and Records Administration).

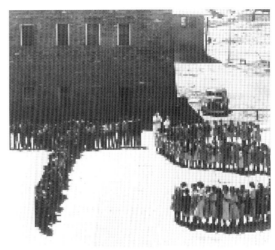

Figure 2.15 "T" stands for trachoma, "S" for sulphanilamide, Trachoma School, Fort Defiance, Arizona, 1941 (from collections of the National Archives and Records Administration).

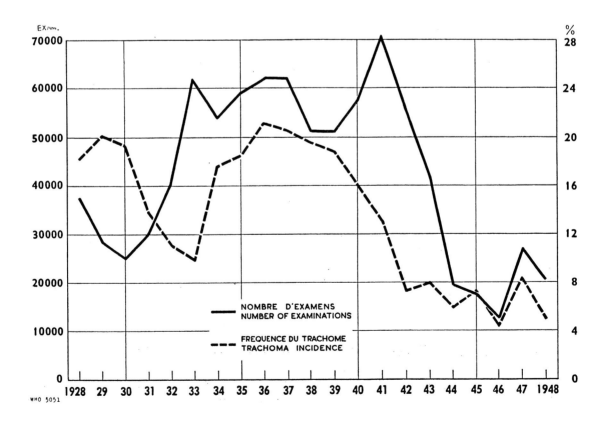

Figure 2.16 Incidence of trachoma in American Indians (WHO 1949 (59); © 1949 WHO, reproduced with permission).

The US Public Health Service established trachoma hospitals in regions such as Kentucky and Tennessee (51) (see Figure 2.13). In other areas like Illinois and Arkansas, a system of permanent field clinics and dispensaries was created. Field nurses held outreach clinics three times a week and provided health education about trachoma and the need to use separate towels. They also gave talks at schools and distributed pamphlets.

Cases of trachoma were treated with copper sulphate and silver nitrate until sulphonamides became available in the late 1930s (6). In 1939 there were some 35,000 cases of trachoma in non-Indian Americans (two-thirds had active trachoma) and 10% were blind (68). Another 25,000 American Indians had trachoma. Siniscal recounts how in Missouri, trachoma caused 25% of the blindness in the 1930s, but by 1955 this had dropped to only 10% (6).

As part of the New Deal in 1935, the American Government turned over trachoma control to the states to administer (74). By the early 1950s trachoma had ceased to be a major problem. Trachoma control activities continued in Illinois for five years after the last active case was detected in 1949 and ceased in Oklahoma and Arkansas in 1955 (6). The trachoma program in Kentucky ended in 1953 when no more cases could be found and all the surgery had been completed (51). The program continued in Missouri in 1953 when only 14 cases were detected (6). In the 1960s the rates of surgery for nasolacrimal duct obstruction and dacrycystitis were supposedly much higher in St. Louis (in the middle of the old trachoma belt) than in other parts of the USA.

Trachoma continued to be a problem in the Indian populations in Arizona and New Mexico and the Indian health service re-established trachoma control units in 1965 (79). Intense interventions, including the community-wide distribution of sulphonamides, with improving socio-environmental conditions led to a decline in the occurrence of trachoma (80) (see Figures 2.14, 2.15). However, trachoma was still reported occasionally in Indian communities until the 1980s (81) (see Figure 2.16).

It is interesting to reflect on how much time and effort was spent on the eradication of trachoma in the USA when, in reality, so few people were

affected. A similar observation can be made for the UK. This gives us an important benchmark to compare monitoring and evaluation targets in the current endemic areas. There was no argument that a prevalence of less than 5% or 10% was not important and treatment activities could be just stopped; in these developed countries "every last case" had to be eliminated.

France

Trachoma is thought to have existed in southern France from Roman times and was further spread by pilgrims in the Middle Ages (24). Although the French Army was severely affected by trachoma during the Egyptian campaign in the early 1800s, the disease did not become a major problem in the civilian population in France, although it was quite widespread. In 1900 the prevalence of trachoma in Paris was 1.7% but most trachoma was evident along the Mediterranean coast (15). The rates of occurrence in Marseilles in 1929 were between 2% to 5% (58) and much of this occurred in immigrant workers from French North Africa. Another focus of infection was the industrial area around Lille which also had a prevalence of trachoma between 2% to 4%. Here it was related to migrant workers from North Africa and Poland. It is interesting to note that in 1884 the rates of trachoma reported for Lille were 50% (82).

Comprehensive recommendations for the management of trachoma were developed and widely circulated in France (24,73). Although French ophthalmologists were not confronted with high levels of trachoma at home, they undertook outstanding work in their colonies, particularly in North and West Africa. The work of Nicolle, Morax, Andre Cuenod (d. 1954) and Roger Nataf (1901–86) is particularly noteworthy.

Japan

It is unclear when trachoma was first recognised in Japan but in the 14th century it was known as "borome" (wretched eye) (54). Some have commented that it was not documented before the middle of the 1800s when Japan reopened trade with the West (9). In 1897, just after the Sino Japanese War (1894–5), the prevalence of trachoma in Tokyo is reported to be 14% and between 25% to 75% of eye patients had trachoma (15) as infected soldiers returned home from Korea and Manchuria (54) (see Figure 2.17).

In 1919 the Trachoma Control Law called for the entire population to be periodically examined and between 7 million to 10 million people were examined each year (9). The Japan Trachoma Society was established to co-ordinate this activity and provide training and guidelines. All men were examined at the age of 19 and again, one year later, when they were called up for military service. All schoolchildren, teachers and those with close occupational contact with others such as nurses and hairdressers were examined every year. Any person who was diagnosed with trachoma was treated (at no charge for the poor) and they and their relatives were given proper hygiene instruction (4). In 1929 the population prevalence was reported to be 13% (58). Trachoma Prevention Day was later marked with educational films and lectures and eventually became the Japanese World Sight Day and is still celebrated on 10 October ("10/10").

With the rapid social change and economic development in Japan, the number of people with trachoma had fallen dramatically in the 1950s, even given the disruption of activities during the Second World War (1939–45) (83) (see Figure 2.18). The amount of blindness due to trachoma had fallen from about 15% of blindness in the 1930s to 0.1% in 1974 (84). In 1983 the Trachoma Control Law was repealed and the Japan Trachoma Society became the Japanese Society for the Prevention of Blindness.

USSR

At the start of the 20th century Russia had the highest rates of trachoma of any European country (15). Trachoma had been thought to exist in the Crimea "from time immemorial". In the early 20th century trachoma was thought to be present throughout the Soviet Union (59) and in the 1920s, the reported rates of trachoma ranged from 6% in Russia to 15% to 20% in the Central Asian Republics, with some areas as high as 86% (58). The first Ophthalmological Congress of the Soviet Union (1926) established guidelines for new dispensaries and "flying columns" to be created to control trachoma. Enabling legislation was passed in 1927 that authorised health authorities to examine anyone thought to be at risk of having trachoma and to compel infected persons to

undergo treatment (59). The specific trachoma intervention program was enhanced in 1938 when trachoma was made a notifiable disease. The program continued through and after the Second World War (52). Trachoma control was again included in Stalin's fourth five-year plan in 1946.

The USSR campaign was designed on the model developed in Egypt by MacCallan and his colleagues. It involved the establishment of ophthalmic hospitals, some stationary and some mobile, and numerous local and regional school dispensaries (52). The ophthalmologic co-ordinating centres provided eye care services but also provided training, liaison and co-ordination for those working in regional and village programs. Regional ophthalmologists co-ordinated field activities that were predominantly carried out by village physicians and trained assistants. Regional health education campaigns were conducted with the emphasis on the eradication of trachoma as a societal disease of the collective.

Good progress was made with general health education campaigns, case identification, treatment of cases with copper sulphate and silver nitrate (and later the sulfa drugs), and socioeconomic development. The advent of tetracycline in the 1950s led to a speedy elimination of trachoma in most areas and similar programs were initiated in Yugoslavia, Hungary, Poland and Rumania.

Thailand

Trachoma has been a major problem in Thailand, particularly in the central and north-east areas. These areas are extremely dry and dusty with poor water supply and are very similar to adjacent areas in Myanmar and Cambodia. Trachoma was known as "Ta Nam" (watery eye) (54). A vertical trachoma control program was started with WHO support in 1959. Having started as a pilot project in one province, Korat, it extended in 1967 to cover nine provinces in the north-east region. Household surveys were performed with door to door registration and examination of all family members. Health education was promoted through community and school meetings and specific training of medical and non-medical support personnel was provided. Individual topical tetracycline treatment was administered by community volunteers and trichiasis surgery was performed at subcentres by mobile teams.

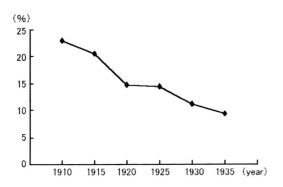

LEFT **Figure 2.17** Trachoma prevalence in Japanese military conscripts (Konyama 2004–2005 (54), reproduced with permission from Wolters Kluwer, France).

BELOW **Figure 2.18** Trachoma prevalence in Japanese schoolchildren (Konyama 2004–2005 (54), reproduced with permission from Wolters Kluwer, France).

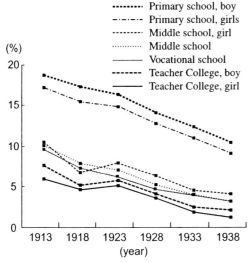

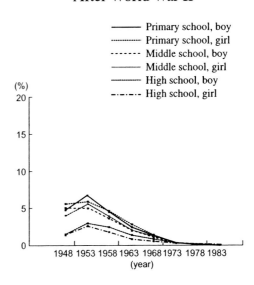

This continued as a vertical program until 1976, by which time trachoma rates were falling, and Thailand had started to develop a primary health care model. The trachoma program was considered a prototype for primary health care and led directly to the development of a primary eye care system (54). The screening of all schoolchildren for trachoma continued as did individual treatment.

When the program started, active trachoma rates were of the order of 20% with 66% of the population showing some signs of trachoma (54). There was not a clear gender difference and trachoma was responsible for 9% of blindness. During this period there was considerable community development and by 1984, the prevalence of trachoma in children had fallen to 0.6%, and trichiasis rates were 0.2%. Based on

these data, the Ministry of Public Health ceased trachoma services in primary and secondary schools and replaced this with a refraction service for schoolchildren. Until that time, all schoolchildren were still routinely examined for trachoma. The work in Thailand is a wonderful example of a successfully planned vertical intervention campaign against trachoma that became integrated into the ongoing primary health care system during its consolidation phase.

There is neither enough time nor is it my intention to document trachoma trends in every country. I have briefly considered a few countries to give an outline of the way trachoma has been managed and disappeared. The unusual situation in Australia will be dealt with in more detail in chapter ten.

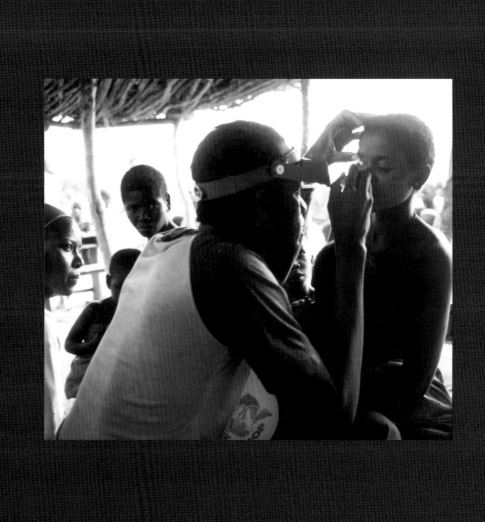

CHAPTER THREE

Clinical diagnosis

*A blind man on a galloping horse on a dark night without
a light can diagnose trachoma*
FRED HOLLOWS, 1976

If the diagnosis were clear and precise, no rules would be required
JULIUS BOLDT, 1904

IT SEEMS UNIVERSALLY accepted and recognised over time that however defined, trachoma has two major phases: active or inflammatory trachoma and cicatricial or late trachoma. Active trachoma is characterised by an inflammatory response associated with the variable presence of demonstrable infection. The inflammation can vary in intensity but when severe, it leads to tarsal scarring and corneal pannus. Cicatricial trachoma is marked by structural change in the lid with tarsal scarring and trichiasis. In this case, inflammation is variable and chlamydia are infrequently seen.

In an endemic area, a well-established case of active trachoma can be very easy to diagnose. I first started trachoma fieldwork in Port Augusta, South Australia, in 1976. On our second day in the field, young schoolboys whom we examined the day before, were everting each other's lids and examining for trachoma. The difficulty with diagnosing active inflammatory trachoma in an endemic area is not so much in making the diagnosis in established cases, but the differentiation of borderline cases from normal, or sometimes, distinguishing cases of severe inflammatory trachoma from acute bacterial or viral conjunctivitis. The detection of trichiasis *only* requires careful examination. However, the diagnosis of trachoma can be much more difficult to make in areas of low endemicity, although severe tarsal scarring, corneal pannus with Herbert's pits and upper lid trichiasis are almost pathonomonic in any setting.

The key sign in active trachoma is the "trachoma follicle", that is, lymphoid follicles or germinal centres in the superior tarsal conjunctiva. However, the intense diffuse inflammatory infiltrate that surrounds the follicles causes tissue damage that leads to scarring and the subsequent lid changes, trichiasis and eventual blindness. Although the presence of superior tarsal follicles is used as the primary diagnostic feature in the grading of active trachoma, it is the intense inflammation shown by conjunctival inflammatory thickening and papillae that reflects the critical process in the pathogenesis. In this regard, when we grade trachoma, we may have been "hoodwinked" by the follicles.

The ancient classification of trachoma

Although trachoma was well recognised in ancient Egypt and China, we have no written descriptions of its clinical evolution. The ancient Greeks and Romans were familiar with trachoma and knew it well, both as a purulent ophthalmia (or lippitudo) and as a cause of the subsequent trichiasis (trichosis). All the surviving ancient medical texts that deal with ocular disease include descriptions of trachoma and its treatment (10).

Hippocrates first recorded the terms "ophthalmia" and "trichosis" (in 400 BC) and compared the changes of the thickened lid to a cut open black fig—both thickened, red and studded with white dots. The Greco-Roman encyclopaedist surgeon Celsus described the roughness of the lid in 14 AD and called the disease "rough eye lids" (aspritudo oculorum palpebrarum) or aspritudo for short. This seems to refer to the changes of active trachoma, but may also have been used to refer to the roughened surface of the tarsus caused by scarring when viewed by the naked eye. The Greek translation of aspritudo is "trachoma", a term first used by Discorides (~60 AD).

A book called De Oculis by Claudius Galerus appeared long after Galen's death in 201 AD. Although attributed to Galen, this book is thought to be a collection of Greek writings put together by an Arabian author (10). Trachoma is described as having four stages. These stages were "itchy eye", "rough", "scarred" and "trichiasis". These four

stages were more fully described by Aetius of Amida (540 AD) and subsequently repeated by many authors. This grading seems to have been widely used around the Mediterranean and was still used in the Middle Ages (21). The Arabian ophthalmologist Ali Ibn Isa of Baghdad (~1000 AD) used the term "sarab" (scabies) in the eye in his classic textbook and this term became widely used. This term was also taken up by medieval Europe as the Arabic texts were first translated to Latin and then from Latin into the vernacular (18).

The 19th century

In the excitement generated by severe purulent conjunctivitis spreading in epidemic proportions and the frequent corneal ulceration that characterised Ophthalmia aegypticus in the early 1800s, the ancient classification was either forgotten or swamped. Vetch was familiar with the ancient texts and treatments and quoted them (16). However, most military surgeons who accompanied the French and British forces in Egypt were not trained in ophthalmology and would not be versed in such matters. Their job was to treat the wounded and sick. As we have seen, most ophthalmologists, such as Mackenzie in his landmark textbook, concentrated almost entirely on the acute manifestations of the ophthalmia (29). They classified the type and severity of the conjunctival discharge, almost infinite variations in ocular pain to which great diagnostic importance was attached, and the degree of corneal involvement, although conjunctival scarring and trichiasis were clearly recognised as late complications.

Mackenzie based much of his material on the work of the British military physician John Vetch, who had written a very interesting monograph detailing his experiences with the Egyptian ophthalmia (16). In his introduction Vetch does refer to the ancient writers, Hippocrates, Aetius and Paullus of Aegetius, as well as Celsus and Avincenna. He differentiated the Egyptian ophthalmia as the "lippitudo of the Ancients" from ocular gonorrhea and stressed the importance of conjunctival "granulations" under the upper lid (see Figure 3.1). This led to the use of the term

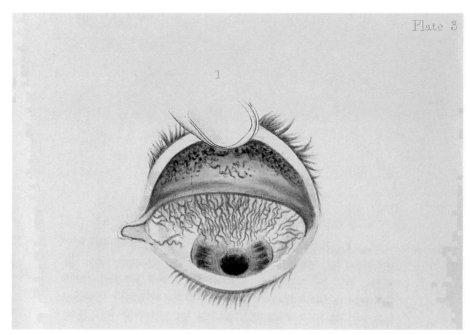

Figure 3.1 Granular conjunctivitis. "Represents a granular state of the conjunctiva of the upper lid, with the first effects by the pressure upon the globe; the inflammation occasioned by the pressure being indicated by the reddened appearance of the subjacent conjunctiva, and the haze of the upper part of the surface of the cornea" (Morgan J. Lectures on Diseases of the Eye. 2nd ed. London: Samuel Highley, 1848).

"granular conjunctivitis" and the granulations were to be distinguished from papillae. Bendz in Copenhagen undertook histologic studies and described the granulations as "collections of lymphoid cells" (85). He identified them as lymphoid follicles and pointed out the similarities between the conjunctival follicles and Peyer's patches in the intestinal mucosa. He differentiated the granulations into "glandular" granulations (or follicles) and "papillary" granulations. Other granulations may include post trachomatous degenerations and concretions that may be seen as calcified inclusions or grains of sand in scarred lids. By the end of the 19th century, the term "follicle" was widely used.

Boldt gives an interesting description of the progressive change in the definition in trachoma that was used by the Prussian Army in the 19th century (15). These changes reflected what was happening elsewhere in Europe. From 1815, all soldiers with contagious ophthalmia were sent home after all pain, inflammation and discharge had "passed off". Their commanding officer was first to notify the district council of a soldier's discharge. Contagious ophthalmia was not defined further, although any recruits with severe contagious ophthalmia were rejected. Men with mild cases of ophthalmia were still recruited.

As Boldt states "an extraordinary difference of opinion often arose over the passing of recruits between the army surgeons and the medical officers" (15). In one instance, 328 possible recruits were initially rejected because of trachoma, but none was thought to have trachoma when they were re-examined. Boldt points out the clinical difficulty of making a precise diagnosis, the occurrence of doubtful cases, the seriousness of the consequences of missing a case of purulent conjunctivitis that could spark an epidemic, and the possibility that potential recruits might aggravate "any slight conjunctivitis" to deliberately avoid conscription. We still encounter similar difficulties today, especially in low prevalence areas.

In 1863, the Prussian Army further defined infectious diseases of the eye to recognise the following conditions: primary granulations, granular conjunctivitis, acute blennorrhoea, chronic blennorrhoea and secondary granulations.

By 1880 a large controversy raged between the so-called "Unitarians" and the "Dualists" (15). By this stage what we now know today as inclusion conjunctivitis (primary granulations, or mild follicular conjunctivitis) was seen to have many similarities with trachoma, but it was self-limiting and did not lead to the chronic blinding sequelae of trachoma. The Unitarians believed that both inclusion conjunctivitis and trachoma were manifestations of the same disease. The Dualists believed they were two quite separate diseases. The Unitarians tended to work in endemic areas whereas the Dualists tended to work in areas where endemic trachoma had become rare (15). This controversy continued to involve intense debate throughout the 1930s and 1950s. It was partially resolved when chlamydia was cultured in 1957, but this issue also underlies the current discussion of reinfection and persistent infection.

The presence of follicles on the upper tarsus was used as the key determining sign between trachoma and inclusion conjunctivitis or follicular conjunctivitis. In 1880, the Prussian Army issued new regulations. The Dualists had prevailed and recruits could be accepted with acute or chronic conjunctivitis with only moderate discharge, slight cases of follicular conjunctivitis with a normal upper tarsal plate, or those with primary granulations (follicles but without appreciable conjunctival oedema or thickening). Presumably

new soldiers were hard to find after the Franco-Prussian Wars and so pragmatically the criteria were weakened.

During this time, Eduard Raehlmann (1843–1917) had reported his extensive histological studies showing the similarity of inclusion conjunctivitis, primary granulations and trachoma (86) (see Figure 3.2). This lent further weight to the Unitarians who prevailed when the Prussian Army regulations were rewritten by von Hippel in 1893. Now recruits with any follicles in the upper lid were excluded (15). The concurrent development of bacteriology and the ability to positively identify gonococcus greatly clarified the confusion between the blennorrhoeic, catarrhal and granular forms of conjunctivitis that had previously confused the diagnosis of acute or active trachoma from other forms of acute ophthalmia.

On the basis of his histological studies, Raehlmann also described trachoma as having four stages (86). The first, Acute Trachoma, had follicles present as part of an acute conjunctivitis.

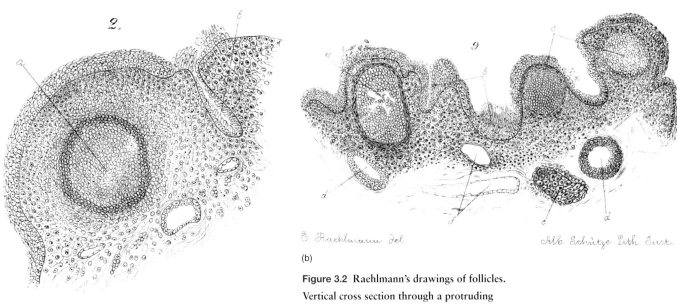

(a)

(b)

Figure 3.2 Raehlmann's drawings of follicles. Vertical cross section through a protruding crease of a mucous membrane
(a) young follicle with a closed capsule of hematoxylin of marked colouring cells
(b) gland depression (Raehlmann 1883 (86)).

This then progressed to Chronic Trachoma of which there were three further stages. The first chronic stage ("Stage 2") was characterised by an increase in the number and size of follicles, the marked development of papillae and the appearance of superior corneal pannus. The next stage ("Stage 3") was characterised by degeneration with the destruction of follicles and early tarsal scarring. The final stage of Chronic Trachoma ("Stage 4") featured cicatrization, as the lid became pale and was no longer swollen, with the ultimate development of entropion and trichiasis. In untreated cases, up to two-thirds of those infected would develop trichiasis or some corneal changes, and 5% would develop dacryocystitis.

Boldt was convinced that the development of conjunctival and tarsal scarring was essential for the healing of trachoma. Scarring destroyed the "adenoid tissue" or follicles which provided "the ground on which trachoma developed". He succinctly states " No scarring, no cure" (15). Although he also observes "The greater and deeper the diffuse infiltration and follicle formation, the more marked the subsequent scarring" (15).

However, despite having described the stages proposed by Raehlmann and the histologic studies that underpinned it, Boldt, a military surgeon with an eye on the military consequences (15), recommended grading or grouping of trachoma cases into four classes following the plan of Hirschberg (87) and Greeff (88):

A Suspicious cases.

B Mild cases with moderate hypertrophy of the conjunctiva and a few follicles in the tarsus.

C Moderately severe cases, showing many follicles in both lids and marked lid swelling.

D Severe cases which already showed cicatricial sequelae such as tarsal scarring, pannus, entropion and trichiasis.

The presence of distinct thickening and infiltration of the tarsal conjunctiva or papillary hypertrophy was regarded as essential for the diagnosis of trachoma (classes B and C).

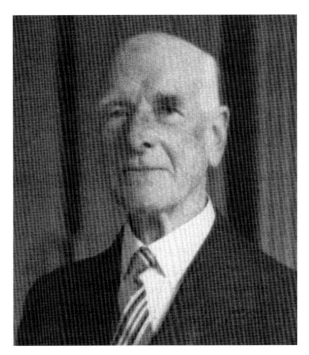

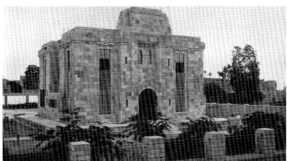

TOP **Figure 3.3** AF MacCallan (Duke-Elder 1965 (412)).

BOTTOM **Figure 3.4** The Memorial Ophthalmic Laboratory, Giza, Egypt (MacCallan 1936 (4)).

MacCallan Classification, 1908

In 1903 a British merchant banker who had financed the building of the original Aswan Dam, Sir Ernest Cassel (1852–1921), donated £40,000 to the Egyptian Government to establish a program to address eye disease in Egypt and to train local doctors in ophthalmology (30). Arthur Ferguson MacCallan (1873–1955), an ophthalmologist from Moorfields, went to Egypt to start this program (see Figure 3.3). This program used both mobile and permanent eye hospitals and soon started school treatment

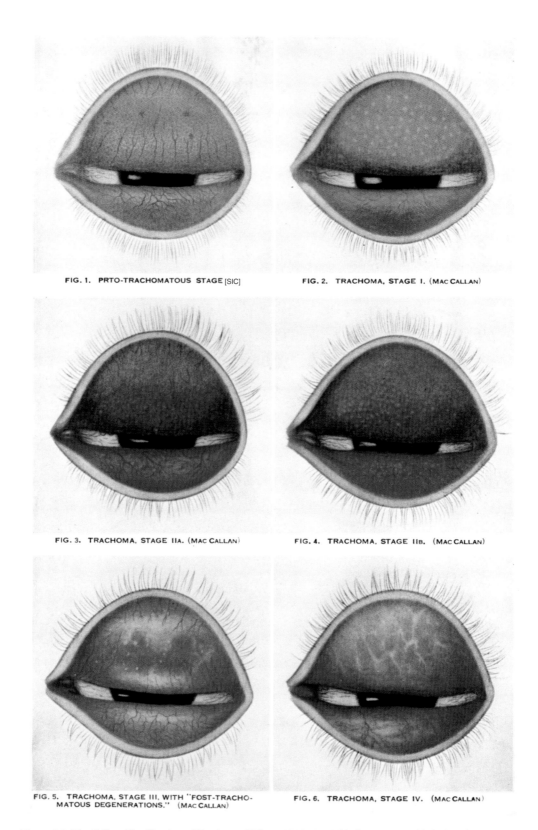

FIG. 1. PRTO-TRACHOMATOUS STAGE [SIC]

FIG. 2. TRACHOMA, STAGE I. (MAC CALLAN)

FIG. 3. TRACHOMA, STAGE IIA. (MAC CALLAN)

FIG. 4. TRACHOMA, STAGE IIB. (MAC CALLAN)

FIG. 5. TRACHOMA, STAGE III, WITH "POST-TRACHO-MATOUS DEGENERATIONS." (MAC CALLAN)

FIG. 6. TRACHOMA, STAGE IV. (MAC CALLAN)

Figure 3.5 MacCallan Classification of Trachoma (Wilson 1932 (32). This figure was published in the American Journal of Ophthalmology, Vol 15, Wilson RP, Ophthalmia Aegyptica, 397–406, © Elsevier (1932)).

Table 3.1: MacCallan Classification of trachoma (89)

Trachoma I, seen typically soon after infection has occurred.

Trachoma II*a*, in which follicles predominate.

Trachoma II*b*, in which a papillary hypertrophy coexists with the follicles. *This subdivision may be split up into trachoma II*b'* and trachoma II*b"*. Trachoma II*b'* is unmixed trachoma; trachoma II*b"* is trachoma complicated by spring catarrh.

Trachoma II*c*, trachoma complicated by chronic gonococcal conjunctivitis.

Trachoma III, in which cicatrization is beginning.

Trachoma IV, in which cicatrization is complete.

*This further subdivision was added in 1913.

programs. After the end of the First World War, the Memorial Ophthalmic Laboratory was built at Giza with support from the Imperial War Graves Commission (4) (see Figure 3.4).

In 1908 MacCallan published his classification system that was to become the standard classification worldwide (89). He subsequently acknowledged this as a natural development of the system previously described by Raehlmann (25). By 1913, his apparently simple four-stage classification actually contained eight stages or sub-stages (see Table 3.1 and Figure 3.5). MacCallan optimistically states "with a comparatively small amount of experience, most cases of trachoma can be placed easily in one or other of these stages. Some cases are borderline between two stages and may be so indicated, eg trachoma I to IIa or trachoma IIa to III". He further states that "unmixed trachoma is always a chronic disease. It frequently commences with acute manifestations or exhibits acute exacerbations, but these are the result of superadded infections with well-known bacteria" (25).

The MacCallan Classification was soon taken up by others. Ernest Fuchs (1851–1930) in Vienna and Edmund Landolt (1846–1926) in Paris both visited MacCallan in Egypt before 1914, and they took his grading back to their clinics where they adopted and promoted it, as did Cuenod and Nataf in Tunis and other leaders in the field. It

became the standard classification for English and French ophthalmologists (73). In fact, the MacCallan Classification was the world standard for over 60 years.

However, the MacCallan Classification had many shortcomings. In 1967 Ida Mann (1893–1983), a distinguished British ophthalmologist who after migrating to Australia did extraordinary work in outback Australia and the Pacific Islands, wrote "We now realise that the old concept of a clearcut clinical entity running a known course divisible into stages through which each case passes, is largely untenable"(90). Again in 1975, Barrie Jones (1921–), a New Zealander who was the first Professor of Ophthalmology in London, suggested that the MacCallan stages of trachoma:

> have come to offer a barrier to elucidation for they tacitly suggest that the disease runs a single cycle and on their own they give no quantification of the intensity of active inflammation, nor a sufficient description of the scarring that leads to the evolution of trichiasis and entropion. The most urgent requirement is to appreciate that the disease is frequently a multi-cyclic infection (91).

The World Health Organization (WHO) was established after the Second World War. Trachoma was one of the high priorities that it inherited from the preceding League of Nations. The first WHO Expert Committee on Trachoma met in 1952 (20). They adopted the MacCallan Classification as the standard for use in administrative documents and for collecting national level data, but as we will see below, they also created a much more detailed and precise grading scheme for "clinical and scientific" use. They developed a complicated coding system to further specify the presence of follicles, papillae and scars and to grade their severity (see Table 3.2). They also advocated recording the presence and extent of corneal vessels and corneal infiltrate.

In 1962, the third Expert Committee reviewed the grading system and proposed further changes (49). They suggested the term "TrD" (trachoma dubium) be used for clinical signs suggestive of an early conjunctival response to invasion by a trachoma virus. They suggested another new category of "ND" (not determined) to indicate doubt as to whether more advanced lesions were

Table 3.2: WHO Expert Committee on Trachoma First Report 1952 (20)

Note: in administrative documents, only the indications of the basic stages of trachoma should be used.

Examples

Tr I = trachoma at onset

Tr II = established trachoma (including florid forms)

Tr III = cicatrizing trachoma

Tr IV = cicatrized or healed trachoma

Note: for documents requiring more precise clinical and scientific recording of observations, additional symbols should be used.

(1) Stages of trachoma (Tr I, Tr II, Tr III, Tr IV)

(2) Presence of an associated disease, mixed form (M)

(3) Indication of verification of cure by a recognised test (v)

(4) Presence of scars (C)*

(5) Presence of follicles (F)* or of prefollicular lesions (prF)

(6) Presence of papillae (P)*

(7) Presence of corneal vessels (V)**

(8) Infiltration of the cornea (i)**

* to be graded by severity of the lesions

** to be graded in mm

trachomatous or not. A further classification of "PrTr" (or proto-trachoma or pre-follicular trachoma) was also added. These changes added further complexity to the MacCallan Classification, but did not address the above shortcomings by Mann and Jones.

Workers in the field also made their own adjustments to the MacCallan Classification. For example, Roger Nichols and the Harvard group working in Saudi Arabia graded individuals as being normal, or having hyperemia, muco-purulent conjunctivitis, or stages II, III or IV of trachoma (92). However, the MacCallan system was well embedded and continued to be described in textbooks and in WHO publications until 1981. It was still in use in reports appearing as recently as 1997 (93).

World Health Organization trachoma classifications, 1952–62

The World Health Organization Expert Committees on Trachoma brought together experts on trachoma from all parts of the world. Membership of the four Expert Committees held between 1952 and 1966 changed somewhat and each member brought their own particular experience and hobby horses. The first Committee (1952) reinforced the status quo and the MacCallan Classification, but as mentioned they suggested a new level of complexity and sub-specification for researchers (Table 3.2) (20).

The second Committee (1956) was more preoccupied with setting a research agenda for trachoma (33). They established the criteria needed to make a clinical diagnosis and insisted that at least two of the following signs be present: follicles (conjunctival or limbal), epithelial keratitis in the

Figure 3.6 Clinical stages of trachoma (Cuenod & Nataf 1934 (97), reproduced with permission from Elsevier Masson).

Early "pure" trachoma (Tr I) – see page opposite

Fig 1. Early trachoma in eight-year-old child: to the naked eye, the conjunctiva presents some "white-yellowish" points composing "granulations" that at this initial stage only project a little.

Fig 2. A small portion of the tarsal conjunctiva of the upper eyelid. The vascular system of the tarsal conjunctiva is very blurred, as though covered by a veil. The follicles appear as "half-blisters", lightly covered and opalescent, with vessels between and around them that seem to come from normal vessels. In addition, one can see on the surface of the conjunctiva the flowering bouquets of the neo-vascularisation raising perpendicular to the conjunctival plane. The upper border of the tarsus and the superior tarsal conjunctiva in addition to follicles also show darker papillae with poorly defined contours. They create a mosaic of papillae around the follicles. In general, the follicles seem to be situated at the bifurcation of the normal tarsal vessels.

Fig 3. An early trachoma follicle: this follicle is characterised by a defined, raised, half-blistered bulge; opalescent but nearly translucent through which one can discern a network of normal conjunctival vessels. This hemispherical bulge has imprecise contours and is surrounded by vascular plumes that rise from the normal network of vessels. Some of these vascular plumes give branches that cross the surface of the follicle and some may penetrate them. The vascularisation of the follicle is essentially at the periphery and on the surface, the trunks of the small capillaries wind over the surface, and only the terminal branches penetrate the follicles. This is the opposite of what is seen in papillae that usually have one, or sometimes two, central vascular trunks with terminal branches that expand on the surface.

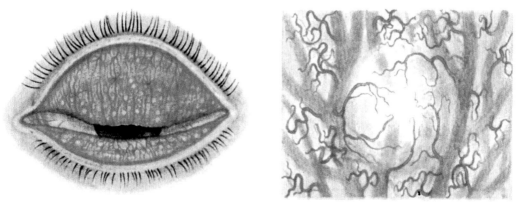

Fig. 1

Fig. 3

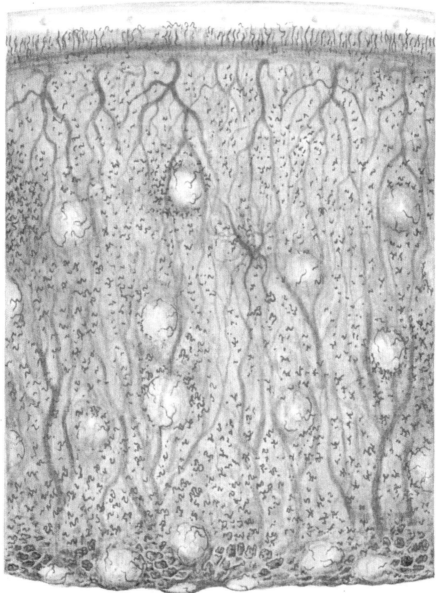

Fig. 2

Figure 3.6 *See legend opposite*

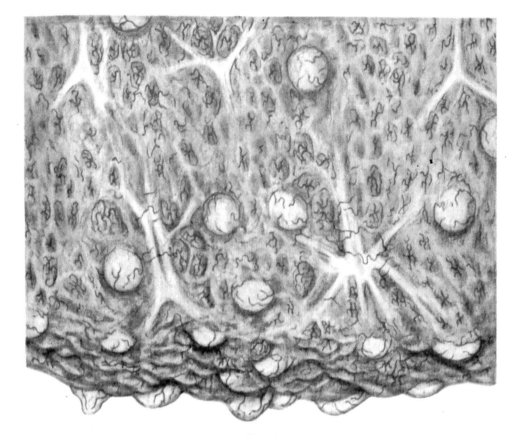

Fig. 1

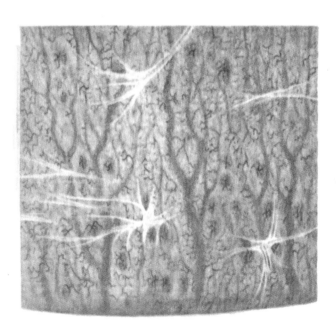

Fig. 2

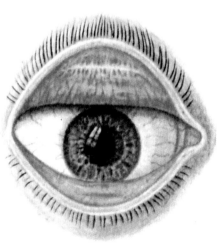

Fig. 3

Figure 3.6 *Continued–see legend opposite*

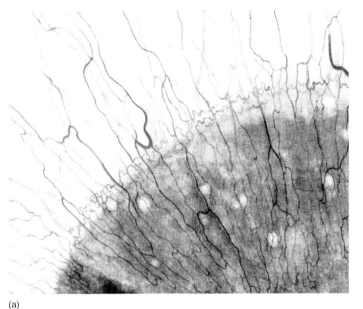 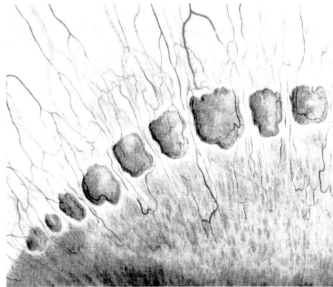

(a)   (b)

Trachomatous pannus – see above

(a) Trachomatous pannus in a developing stage: biomicroscopy clearly confirms that trachomatous pannus merits the name of a "Vasculo-granular Veil". The superior third of the cornea shows an extensive infiltration. Instead of stopping at the limbus, the vessels of the bulbar conjunctiva continue directly towards the centre of the cornea, perpendicular to the limbus.

These vessels stop at the limit of infiltration and anastomose, making vascular arcades and loops. Studies of early pannus indicate that the infiltration precedes this vascularisation of the infiltrated zone and that focal inflammatory condensations are usually situated at the points of vascular branching.

These focal collections more or less crimp the vessels; they are lightly covered by the corneal epithelium and constitute true follicles, some are vascularised and clearly resemble the trachoma follicles of the conjunctiva. Beyond the zone of infiltration and in the healthy cornea there are more or less isolated focal points of infiltration that seem to precede the infiltration and the vascularised pannus.

(b) Trachomatous pannus and limbal changes: the cornea presents a thinned pannus; the "veil" has regressed. The infiltration is gray and transparent in the upper third of the cornea; with very fine vascularisation. All along the superior arc of the limbus is a veritable chain of small excavations of varied shape and size, with a transparent base that more or less crimps the fine vessels. These are the "limbal ocelles" of Bonnet or Herbert's Pits that are the remainder of the follicles that occur in trachomatous pannus and particularly the limbal follicles (the Sago limbus of Bonnet) that have now healed and now are empty.

Trachoma scarring – see page opposite

Fig 1. Early trachoma scarring (Tr III): the star-like scars are shown as if they mark the position of old follicles. There is still the neat array of papillae and many typically trachoma follicles.

Fig 2. Spontaneous trachoma scarring (Tr IV): a case of trachoma that healed spontaneously that was found while looking for a foreign body under the lid of a high school student in Tunisia. The follicles have gone but there are some residual papillae. The surface of the conjunctiva is seeded with very fine scarring with an irregular "star shape".

Fig 3. Trachoma scarring (Tr IV): Arlt's line is visible with the naked eye. Brilliant white lines can be seen on the palpable conjunctiva. They constitute scarring that extends from Arlt's line throughout the upper eyelid.

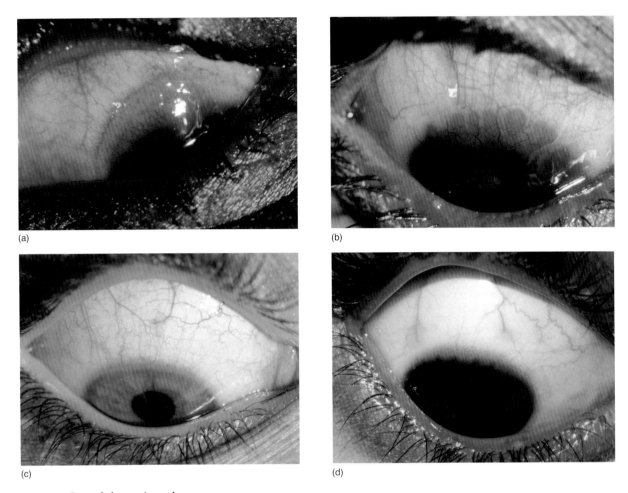

Figure 3.7 Corneal changes in trachoma

(a) the string of small elevated limbal follicles can be seen at the limbus with surrounding pannus

(b) very large limbal follicles clearly displacing the vessels in the limbal pannus

(c) fine residual pannus after the resolution of all inflammation

(d) fine trachomatous pannus with typical Herbert's pits.

upper cornea, superior corneal pannus, or typical conjunctival scarring. They also reaffirmed that trachoma could arise as an acute disease even in the absence of secondary bacterial or viral infection; but they considered such an acute onset to be rare as most cases of uncomplicated trachoma had an insidious onset.

The third Committee (1962) was particularly concerned with the laboratory methods used to diagnose trachoma (49). Since chlamydia was first cultured in 1957, there had been a rapid development in a wide range of laboratory diagnostic tests. The ability to culture chlamydia also opened the way to vaccine development and the Committee developed some guidelines for the design and

parameters for vaccine trials. They also formulated and introduced an index for the clinical grading of severity and gravity that was subsequently further developed (94).

The fourth Committee was also preoccupied with the importance of changes in the superior cornea; the development of micro and macroscopic pannus, subepithelial opacification and superficial punctate keratitis. Phillips Thygeson (1903–2002), the Founding Director of the Francis Proctor Foundation in San Francisco, was a man who made enormous contributions to the field over nearly 70 years. He was also known to hold firm opinions and was one of few people on each of the four Expert Committees. He stated elsewhere that pannus was "an unequivocally essential component of trachoma" (95).

The slit lamp was invented in 1911 by the Swedish ophthalmologist Alvar Gullstrand (1862–1930, Nobel Laureate in 1911) but was not widely used until the 1920s. Prior to this, loupes of up to 10 times magnification had been used to study and describe the corneal changes. The slit lamp facilitated these studies and several detailed studies of the conjunctival and corneal changes appeared (96,97) (see Figure 3.6). This led to an increased awareness of corneal neovascularisation and pannus. In milder cases pannus and corneal changes may only be seen by slit lamp examinations. However in 1904 Major H. Herbert, a British ophthalmologist serving in Bombay had described his characteristic limbal pits (98). Subsequently pannus and Herbert's pits became prerequisites for the diagnosis of trachoma (see Figure 3.7). Detailed studies and drawings of the corneal vascular changes had been made by Rowland Wilson (1896–1981) in Egypt in 1932 (96). Wilson, a New Zealander, had succeeded MacCallan as the Director of the Giza Laboratory from 1926 to 1945.

During the "aetiology" wars fought in the 1930s over claims such as Noguchi's for *B. granulosis*, the presence of corneal changes became the defining criterion for real trachoma for many strong characters. Thygeson had put much store on the fact that the studies of *B. granulosis* had not produced these corneal changes, and he used this fact to argue that *B. granulosis* could not be the causative agent of trachoma. Similar criticisms were laid against any human "volunteer" or animal study that did not generate corneal changes. The third Committee accepted the necessity to precisely monitor and document corneal changes, although they recognised that there was "a difference of opinion in the diagnostic importance of pannus". Some very detailed classification schemes for grading pannus in field studies were devised (99); the proponents developed considerable skill and accuracy, whether using a slit lamp or loupe, and even graded the first millimetre of pannus into quarter segments (100). However, the detailed grading of pannus ultimately proved to be of little practical use.

The WHO trachoma grading system, 1966–81

The fourth WHO Expert Committee (now a Scientific Group) finally tackled the issue of trachoma grading head on in 1966 (50). Although they did not actively condemn the MacCallan Classification, they did introduce a new grading system. The new system came in two forms: A could be used for a full examination which required the use of a slit lamp and the staining of the cornea, and B was a minimal examination using the naked eye or a binocular loupe considered suitable for field studies. Twenty signs were to be graded for the slit lamp exam and eight were used in the minimal exam. Most signs were graded from 0 to 3, although some were graded from 0 to 2, 4 or 5 (see Table 3.3) (50). The grading of these signs, in some cases 22, proved exceedingly tedious to perform in 16 fields and highly complex to analyse. The concepts of grouping signs to give measures of intensity, severity and gravity were further refined. Although the intensity index proved useful and all signs were further refined, it seems that the gravity index was only used by its originators.

This Scientific Group also spent considerable time discussing the issues of distinguishing trachoma, inclusion conjunctivitis and ocular infection with the lymphogranuloma venerum (LGV). All three diseases were caused by chlamydia and although agreeing on the different clinical features of each "syndrome", this Scientific Group recommended continuing research into this issue.

Subsequently, further refinements and modifications to the trachoma grading system were put forward by the staff of the WHO Trachoma Program. In 1967, Fakhry Assaad and Peter Maxwell-Lyons more fully developed the concept of the aggregation of signs of trachoma into cardinal signs for diagnosis, signs that indicated the intensity of the disease and the gravity or likelihood of visual loss (see Table 3.4) (101).

The next development in 1973 was the publication of a new WHO grading system by Mario Tarizzo (d. 1980), then Director of the WHO Trachoma Program (102). This revised the 1966 WHO Scientific Group Classification and

Table 3.3: Fourth WHO Scientific Group on trachoma 1966 (50)

Methods of scoring and recording trachoma

A. *Full examination* (using available diagnostic aids: major biomicroscope and staining of cornea) practicable only in detailed studies of small groups.

B. *Minimal examination* (using naked eye of binocular loupe) practicable in large-scale studies (*****Denotes signs to be collected).

Physical sign	Degree of involvement	Score [1]
Ptosis	Detectable	1
	Definite, but not completely covering the pupil	2
	Covering the pupil	3
Sinuous outlines of the upper lid border (Herbert's sign)	Present	1
Exudate (observed without previous cleaning)	Minimal	1
	Moderate, but lids not stuck together	2
	Lids stuck together	3
Pre-auricular lymph nodes Size	Just palpable	1
	Easily palpable (but not detected by observation)	2
	Visibly enlarged	3
Tenderness	Slight, elicited on palpation	1
	Moderate, elicited on palpation (patient resenting palpation)	2
	Severe, associated with pain	3
Hyperaemia of bulbar conjunctiva	Circumcorneal flush or slight extension from the fornices	1
	Patchy	2
	Total, with or without minute haemorrhages	3
Oedema of upper lunula [2] (Wilson's sign)	Detectable by major biomicroscope	1
	Detectable by the naked eye of binocular loupe	2
	Bulbar chemosis	3
* *Conjunctival follicles* [3] Upper tarsal conjunctiva	Involving < ⅓ of surface area	1
	Involving ⅓ to ⅔ of surface area	2
	Involving the entire surface area (not confluent)	3
	Total confluent involvement (Stellwag's sign)	4
Upper fornix	Slight involvement	1
	Moderate or marked involvement but not confluent	2
	Total confluent involvement	3
Semilunar folds	Slight involvement	1
	Moderate or marked involvement but not confluent	2
	Total confluent involvement	3
Bulbar conjunctiva	Presence of follicles	1
Lower tarsal conjunctiva and fornix	Involving < ⅓ of the surface area	1
	Involving ≥ ⅓ of the surface area short of total involvement	2
	Involving the entire surface area	3
* *Diffuse cellular infiltration and papillary hyperplasia* (upper tarsal conjunctiva)	Minimal; major biomicroscope needed for recognition, normal vessels not obscured	1
	Moderate; recognisable by the naked eye or binocular loupe, normal vessels appear hazy	2
	Pronounced; conjunctiva thickened and opaque, normal vessels obscured	3

Table 3.3: *continued*

★ Conjunctival scars	Deviation of upper tarsal conjunctival vessels, and/or fine scattered superficial scars in upper tarsal conjunctiva, or scars of any severity or extent in other conjunctival sites	1
	Moderate readily recognisable scarring with no shortening or distortion of the upper tarsus	2
	Dense scarring of the upper tarsal conjunctival tissue	3
	Trichiasis and/or entropion	4

★ Limbus and cornea:
★ Pannus
Vessels (measured from the upper limbus)

Micropannus	0.5 – <1.0 mm extension beyond normal limbal opacity, as demonstrated by direct focal illumination	1
	1.0 – <2.0 mm extension	2
★ Macropannus	2.0 – <4.0 mm extension	3
	4.0 – <6.0 mm extension	4
	6.0 mm or more extension	5
★ Infiltration just beyond corneal vessels	Minimal infiltration recognisable only by major biomicroscope	1
	Infiltration barely recognisable by naked eye or binocular loupe	2
	Dense opacification	3
★ Limbal follicles	One to three typical follicles	1
	More than three, but not involving entire upper lunula	2
	Entire upper lunula involved	3
	Cornea encircled or two rows of follicles above	4
★ Herbert's pits	One to three typical pits	1
	More than three but entire upper lunula not involved	2
	Entire upper lunula involved	3
	Cornea encircled or two rows of pits above	4
★ Corneal scars	Minimal, resulting in slight or no visual loss [4]	1
	Moderate visual loss, pupillary area involved	2
	Resulting in gross visual loss in one eye	3
	Resulting in gross visual loss in both eyes (economic blindness)	4

[1.] If the physical sign has been looked for but not detected this should be indicated by a "0"; if the physical sign has not been checked (for example, pannus in very young children) this should be denoted by a blank.

[2.] The term "upper lunula" is used to denote the crescentic semi-opaque zone at the limbus extending from 12 o'clock to 3 o'clock with its widest portion, up to 2.5mm, at the 12 o'clock position (Busacca, A. (1952) *Biomicroscopie et histopathologie de l'oeil*, Zurich).

[3.] These scores apply to immature follicles. It is also necessary to record the presence of mature follicles. If these are present, the follicle score given for the site will be *multiplied by the factor of 2*.

[4.] Assessed by objective examination.

Table 3.4: The physical signs of trachoma used for the diagnosis, intensity and gravity of the disease, WHO, 1966 (101)

Diagnosis (cardinal signs)	Intensity	Gravity
	Ptosis	
	Herbert's sign	
	Exudate	
	Lymphadenopathy	
	Hyperaemia	
	Lunular edema	
	Papillary hyperplasia	
Follicles	Follicles	Follicles
Cicatrization		Cicatrization
Pannus (active or healed)	Pannus	Pannus
		Corneal scars
Limbal follicles or Herbert's pits	Limbal follicles	

Table 3.5: Intensity of inflammation, WHO, 1981 (107)

Intensity	Follicles	Papillae	Key sign
Severe	F_3 (or F_2 or F_1)[1]	P_3	P_3
Moderate	F_3	P_2	F_3
Mild	F_2	P_0, P_1 or P_2	F_2
Trivial (insignificant) or absent	F_0 or F_1	P_0, P_1 or P_2	F_0 or F_1

[1] The follicles may be obscured by severe papillary hypertrophy and diffuse infiltration (P_3)

recommended the use of only nine signs to grade trachoma: upper tarsal follicles (1–4), upper tarsal diffuse cellular infiltration and papillary hyperplasia (0–3), upper tarsal conjunctival scars (1–4, with 4 being trichiasis or entropion), micropannus (graded 0–2), macropannus (graded 3–5), corneal infiltration (0–3), limbal follicles (0–4), Herbert's pits (0–4), and corneal scars (0–4). Although mention was made of the fourth Scientific Group's use of signs to describe relative intensity and relative gravity, a new definition of grave lesions (disabling and/or potentially disabling) was given as F_3C_1, F_2C_2, C_3, trichiasis, pannus 4+mm or corneal opacity. Severity was now to be expressed as the average (or the sum) of the grading of all signs except for papillae, limbal follicles and Herbert's pits. The MacCallan Classification with the use of TrD for trachoma dubium continued to be recommended.

In Australia, Fred Hollows (1929–93) and the National Trachoma and Eye Health Program (NTEHP) team developed a somewhat similar grading scheme in 1975, although they graded only seven signs, for the first time, one of which was specifically trichiasis (103). The NTEHP graded the presence of superior tarsal follicles, papillae and scarring, and Herbert's pits, limbal follicles and trichiasis, all on a scale of 0–3 except pannus, which was graded 0–5. This group graded with loupes and a hand torch. This grading was simple to use, had good reproducibility both among observers and between observers and was widely used in Australia (103).

The NTEHP constructed two scales to report their data, one for follicular trachoma and one for cicatricial trachoma. Severe follicular trachoma (FTA) was defined by upper tarsal or limbal follicles 3 or papillae 3 in the presence of limbal or tarsal follicles. Intermediate follicular trachoma (FTB) was present with follicles graded 1 or 2. Severe cicatricial trachoma (CTA) had trichiasis, 5mm pannus or scarring 3, intermediate (CTB) scarring 2 or pannus 3 or 4, and a third category (CTC) for lesser scarring, pannus and Herbert's pits.

Chandler Dawson (1930–), who became the fourth Director of the Proctor Foundation, and a group working in Tunisia, further developed the idea of assessing the severity of infection and developed an intensity scale based on the WHO grading system (104). Their intensity of

Table 3.6: WHO Trachoma Grading, 1981 (107)

The scores for upper tarsal follicles (F) are:

F_0	No follicles
F_1	Follicles present, but no more than five in zones 2 and 3 together
F_2	More than five follicles in zones 2 and 4 together, but less than five in zone 3
F_3	Five or more follicles in each of the three zones.

The scores for upper tarsal papillary hypertrophy and diffuse infiltration (P) are:

P_0	No follicles
P_1	Minimal: individual vascular tufts (papillae) prominent, but deep subconjunctival vessels on the tarsus not obscured
P_2	Moderate: even more prominent papillae, and normal vessels appear hazy, even when seen by the naked eye
P_3	Pronounced: conjunctiva thickened and opaque, normal vessels on the tarsus are hidden over more than half of the surface.

Conjunctival scarring (C):

C_0	No scarring on the conjunctiva
C_1	Mild: fine scattered scars on the upper tarsal conjunctiva, or scars to other parts of the conjunctiva
C_2	Moderate: more severe scarring but without shortening or distortion of the upper tarsus
C_3	Severe: scarring with distortion of the upper tarsus.

Trichiasis and/or entropion (T/E):

T/E_0	No trichiasis or entropion
T/E_1	Lashes deviated towards the eye but not touching the globe
T/E_2	Lashes touching the globe but not rubbing on the cornea
T/E_3	Lashes constantly rubbing on the cornea.

Corneal scarring (CC):

CC_0	Absent
CC_1	Minimal scarring or opacity but not involving the visual axis, and with clear central cornea
CC_2	Moderate scarring or opacity involving the visual axis, with the pupillary margin visible through the opacity
CC_3	Severe central scarring or opacity with the pupillary margin not visible through the opacity.

inflammation scale had four categories (see Table 3.5) (107). They also developed a better definition of the signs and zones of the tarsus. Barrie Jones, who was familiar with this work, also used this scale in his studies in Iran (105). This grading system provided the basis for the 1987 simplified grading. However, the refined WHO grading system became quite widely used and is still used in some research (106). It has a broader range of categories and is more useful than subsequent simplified grading for detailed studies, especially those comparing the presence of infection with clinical disease.

The grading of the intensity of inflammation was further promoted in a revised WHO Trachoma Grading Manual published in 1981 (107). This new manual simplified the grading to use just five signs, upper tarsal follicles (F graded 0–3), upper tarsal papillary hypertrophy and diffuse infiltration (P 0–3), conjunctival scarring (C 0–3), trichiasis and/or entropion (T/E 0–3) and corneal scarring (CC 0–3)

(see Table 3.6) (107). It defined three zones in the everted upper lid (see Figure 3.8). The manual contained useful figures and photographs. The four stage MacCallan Classification was again described in this publication.

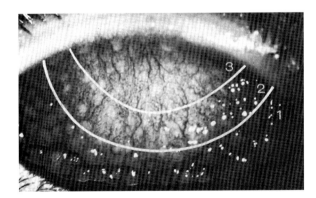

Figure 3.8 WHO 1981 Grading Classification introduced three zones in the everted lid. Follicles within zones 2 and 3 were to be graded. (Dawson CR, Jones BR, Tarizzo M, 1981 (107) © 1981 WHO, reproduced with permission).

Table 3.7: WHO simplified grading for trachoma 1987 (112) (see Figure 3.10)

Trachomatous inflammation – follicular (TF): the presence of five or more follicles in the upper tarsal conjunctiva (Plate 1B)

Follicles are round lumps or spots that are paler than the surrounding conjunctiva. In the grading systems discussed here, follicles must be at least 0.5mm in diameter, ie at least as large as those shown

Care should be taken to distinguish follicles from spots due to small scars and from degenerative deposits in the conjunctiva. Small scars are not round, but have angular borders with sharp corners, whereas follicles have rounded edges that are not sharply defined. Degenerative deposits include conjunctival concretions that are yellow or white opaque masses with clear-cut edges, as well as cysts that appear as clear bubbles in the conjunctiva.

Trachomatous inflammation – intense (TI): pronounced inflammatory thickening of the upper tarsal conjunctiva that obscures more than half of the normal deep tarsal vessels

The key feature of this grade of trachoma is the pronounced inflammatory thickening, which is defined as being present when, in more than half the area of the tarsal conjunctiva, the large deep tarsal vessels are not visible because they are obscured by inflammatory infiltration of follicles. In severe trachomatous inflammation, the tarsal conjunctiva appears red, rough and thickened. This is due to diffuse inflammatory infiltration, oedema, or enlargement of vascular tufts (papillary hypertrophy); also there are usually numerous follicles, which may be partially or totally covered by the thickened conjunctiva. Inflammatory thickening and opacification of the conjunctiva should not be confused with that caused by scarring, especially diffuse fibrosis or formation of a fibrovascular membrane.

Trachomatous scarring (TS): the presence of scarring in the tarsal conjunctiva

Scars are easily visible as white lines, bands, or sheets (fibrosis) in the tarsal conjunctiva. Characteristically, they are glistening and fibrous in appearance, with straight, angular or feathered edges. Scarring, especially diffuse fibrosis, may obscure the tarsal blood vessels, and so must not be confused with diffuse inflammatory thickening.

Trachomatous trichiasis (TT): at least one eyelash rubs on the eyeball

Evidence of recent removal of inturned eyelashes should also be graded as trichiasis.

Corneal opacity (CO): easily visible corneal opacity over the pupil

This sign refers to corneal scarring that is so dense that at least part of the pupil margin is blurred when viewed through the opacity. The definition is intended to detect corneal opacities that cause significant visual impairment (less than 6/18 or 0.3 vision), and in such cases the visual acuity should be measured if possible.

Method of examination

The examination should normally be performed with binocular loupes (x2.5) and adequate lighting (either daylight or a torch). If appropriate, loupes of higher magnification or a slit lamp (biomicroscope) can be used, but the same optical aid and level of magnification should be used for all examinations. The grading obtained with a higher magnification may not necessarily be directly comparable to that with x2.5. Eyes should be examined first for inturned eyelashes (TT), and the cornea then scrutinized for opacities (CO). In order to check for inturned eyelashes, the upper lid should be pushed upwards slightly to expose the lid margins. The upper eyelid should then be examined for inflammation (TF and TI) and scarring (TS). Each eye must be examined and assessed separately. Clinical signs must be clearly seen in order to be considered present. If in doubt, a sign should be regarded as absent.

The WHO simplified grading system, 1987

In the early 1980s, various attempts were made to use these grading systems and to codify them into a single system for field studies and research (108,109,110). We developed a simplified grading system for our field studies and although there was good intra-observer agreement, the agreement was less consistent (111). However, it became increasingly apparent that the existing grading schemes were confusing, lacked clear descriptions and were not really suitable for field use. They also collected a lot of information that was of little value and much of which was never analysed or presented. Why go to all that effort to collect data that were never used?

Dr Bjorn Thylefors had taken over as Director of the WHO Prevention of Blindness Program that evolved out of the WHO Trachoma Program in 1977. Thylefors put together a group of "experts" that came to include Dawson, Jones, Daghfous, Pararajasegararan, Lwin, West and myself (see Figure 3.9).

The first stage was to refine the number of signs that were being graded and five were finally

RIGHT **Figure 3.9** Field testing the prototype WHO simplified grading, (from left to right) Chan Dawson, M Hassayoun, MT Daghfous, driver, Bjorn Thylefors, Fetuhri Chadgrah, Barrie Jones, Tunisia 1985.

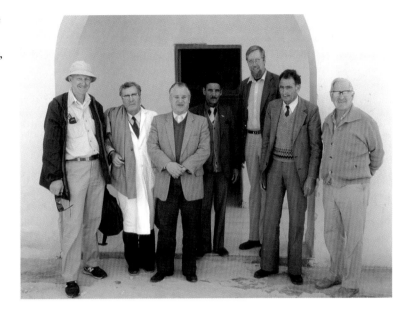

BELOW **Figure 3.10** WHO Simplified Trachoma Grading card (WHO 1987; © 1987 WHO, reproduced with permission).

TRACHOMA GRADING CARD

- Each eye must be examined and assessed separately.
- Use binocular loupes (x 2.5) and adequate lighting (either daylight or a torch).
- Signs must be clearly seen in order to be considered present.

The eyelids and cornea are observed first for inturned eyelashes and any corneal opacity. The upper eyelid is then turned over (everted) to examine the conjunctiva over the stiffer part of the upper lid (tarsal conjunctiva).

The normal conjunctiva is pink, smooth, thin and transparent. Over the whole area of the tarsal conjunctiva there are normally large deep-lying blood vessels that run vertically.

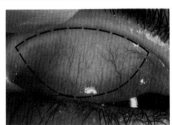

Normal tarsal conjunctiva (x 2 magnification). The dotted line shows the area to be examined.

TRACHOMATOUS INFLAMMATION – FOLLICULAR (TF): *the presence of five or more follicles in the upper tarsal conjunctiva.*

Follicles are round swellings that are paler than the surrounding conjunctiva, appearing white, grey or yellow. Follicles must be at least 0.5mm in diameter, i.e., at least as large as the dots shown below, to be considered.

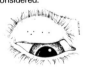

TRACHOMATOUS INFLAMMATION – INTENSE (TI): *pronounced inflammatory thickening of the tarsal conjunctiva that obscures more than half of the normal deep tarsal vessels.*

The tarsal conjunctiva appears red, rough and thickened. There are usually numerous follicles, which may be partially or totally covered by the thickened conjunctiva.

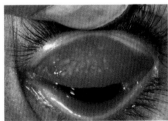

Trachomatous inflammation – follicular (TF).

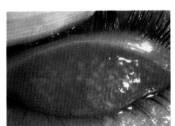

Trachomatous inflammation – follicular and intense (TF + TI).

TRACHOMATOUS SCARRING (TS): *the presence of scarring in the tarsal conjunctiva.*

Scars are easily visible as white lines, bands, or sheets in the tarsal conjunctiva. They are glistening and fibrous in appearance. Scarring, especially diffuse fibrosis, may obscure the tarsal blood vessels.

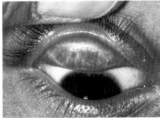

Trachomatous scarring (TS)

TRACHOMATOUS TRICHIASIS (TT): *at least one eyelash rubs on the eyeball.*

Evidence of recent removal of inturned eyelashes should also be graded as trichiasis.

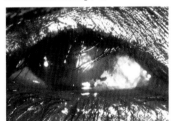

Trachomatous trichiasis (TT)

CORNEAL OPACITY (CO): *easily visible corneal opacity over the pupil.*

The pupil margin is blurred viewed through the opacity. Such corneal opacities cause significant visual impairment (less than 6/18 or 0.3 vision), and therefore visual acuity should be measured if possible.

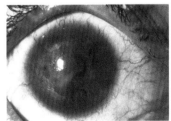

Corneal opacity (CO)

TF:– give topical treatment (e.g. tetracycline 1%).
TI:– give topical and consider systemic treatment.
TT:– refer for eyelid surgery.

**WORLD HEALTH ORGANIZATION
PREVENTION OF BLINDNESS AND DEAFNESS**

Support from the partners of the WHO Alliance for the Global Elimination of Trachoma is acknowledged.

Table 3.8: Key measures for assessing the importance of trachoma in a community, WHO, 1987 (128)

The proportion of trachoma inflammation (TF, with or without TI) amongst children less than 10 years old
This demonstrates how widespread the infection is in the community.

The proportion of intense trachomatous inflammation (TI) in children less than 10 years old
This demonstrates how severe the disease is in the community.

The proportion of conjunctival scarring (TS)
This demonstrates how common trachoma was in the past.

The number of people with trichiasis (TT)
This indicates the immediate need to provide surgical services for lid correction.

The proportion of people with corneal opacity (CO)
This demonstrates the impact of trachoma in the community in terms of visual loss.

selected: tarsal follicles, inflammatory thickening, tarsal scarring, trichiasis and corneal opacity. These signs assessed active trachoma (established and severe), cicatricial trachoma (established and late) and corneal scarring (a surrogate for vision loss) as a measure of the impact of trachoma. Each sign was to be graded present or absent and each was mutually independent.

The next step was to devise both verbal and visual criteria to define each sign. This is a difficult task because the skill in grading trachoma involves pattern recognition more easily learnt from patients, photographs or other visual images, rather than the written word. With a working set of definitions and photographs, extensive observer trials were held in Tunisia. The results were quite good except for the sign TI that did not have good reproducibility. The definition of TI was revised, further observer trials were successfully conducted in Burma, and the simplified grading system was finalised and published in the WHO *Bulletin* in 1987 (see Tables 3.7 and 3.8 and Figure 3.10) (112,128).

At the same time, a study from Tanzania showed that the grading system could be learnt quickly by ophthalmologists and ancillary health personnel (ophthalmic nurses) and was suitable for widespread use in field studies (113). Further studies showed that with the simplified system, there was generally good agreement between the clinical grading performed in the field and the grading of photographs (114,115). This is particularly important for clinical trials and longitudinal studies where it is almost impossible

to control for observer drift when exams are repeated months or years apart. As well, it may be difficult to mask an examiner to the intervention that has taken place. Photographs taken at different times of study subjects can be graded at the same time in a masked fashion to control for both observer drift and observer bias.

The grading of TF (the presence of five or more follicles in the upper tarsal conjunctiva) was based on the 1981 WHO grading of F_2 and F_3. The zone defined for simplified grading was taken to be the same at zones 2 and 3 of the 1985 WHO grading. These zones were derived from the division of the tarsal plate into thirds by the fourth WHO Scientific Group. For the first time, simplified grading set a minimum size of follicles (0.5mm) and provided an illustration with accurately sized dots.

The definition of TS was defined as easily visible scarring. It was intended to be comparable to C_2 in the previous grading. However, field reports suggest this was used only for more severe scarring, possibly because of the fairly advanced scarring shown in the definitional photograph (see Figure 3.11).

TT was intended to approximate T/E_2 of the previous WHO grading. Before then trichiasis had not been graded separately, but served as a sign for the ultimate grade of tarsal scarring. The inclusion of epilation as evidence of trichiasis was new. A further subclassification of TT has been proposed by several authors (116,117).

The definition of CO followed the WHO 1981 grading of CC_2 of corneal opacity, but relied on the

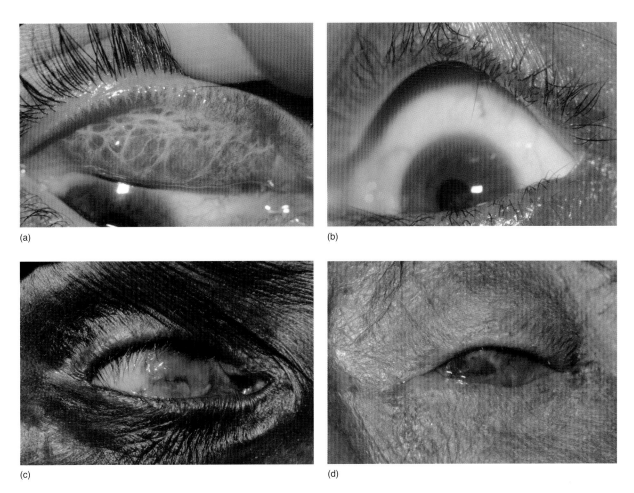

Figure 3.11 Cicatricial trachoma

(a) typical basket weave scarring in the tarsal conjunctiva that already leads to

(b) single lash trichiasis (in the same eye as (a))

(c) advanced trichiasis and dense corneal scarring

(d) broken lashes from epilation and dense corneal opacity.

blurring of the pupil margin for its definition, rather than the converse definition, that the pupil margin was still visible. CO was selected as an indicator of visual impairment and its definition was based on collective experience. I was unaware of a paper at that time which reported 99% of people in Qatar who had central diffuse corneal opacities had visual acuity of < 6/18 (118). Subsequently in Tanzania, 85% had < 6/18 visual acuity (119).

As it happened, during a visit to Australia I had shared the provisional grading criteria we had used in a study (120) with Fred Hollows who liked its simplicity and straightforwardness. He adopted it as a new grading system in Australia, even though the WHO working definition of TI turned out to be unsatisfactory. Subsequently there were some difficulties bringing the grading in Australia into line with the final WHO simplified grading system.

Reflections on the WHO simplified grading system

In general, simplified grading has been taken up with much enthusiasm and has been widely used (121). To my mind, this enthusiasm needs to be tempered in two areas: the grading of TI and the use of the simplified grading system in detailed studies. First, the grading of the sign TI is quite problematic. The key feature of this sign is inflammatory thickening, that is, thickened, red, velvety inflammation and infiltration of the tarsal conjunctiva, often with masses of papillae. TI is a measure of this marked inflammation in the tarsal conjunctiva (see Figure 3.12).

When this sign was developed, an arbitrary decision had to be made as to the extent of the inflammatory thickening required to meet the criteria for the sign to be present. The obscuration of the underlying tarsal vessels was taken as the indicator of the presence of sufficient inflammatory thickening in that part of the conjunctiva to reach the criteria of TI. The initial definition of TI required this degree of thickening to extend over the whole tarsus so that no normal tarsal vessels could be clearly seen. This followed the definition used by the fourth WHO Scientific Group (1966) (Diffuse cellular infiltration papillary hyperplasia; pronounced conjunctiva thickened and opaque, normal vessels obscured (score 3)). With this extreme definition and the need for such extensive inflammatory thickening, only a very small number of people were affected and observer agreement was poor. With the initial definition TI was not a particularly useful sign. The revised definition recommended at least half the tarsal vessels should be obscured, that is, inflammatory thickening of sufficient depth to obscure tarsal vessels had to extend over at least half the area of the tarsal plate. The revised definition was essentially identical to P_3 in the 1981 WHO system. This was more workable and became the final definition.

Unfortunately, many have misunderstood the definition of TI, and have taken the inability to see tarsal vessels, or even just the presence of redness of the lid, to be sufficient to grade TI, without any regard to the presence of inflammatory thickening. This has led to the overgrading of TI. Typically in children one might expect the ratio of TF to TI to

be of the order of 3:1 to 10:1 (122,123), but some studies have reported ratios of 1:1, strongly suggesting overdiagnosis of TI or else severe, unreported epidemics of acute bacterial or viral conjunctivitis. One study specifically looked for adenovirus in children with trachoma in Tanzania. It found 2% had positive polymerase chain reaction (PCR) for adenovirus (124). The conjunctivitis in epidemics of adenovirus is of relatively short duration (about two weeks).

Of more concern is the reported high frequency of TI in elderly people. With densely scarred tarsal plates, the tarsal vessels can be obscured by tarsal scarring. Conjunctival inflammation is also common if there is trichiasis or chronic bacterial conjunctivitis and the conjunctiva will be red. In neither of these cases is obligatory inflammatory thickening required for TI to be graded present. A recent example of the probable misdiagnosis is where 44% of children were reported to have TI, as well as 20% to 30% adults (125). Another example is where TI was seen in 37% of those aged over 15 years and everyone over the age of 35 years (126). The overdiagnosis of TI led to its omission in the most recent revision of the WHO Trachoma Guidelines (127). This may help standardise field assessment, but it does mean that we are totally reliant on follicles, and it de-emphasises the importance of TI as an indicator of the high frequency and load of infection and the high risk of subsequent scarring.

The second area of concern about the misuse of the simplified grading system has been its use in detailed studies, especially those looking at the correlation of infection and clinical signs. This will be discussed in further detail, but when one is using the most sophisticated diagnostic or laboratory tests such as PCR, the assessment of clinical diseases needs to be as detailed and sensitive as possible. One should surely use the 1981 WHO grading system, or possibly the detailed 1962 grading. It seems an elementary mistake to use a simplified grading system for such detailed research analyses. One must remember:

The simplified grading system was developed for use by trained non-specialist personnel to provide reliable information on trachoma and population-based surveys and for the simple assessment of the disease at the community level. Clearly the system gives a less

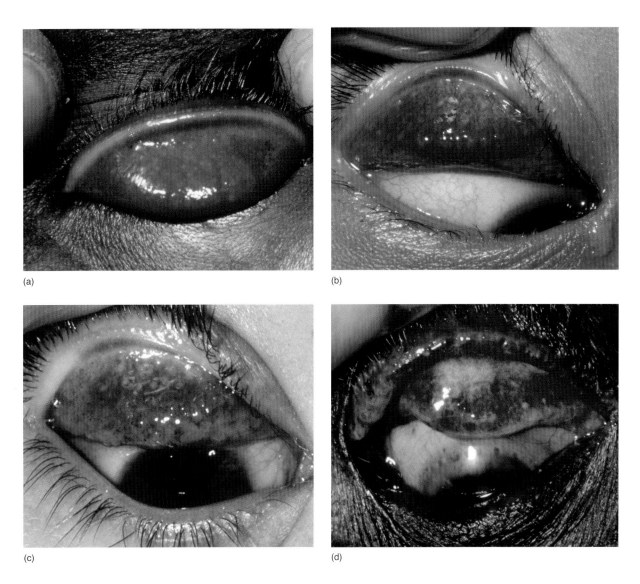

(a)

(b)

(c)

(d)

Figure 3.12 TI is characterised by inflammatory thickening

(a) typical diffuse inflammatory thickening with many follicles (TF and TI)

(b) diffuse red velvety thickening of the tarsal conjunctiva with many small follicles (TF and TI)

(c) very extensive inflammatory thickening with marked accumulation of follicles without much redness (TF and TI)

(d) old scarred eyelid with no inflammatory thickening, although the tarsal conjunctiva is quite red (TS but not TI). This eye also shows marked pannus and a string of pigmented Herbert's pits.

detailed picture of trachoma than more complex methods for use by specialists, but should provide more reliable for less experienced observers (112).

Since the simplified system was published nearly 20 years ago, it has formed the basis of the GET 2020 program of the WHO and SAFE Strategy (127,128). There has been little suggestion for further change or refinement. However, at one time Dawson and co-workers suggested that the definition of TF would be strengthened if it were tightened to be the same as F_3 in the 1981 WHO grading rather than F_2 and F_3, and if TI had been loosened to be equivalent to P_2 and P_3, rather than exclusively P_3 (129). This suggestion was based on their 18 year longitudinal examination of the predictors for scarring and trichiasis in Tunisia, but this has not been further developed.

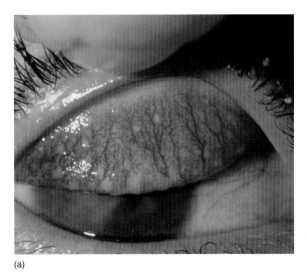
(a)

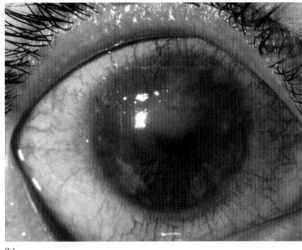
(b)

Figure 3.13 A culture confirmed case of ocular infection with LGV
(a) typical chlamydial follicular conjunctivitis
(b) severe keratitis with a small central ulcer ahead of marked corneal pannus.

2006 changes: a new grading?

As people gained more experience with simplified grading, it became apparent that knowledge of the prevalence of TS was of relatively little practical use, and the prevalence of TI could be quite variable, possibly due to misclassification as discussed above. This led to a further revision by the WHO in 2006 that recommended data be collected on TF, TT and CO only. TF was to be used as the sign of preference in assessing the need for trachoma control programs and monitoring results. TT would indicate people in need of surgery and calculate requirements for surgery. CO would continue to be used as an indicator of the burden of blindness and visual impairment due to trachoma (127). What is needed are some better short-term measurements of the effect of antibiotic control programs (100). Waiting for 20 years to determine changes in corneal scarring or blindness

is not very useful. The obvious intermediate surrogate is the presence of conjunctival scarring in children using either TS or C_2/C_3. This degree of conjunctival scarring incurs a high risk of trichiasis a couple of decades later (129). Testing for infection may prove useful to determine the efficacy of antibiotic treatment because clinical signs may persist long after treatment.

Some 2400 years after Hippocrates, we have gone from regarding trachoma as a relatively simple disease of having a rough lid and later trichiasis, through increasing degrees of complexity, countless hours or decades of intense arguments, disputes and debates, impossible classifications and ever expanding subclassification, using a multiplicity of terms to bring it all back to a definition of a disease with a roughened lid (TF) and trichiasis (TT). Oh, the price of progress!

Differential diagnosis

If it is hard to define what trachoma is, it is equally difficult to define what trachoma is not. The difficulty in establishing the differential diagnosis of trachoma from other forms of infection severely impeded the military surgeons of the early 1800s (see Table 3.9) (35). However, by 1900 a reasonable differential diagnosis could be made, in large part because of the ability to identify many of the bacterial causes of acute and chronic conjunctivitis (see Table 3.10) (15). With the introduction of Giemsa cytology it became much easier to make more specific diagnoses of chlamydial infection. The differential diagnosis set out by MacCallan (4) is instructive (see Table 3.11) (25) and shows an interesting progression from the 1904 list (15).

It was not until chlamydia could be cultured that the causative organism for many of the various forms of follicular conjunctivitis could be confirmed. The third WHO Expert Committee still

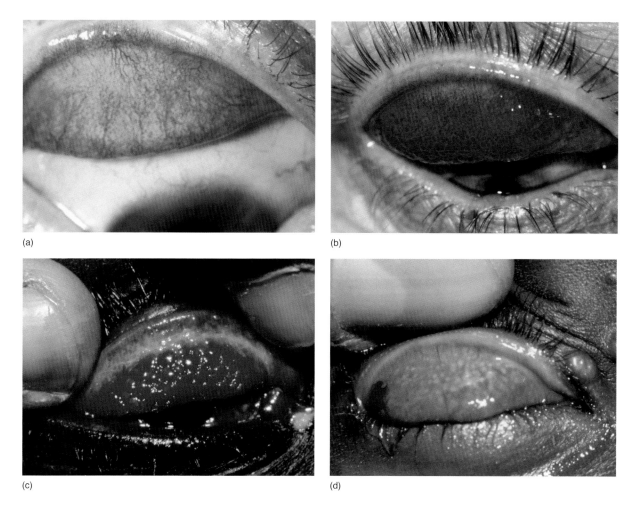

(a)

(b)

(c)

(d)

Figure 3.14 The differential diagnosis of trachoma

(a) epidemic keratoconjunctivitis: a mild case showing a few small follicles

(b) epidemic keratoconjunctivitis showing a more severe reaction with a few small follicles and a marked papillary response

(c) severe vernal conjunctivitis with large cobblestoning

(d) molluscum contagiosum with a marked follicular and papillary reaction.

Table 3.9: Differential diagnosis of trachoma, Piringer 1841 (35)

Characteristics of gonorrheal and Egyptian ophthalmia (trachoma)

Gonorrheal ophthalmia	**Egyptian ophthalmia (trachoma)**
Usually unilateral	Usually bilateral
Onset more rapid	Onset more gradual
Becomes severe more gradually	Becomes severe rapidly
Affects bulbar conjunctiva	Affects palpebral conjunctiva
Mucous is thicker, purulent	Secretion is pale, thinner
Keratitis occurs infrequently	Keratitis is usual
Cornea is destroyed from the surface	Cornea is destroyed from the underside

Table 3.10: Differential diagnosis of trachoma, Boldt 1904 (15)

Acute ophthalmia
   Gonococcal conjunctivitis
   Koch-Weeks conjunctivitis
   Acute conjunctivitis (Staphylococcus, Streptococcus,
      Pneumococcus, Haemophilus)

Follicular conjunctivitis
   Tuberculosis
   Syphilis
   Chronic Morax-Axenfeld infection
   Spring catarrh
   Chronic eye disease (atropine, eserin, zinc)
   Leukaemia and pseudoleukaemia
   Retained foreign bodies, seeds, grains, hairs from
      plants and caterpillars

Artifactitious (especially in military conscripts)

Scarring
   Post gonococcal conjunctivitis
   Post diphtheria conjunctivitis
   Pemphigus
   Blepharoconjunctivitis.

Table 3.11: Differential diagnosis of trachoma, MacCallan 1913 (25)

This subject may be studied in the following subdivisions:

1. Acute conjunctivitis complicating trachoma
   (a) Caused by the gonococcus:
      1. Ophthalmia neonatorum and acute gonococcal
         conjunctivitis of young children
      2. Gonococcal conjunctivitis:
         a. Acute
         b. Subacute
         c. Chronic
   (b) Caused by the diplobacillus of Morax-Axenfeld
   (c) Caused by the Koch-Weeks bacillus
   (d) Caused by other organisms

2. Chronic conjunctivitis

3. Follicular conjunctivitis

4. Spring catarrh

5. Parinaud's conjunctivitis

6. Atropine irritation.

gave a fairly lengthy differential diagnosis (see Table 3.12) (49). Much effort was spent in differentiating the signs of inclusion conjunctivitis from those of trachoma (130). The 1981 WHO manual limited the differential diagnosis to cases of chronic follicular conjunctivitis that were neither caused by chlamydial infection nor by chronic bacterial infection that could often merge into endemic trachoma (107) (see Table 3.13).

It was probably due to the development of better diagnostic tests that the somewhat ephemeral conditions of folliculosis and various chronic follicular keratoconjunctivitities are no longer seen. Perhaps these conditions are now diagnosed as sporadic chlamydial infections or some other more recently recognised cause. Certainly in some cases, chlamydial inclusion conjunctivitis and Moraxella conjunctivitis can persist for more than a month, and LGV conjunctivitis can occur rarely (see Figure 3.13).

Table 3.12: Differential diagnosis of trachoma, WHO 1962 (49)

The following terms of follicular conjunctivitis and follicular hyperplasia are recognised by the Committee:

(1) Acute follicular conjunctivitis

    (a) Inclusion conjunctivitis

    (b) Adenovirus conjunctivitis

        (i) Pharyngoconjunctival fever (in some cases clinical manifestations of systemic disease may be minimal or absent)

        (ii) Epidemic keratoconjunctivitis

    (c) Acute herpetic keratoconjunctivitis

    (d) Newcastle disease conjunctivitis

(2) Chronic follicular conjunctivitis (Axenfeld type)

(3) Toxic follicular conjunctivitis

    (a) Molluscum contagiosum conjunctivitis

    (b) Eserine conjunctivitis and conjunctivitis due to other miotics

    (c) Conjunctivitis with transient follicular hyperplasia due to miscellaneous irritants

(4) Folliculosis.

Tables 3.9 to 3.14 show the changing differential diagnosis of trachoma from 1841 to 2006

Table 3.13: Differential diagnosis of trachoma, WHO 1981 (107)

Differential diagnosis

1. Folliculosis

2. "Toxic" follicular conjunctivitis induced by:

    (a) molluscum contagiosum

    (b) topically applied drugs

    (c) eye cosmetics

3. Bacterial: caused by *Moraxella* species and other bacteria

4. Axenfeld's chronic follicular conjunctivitis

5   Chronic follicular keratoconjunctivitis of Thygeson

6. Parinaud's oculoglandular syndrome.

Table 3.14: Differential diagnoses for follicular conjunctivitis, Wright 2006 (140)

Diagnosis	Distinguishing features
Trachoma	Should be suspected in an area thought to have endemic trachoma. Can be confirmed with laboratory evidence of *C. trachomatis* infection.
Inclusion conjunctivitis	Generally occurs in adults not living in trachoma-endemic areas and is related to the genital strains of *C. trachomatis*.
Viral conjunctivitis	Is a common cause of follicles; it can be distinguished from trachoma by an acute history and the presence of a mucopurulent discharge.
Bacterial conjunctivitis	Bacterial infection, such as *Moraxella*, can be a rare cause of follicle formation.
Hypersensitivity conjunctivitis	Occurs following chronic exposure to drugs or eye cosmetics; a careful history is important.
Vernal conjunctivitis	Is an allergic disorder; patients often have associated atrophy. Symptoms include itchiness, lacrimation, photophobia, foreign body sensation and burning.
Parinaud oculoglandular syndrome	Is a rare ophthalmic condition that may cause follicles; it is associated with cat-scratch fever, tuberculosis, syphilis, lymphogranuloma venereum and glandular fever.

Figure 3.15 The severe purulent discharge associated with gonococcal conjunctivitis.

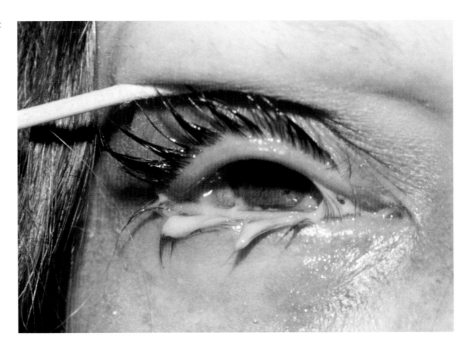

C. psittaci (psittacosis) and *C. felis* (cat scratch fever) can rarely produce chronic follicular conjunctivitis. A more up to date differential diagnosis is shown in Table 3.14. (See Figure 3.14).

One also needs to be aware that the concurrence of acute or concomitant bacterial infection was the cause of so much confusion amongst the various ophthalmias of the 19th century. In any areas with endemic blinding trachoma, bacterial conjunctival pathogens are common (see Figure 3.15).

The reported frequency of bacterial conjunctivitis in cases with trachoma varies widely with the criteria used to define the bacterial infection. Frank purulent conjunctivitis was seen in 2.5% of children with trachoma in Saudi Arabia (92) and mucopurulent conjunctivitis in 16% of children in Lebanon (131). In Southern Tunisia haemophilus species were cultured in 40% of children with trachoma and Moraxella in 16% (132). Another study on the same group of children using Giemsa cytology identified probable haemophilus in 53% of smears, Moraxella-like organisms in 35%, and various cocci

(staphylococcus and streptococcus) in 49% (133). A further analysis of data from these children with trachoma showed that in those who were inclusion positive 83% had severe intense trachoma irrespective of the presence of *H. aegyptius* infection. However, in those who were inclusion negative, 28% had intense trachoma in the absence of *H. aegyptius*, compared to 68% where *H. aegyptius* was seen on Giemsa stains (134).

Twenty-five per cent of children in Egypt have been reported to have a concomitant bacterial secondary infection (135). In Palestine, pathogenic bacteria were cultured from 75% of eyes with moderate to severe trachoma (136). The organisms isolated included staphylococcus aureus, staphylococcus albus and alpha haemolytic streptococcus. Of course, the seasonal epidemics of haemophilus (Koch-Weeks) conjunctivitis and neisseria conjunctivitis in Egypt and Palestine that occur in July to September have been well documented (32,137). In Lebanon these seasonal epidemics have been termed "harvest" (July and August) and "fig" (August and September) conjunctivitis (131). Similar epidemics are reported across North Africa including Tunisia (138) and Morocco (139). Dacryocystitis and dacryoadenitis were found to occur three times more commonly in those with trachoma than those without, and corneal ulceration was four times more common in those with trachoma (136). There was no increased frequency of herpes simplex viral keratitis.

It is important to remember some of the other causes of tarsal scaring that may include severe atopic conjunctivitis, severe molluscum contogiosa, adeno-viral epidemic kerato-conjunctivitis. Severe blepharitis with chalazion can also cause tarsal scarring that may at times be confusing. In each of these conditions, fine corneal pannus may also be evident.

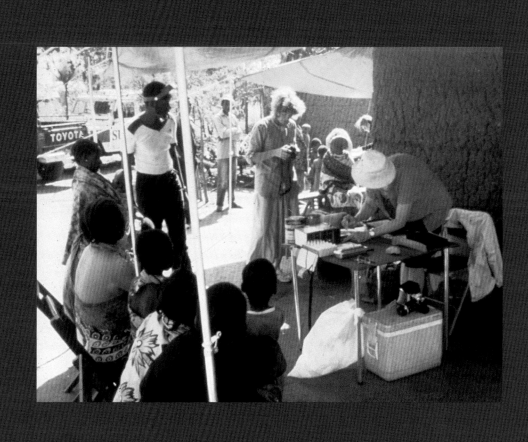

CHAPTER FOUR

Laboratory diagnosis

*In trachoma, the lack of simple, definitive, laboratory diagnostic
procedures suitable for wide application has placed the onus largely and
usually exclusively, on clinical observation*

FAKHRY ASSAAD & PETER MAXWELL-LYONS, 1967

*The laboratory diagnosis of chlamydial infection in general,
and trachoma in particular, has been frustrated by the frequent occurrence
of apparently false negative tests*

HUGH TAYLOR, 1991

MANY STUDIES BY a wide range of people in the early 1800s had shown that ophthalmia (or trachoma) could be transferred by means of inoculation of ocular discharge from one eye to another or from an eye to a urethra (35). For many people, this confirmed the contagious nature of trachoma. However, it was not until Louis Pasteur (1822–95) irrefutably demonstrated the presence of bacteria in the 1860s, that the theory of spontaneous generation was disproved. With the work of Robert Koch (1843–1910) in Berlin that established the germ theory of disease in the 1870s, the notion that trachoma could be acquired from the myasm was finally dispelled. Quickly thereafter, bacteriological knowledge exploded with the rapid identification of a multitude of organisms. Albert Neisser (1855–1916) identified the gonococcus *Neisseria gonorrhea* in 1879, the fourth bacteria to be identified. In 1884 Koch went with Neisser and a French team to Egypt to study cholera where Koch identified the Koch-Weeks bacillus, subsequently renamed *Haemophilus aegyptius*. In 1896 the Morax and Axenfeld bacillus was first identified in Egypt by Victor Morax, subsequently renamed *Neiserria catarrhalis* and then *Moraxella catarrhalis* (141).

Trachoma was considered to be a viral disease, an infectious disease for which a bacteria had not been identified (15). It was suggested it shared many similarities with malaria and may be caused by a plasmodium. Like malaria, it also seemed to have two types: one found in people living in marshes and delta regions and the other associated with dry dusty areas.

65

It was the era-defining recognition by Halberstaedter and von Prowazek in 1907 of Giemsa-stained intracytoplasmic inclusions that finally confirmed the infective nature of trachoma (142). For the first time, this enabled a definitive positive laboratory identification of the trachoma organism, hence the laboratory diagnosis of trachoma. Although Giemsa cytology was essentially 100% specific, it had a low sensitivity, and the issue of the low sensitivity of subsequent tests combined with the inability to demonstrate organisms in every case of clinical trachoma, continues to bedevil the field a century later.

Giemsa cytology

Gustav Giemsa (1867–1948) of the Bernhard Nocht Institute of Tropical Medicine in Hamburg had explored the number of analine dye derivatives developed in Germany at the turn of the century. Austrians Stanislaus von Prowazek (1875–1915), a parasitologist and zoologist, and dermatologist Ludwig Halberstaedter (1876–1949), went to Batavia (Jakarta) with Neisser to study experimental syphilis infections in monkeys. They found trachoma was common and undertook further experimental studies, first infecting orang utans with conjunctival secretions (142). The orang utans developed an acute conjunctivitis with marked tissue swelling but follicles and trachomatous scarring were not reported. However, the infection did spread to the opposite eye and the secretions could be used to infect other orang utans.

Conjunctival scrapings from orang utans were stained with the Giemsa stain and showed the now characteristic blue intracycloplasmic inclusions. Halbestaedter and von Prowazek also recognised small red bodies they called "elementary bodies" (see Table 4.1, Figure 4.1). The blue inclusion body was thought to be a "plastin-like" mantle or cloak that concealed or masked the tiny red elementary bodies. This led to the name Chlamydozoa or "mantled bodies". Similar inclusions and free elementary bodies were seen in scrapings from patients with active trachoma, but were not seen in treated or old cases of trachoma.

In 1907 Nicolle and colleagues in Tunis had already confirmed the infectiousness of this agent in monkeys and they undertook a range of very sophisticated studies in monkeys and humans (143). They showed the agent was small and passed through a fine Berkefeld V filter. It could be destroyed by heating to 50 °C and by drying for one hour at 32 °C.

Karl Lindner (1883–1961), an ophthalmologist in Vienna, had identified the complete life cycle of chlamydia between 1910 and 1913 (144,145). He demonstrated that the inclusion was made of many blue-staining reticular bodies, each of which would condense to form an elementary body. He also undertook experimental infections in baboons (146).

The findings of Halberstaedter and von Prowazek were controversial. Their inclusions could be found in cases of ophthalmia neonatorum and gonococcal ophthalmia, and many questioned the specificity of the conclusions. Subsequently, it was shown that inclusions were present in patients with ophthamia neonatorum, inclusion conjunctivitis and urethritis from whom gonococcus could not be isolated (147,148). In the 1930s Thygeson conducted some quite

---

Table 4.1: Description of chlamydial inclusions by Halberstaedter & von Prowazek (142)

In the Giesma-stained preparations, dark blue, non-homogenous irregular inclusions were visible within the epithelial cells in the light blue protoplasm near the nucleus (first observed by von Prowazek). These initially small round or oval deposits gradually grew larger, assumed a mulberry-like form and, simultaneously with progressive enlargement, underwent an increasing disaggregation which started in the centre. Eventually, they mostly assumed a cap-shaped form over the nucleus.

Within these inclusions red-stained, discrete, very fine particles appear, which rapidly multiply, displacing the blue-stained masses and gradually causing their disappearance. Finally, they occupy the greater part of the protoplasm, whereas the blue-stained substances are evident only as small islands between them. In the smears one can also observe free particles besides the cells. In some animals these inclusions disappeared after about a week and reappeared several days later.

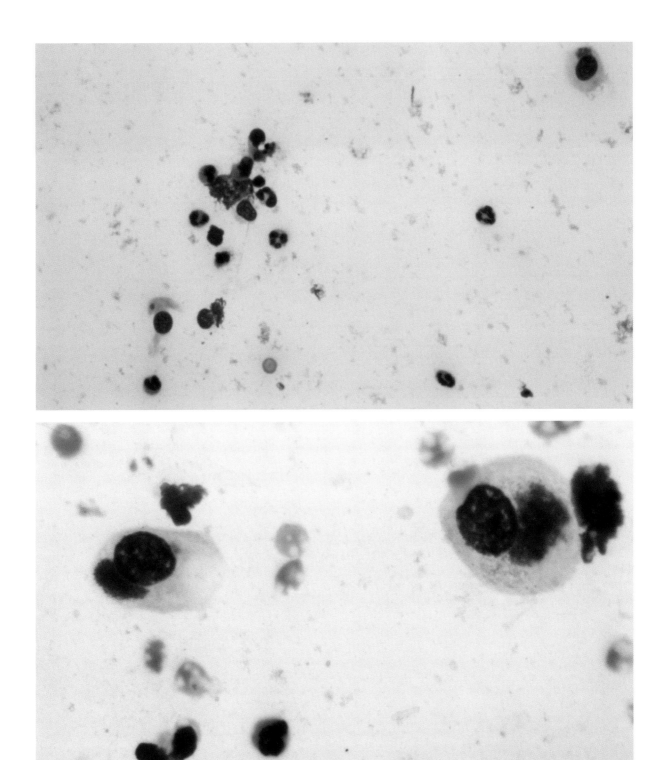

Figure 4.1 Giemsa cytology

TOP low power view to show an epithelial cell with an inclusion and the mixed inflammatory cellular exudate with both lymphocytes and polymorphs

BOTTOM high power view to show intracytoplasmic inclusions in epithelial cells, again with a mixed inflammatory infiltrate.

extraordinary experiments, preparing sterile filtered preparations of purified elementary bodies from children with trachoma and infected human volunteers and baboons (149,150). This confirmed that elementary bodies from the inclusions of chlamydiae could be transmitted to cause infection.

Giemsa cytology became the standard laboratory test for trachoma and it is hard to estimate how many hundreds of thousands of hours microscopists have spent carefully scanning slides for the elusive inclusions. Typical smears, for example, may have 500 to 5000 cells, but might only include one or two inclusions (151). Some laboratories accepted slides with as few as 50 cells (131). Although there were multiple steps in the collection and processing of a Giemsa smear where mistakes could be made, the single most critical component was the skill, experience and patience of the cytologist.

In addition to epithelial cells and inclusions a range of inflammatory cells and bacteria can be recognised with Giemsa cytology. The cells include Polymophonuclear neutrophils, small and medium lymphocytes, plasma cells, blastoid cells, Leber cells (macrophages with cytoplasmic debris) and multinucleated epithelial cells (133). The bacteria include Haemophilus species, streptococci, pneumococci, Neisseria, staphylococci and diphthesoids (152). Methods to improve the sensitivity of Giemsa cytology were attempted including scoring of the inflammatory cells contained in the smear (153). The intracytoplasmic inclusions could also be stained with iodine and iodine staining was advocated by some investigators as a cheaper alternative, although this reduced the sensitivity even further (152).

Bacillus granulosis

Many people from countries around the world continued to attempt to culture and identify chlamydial organisms that could be seen in Giemsa-stained inclusions. Over time, different bacteria were described, but until the 1950s none of the claims were substantiated. Perhaps the most notable of these was the discovery of *Bacillus granulosis* by Noguchi.

Hideyo Noguchi (1876–1928) was a

distinguished virologist at the Rockefeller Institute. The Noguchi Memorial Institute for Medical Research in Accra, Ghana, is named after him. In 1927, he isolated a new bacterium from the eyes of American Indians with trachoma in New Mexico (154). Noguchi initiated extensive studies in a variety of primates. He also shared his isolate with other laboratories (154), but unfortunately died the following year in Ghana while studying yellow fever. His work was continued by colleagues for some time and others tried to repeat his work elsewhere. There was uncertainty as to whether the minute organism was a Gram-positive or Gram-negative bacillus, and various attempts to induce trachoma in orang utans, chimpanzees and rhesus monkeys by others were mostly unsuccessful or not repeatable. For example, samples of the organism sent to Egypt were found to be ineffective and others could not identify *B. granulosis* from patients with trachoma (4). By 1935 researchers had discarded the notion that *B. granulosis* was the cause of trachoma (155).

It is instructive to look at this episode because it shows some of the difficulties of working with trachoma, casts some light on the relation between infection and disease, and shows the role forceful personalities can play in shaping current and future perceptions. Noguchi was a careful and respected researcher in a leading laboratory. He went to considerable lengths to collect specimens from Indian children in Albuquerque with Stage II (active) trachoma (154). He had assistance from Dr Francis Proctor (1864–1936) and the Indian Medical Service. The organism he isolated was difficult to grow and grew best in a semi-solid leptospira medium. To confirm the pathogenicity of *B. granulosis*, he used a monkey model. The monkeys were infected by subconjunctival injections of *B. granulosis* into the upper fornix followed by scarification of the conjunctiva. Twenty-one of 25 monkeys developed at least "mild subacute" conjunctivitis, which Noguchi claimed to be trachoma, but the elusive organism could only be re-isolated occasionally, one to five months after inoculation. Several attempts were made to inoculate two chimps and an orang utan but the results are difficult to interpret.

The drawings Noguchi made of the upper lid show follicles in the upper fornix, but none on the tarsus (see Figure 4.2). Later the tarsi were actually removed for histology so further observations were confined to the fornix conjunctiva. Superior fornix follicles in monkeys are common; they are a non-specific sign of conjunctival inflammation and once induced, may remain for months or years in otherwise "quiet" eyes. To my mind, Noguchi had not produced disease that looked anything like trachoma. A second problem Noguchi faced was tuberculosis in his monkey colony. In different studies he notes some 10% to 15% of his monkeys died from tuberculosis. It is impossible to determine what impact this may have had on his findings.

Robbins summarised more than 100 papers published between 1927 and 1935 on *B. granulosis* (155). Sixteen laboratories confirmed Noguchi's isolation of *B. granulosis* from trachoma but in many papers, the work was not well described or substantiated. Another 15 laboratories could not repeat the work. Interestingly, Thygeson was listed in each group with different collaborators. There were eight reports of successful infection in monkeys and two reports of failure, one by Wilson in Egypt and another by Proctor, Finnoff and Thygeson. Finally, Robbins lists 23 reported attempts to infect human volunteers; only one volunteer became infected and was graded as Trachoma Stage III by Proctor. Thygeson reported that another boy developed trachoma after inoculation (149).

Robbins concluded that Noguchi had isolated a previously unknown organism from cases of trachoma. This organism induced a "granular conjunctivitis" in monkeys that was not identical to trachoma and that human experiments had been failures. For these reasons *B. granulosis* could not be considered the cause of trachoma (155).

This controversy around *B. granulosis* generated a lot of intensity and finally it was accepted that the initial observations were flawed. However, the key finding that was used to discredit the animal studies was the absence of corneal changes. The paramount importance of the presence of corneal changes in trachoma was subsequently transferred to the clinical grading of trachoma and included in the WHO grading systems of the 1950s, 1960s and 1970s. It was finally discontinued in the 1980s. Even when chlamydia was cultured in 1957, monkey experiments were dismissed because single

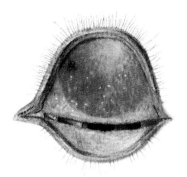

Figure 4.2 Conjunctivae of *Macacus rhesus* 8 24 days after inoculation with culture. Follicles can be seen in the upper fornix bordering the tarsus but only some encroaching on the superior tarsus (Noguchi 1928 (154); Reproduced from Journal of Experimental Medicine, 1928,48:1–53 © 1928 Rockefeller University Press).

inoculations did not lead to marked pannus or chronic disease. The notion that a single infection would lead to blindness in trachoma was eventually proven to be inappropriate, as the importance of repeated episodes of reinfection became recognised.

Chlamydial culture

The second major revolution in the identification of chlamydia occurred in Beijing in 1957 when T'ang Feifan (1897–1958), Chang (Zhang) Xiaolou (1914–90), Huang Yuantong (1924–) and Wang Keqian (1923–) from Tong Ren Hospital (see Figure 4.3) successfully isolated the trachoma "virus" in a chick embryo (156). They reported the isolation of three strains of chlamydia obtained from humans with trachoma.

Four innovations made the Chinese breakthrough possible. First, they inoculated their samples into the egg yolk of the embryonated egg, rather than the chorio allantoic membrane. Other workers had assumed that because chlamydia infected epithelial cells, if they were to grow in an egg culture they would grow in the chorio allantoic membrane not in the yolk sac, although the yolk sac culture of LGV had been in use for some time (157). Their second innovation was the concomitant use of penicillin and streptomycin. Fortuitously, these antibiotics were essentially ineffective against chlamydia, but they prevented bacterial contamination that would otherwise have

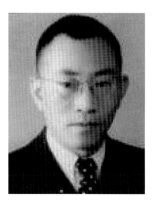 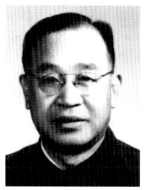 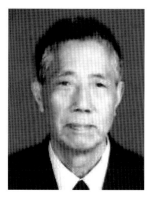 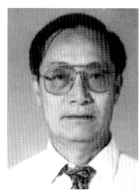

Figure 4.3 The Chinese scientists credited with the first reliable culture of chlamydia
FROM LEFT TO RIGHT Dr T'ang, Dr Chang, Dr Huang, Dr Wang, (courtesy, Hu Ailian).

overgrown the chlamydia and destroyed the embryo. Bacterial contamination had been a major barrier in attempts to culture chlamydia. Third, they incubated the eggs at 35 °C, the temperature of the conjunctiva, rather than 37 °C. Finally, T'ang used repeated blind passage where the contents of one inoculated egg were reinoculated into new eggs. The repeated passaging of material increased the likelihood of finally obtaining a positive culture.

Having isolated chlamydia, T'ang and colleagues immediately undertook a series of experiments to characterise the new organism. They assessed its physical characteristics and tested its susceptibility to heat, pH change, drying, freezing, freeze-thawing and various chemical inactivation methods, including glycerine, alcohol and formalin. They also tested its susceptibilities to the range of available antibiotics and identified its susceptibility to sulphonamides and tetracycline. They conducted animal experiments and infected mice, rabbits, guinea pigs, pigeons and hens without success. They were able to produce acute, inclusion-positive conjunctivitis in rhesus monkeys that developed a self-limited acute conjunctivitis within seven to 10 days, lasting two to three months. Two of their seven monkeys had inclusions on Giemsa stain (156). They performed preliminary studies with tissue culture of conjunctival epithelium but these were unsuccessful. They initiated toxicity studies by injecting mice with chlamydia intravenously or into the brain. They subsequently reported the

successful infection of volunteers with cultured material (158).

The culture of chlamydia was an amazing breakthrough and in a noteworthy spirit of international collaboration, the Chinese shared specimens so that Collier and his group in London were soon able to grow chlamydia, and subsequently cultured new isolates from The Gambia (159). Similarly, within a few years groups around the world were growing new isolates.

However there is another part to this story. In 1937, Atilis Macchiavello, a Chilean consultant epidemiologist working with the Pan American Sanitary Bureau in Lima, Peru, developed a new stain (Macchiavello Stain) that detected both rickettsia and chlamydia (160). In 1943, he obtained conjunctival scrapings from a 17-year-old Ecuadorian student with typical Stage II trachoma and inoculated this into the yolk sacs of seven eggs (161,162). Despite contamination in a number of eggs, infection that developed in the remaining eggs showed characteristic intracellular inclusions, reticulate bodies and free elementary bodies. This material remained sterile in bacterial culture and could be passaged serially. A six-year-old child was experimentally infected and developed acute conjunctivitis within six days, and by three weeks had started to develop corneal vascularisation. The child was treated with sulphonamides with a reduction of symptoms within four days, was essentially normal at two months and completely cured at one year. Inclusions were identified in conjunctival scrapings at day 10 and the agent was re-isolated by egg culture.

These exciting experiments were overlooked by other workers in the field. They were published in Spanish during the middle of the Second World War from a relatively peripheral centre by someone who was not known to be working in the field. However, a summary of these findings was published in English after the war in 1948 (163). Two groups picked up this work and confirmed the findings (164,165). To reduce contamination of the eggs, the Egyptian group first inoculated the eyes of baboons and grivets with trachoma scrapings (165). They then took further scrapings from the infected monkeys that were used to inoculate eggs. By using serial passage from monkey to egg to monkey, they were able to serially pass the organism multiple times. Without antibiotics attempts at repeated egg passage would rapidly become infected. When infected with the cultured organism, monkeys developed a typical follicular conjunctivitis at about 14 days.

Unfortunately the work of Macchiavello was not fully accepted. The report was considered incomplete and the number of experiments was relatively small (148). Further, Macchiavello did not or could not share his isolate with other laboratories for confirmation. His impressive results failed to receive the attention they probably deserved. In 1956, the second WHO Expert Committee formulated the following criteria to validate the isolation of chlamydia: typical inclusions needed to be demonstrated on serial cultures, the agent needed to induce experimental trachoma in monkeys, a serologic relationship between the cultured virus and trachoma needed to be established and finally human infection experiments were required (33).

In contrast, the work of the Beijing group was undoubtedly aided by the use of streptomycin. They were able to produce large quantities of chlamydia in the laboratory and undertook an impressive range of studies to characterise their organism. However, they did not initially undertake the human experimental infections until later. Moreover, they were able to provide their isolate to other workers in the field, particularly to the group working in London, who rapidly extended this

work and isolated further strains. Although Macchiavello may have been the first to culture chlamydia, it was the work of T'ang and colleagues that really changed perceptions in the field. The ability to culture chlamydia led to an explosion of research activity. Work progressed at a rapid pace to develop serology testing and vaccines, refine the culture method, study the life cycle including studies with the newly available electron microscope, and assess growth characteristics and further antibiotic susceptibility studies. A whole new research field had thus been initiated.

There was a lot of confusion about nomenclature and the general recognition of similarity, but also significant differences between trachoma and inclusion conjunctivitis, as well as with psittacosis and lymphogranuloma venereum. Terms such as paratrachoma, TRIC (Trachoma and Inclusion Conjunctivitis) agents and Bedsonia, were used sequentially before the general term chlamydia was finally widely accepted (see chapter five).

Tissue culture methods

Although considered an outstanding technical advance, embryonated or fertilised egg culture was extraordinarily tedious, difficult, expensive and slow. It required careful attention and considerable laboratory skill. Laboratories performing egg culture would have dozens of fertile eggs delivered each week. After inoculation on day six, eggs were examined and "candled" each day until harvesting at nine to 13 days. Often two further blind passages were performed before a specimen was declared negative and laboratory accidents were difficult to avoid.

Researchers looked for other ways to grow chlamydia. The first effective tissue culture method was described by Gordon and Quan from the Naval Medical Research Institute in Bethesda (166). They used a monolayer of McCoy cells irradiated to prevent further multiplication. McCoy cells were a transformed mouse fibroblast line. Glucose had been added to the media to make the elementary bodies (EB) "more sticky" and after inoculation, cells and culture medium were centrifuged to bring the chlamydia into contact with the monolayer's cell surface to facilitate cell adhesion and EB uptake. With a series of minor modifications, this became the standard tissue culture method. Tissue culture was shown to be at least as sensitive as egg culture, but much cheaper and more convenient. It was also faster and less susceptible to bacterial contamination.

Over time, other modifications to tissue culture included the use of HeLa cells, a human cell line of cervical origin, the use of idoxuridine or cyclohexamide instead of irradiation to inhibit cell division, the change from vials to microtitre plates and the use of DEAE-dextran instead of glucose to improve EB adhesion (see Figure 4.4).

Various stains were used to identify infected cells. Iodine was used initially, but both polyclonal and monoclonal immunoperoxidase and immuno-fluorescence detection have also been used (see Figure 4.5).

A positive culture isolation is definitive proof of the presence of viable chlamydia and for this reason culture was regarded as the "gold standard" for chlamydial detection. However, culture methods have a finite sensitivity and some 10 to 100 EB may be required to be inoculated to obtain one inclusion. Specimens for tissue culture need to be carefully stored and shipped, and strict attention paid to the maintenance of a continuing cold chain of storage from the field to the laboratory. Tissue culture is susceptible to inhibition and infection and multiple blind passages may be required before a particular culture becomes positive. At times, non-viable EB can be seen in negative cultures. Blind passage may increase the positive isolation rate. Using up to six blind passages 84% of cultures were positive on the first passage, 10.2% on the second, 4.7% on the third, and 1.1% on the fourth to sixth passage (167). DFA and PCR studies have confirmed that specimens that only become positive after multiple blind passages have lower numbers of EB than those specimens that are positive on the first passage (167,168).

Culture is still a relatively slow procedure requiring several days to obtain an initial result and longer for each blind passage. It requires specially equipped laboratories with specially trained and skilful staff. Although tissue culture became the standard in reference and research laboratories, it was not widely used outside these dedicated facilities.

Serology

The first serologic diagnostic test for chlamydia was developed in the 1930s (169). It was a complement fixation assay that used a group specific polysaccharide antigen prepared from cultures of either the psittacosis agent or LGV. Although regarded as an advance at the time, it had poor specificity because of broad cross reactivity. It was not widely used for trachoma, but was used quite extensively for psittacosis and LGV diagnoses (170). When more specific tests were developed complement fixation was rapidly superseded. The Frei Test (a skin test) was developed to diagnose LGV. It used LGV heat-inactivated antigen initially obtained from LGV discharge and later cultured in monkey or mouse brains (170).

The ability to culture chlamydia also provided antigen and paved the way for a new range of serologic tests (50). Many laboratories started to develop their own serology assays including neutralisation tests using serum, and micro-agglutination tests using purified elementary bodies. Other work included skin testing with elementary body preparations. A radio isotope precipitation (RIP) test was subsequently developed that used group specific antigen, which was more sensitive than the complement fixation test (105,171).

The development of the micro-immunofluorescence assay (microIF) by San Ping Wang (1920–2001) in Seattle revolutionised chlamydial serology. This test was first explained in detail with a series of papers at the 1970 Symposium on Trachoma held in Boston (172,173,174,175) and expanded in 1977 (176).

A range of type-specific polyclonal antibodies had been developed by Wang. He used these to serotype different strains of chlamydia. Wang and Grayston identified the four classical trachoma strains, A, B, Ba and C, as well as the three most common genital strains: D, E and F and the three LGV strains: L_1, L_2 and L_3. Wang's microIF classification of serotypes was an order of magnitude more sophisticated than the classification being developed by the Harvard group who had identified only three types of chlamydia (177). The ability to serotype chlamydia also made redundant ongoing attempts to classify chlamydia by antigen identification using gel

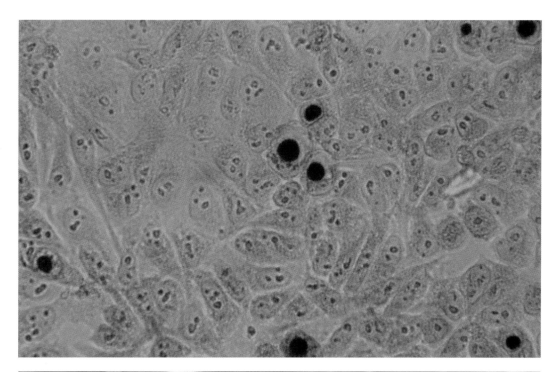

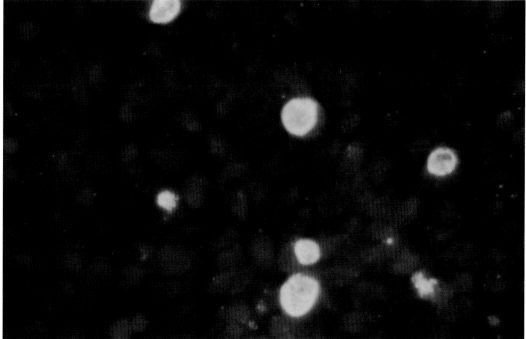

Figure 4.4 Chlamydial inclusions in tissue culture
of cyclohexamide treated McCoy cells
TOP stained with iodine stain
BOTTOM stained with fluorescent monoclonal
antibody.

RIGHT **Figure 4.5** Plating out a chlamydial
culture in a microtitre plate.

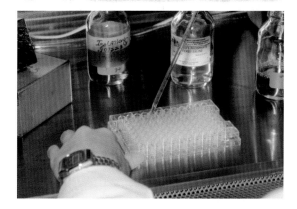

diffusion, mouse toxicity testing and other studies.

In addition, Wang and co-workers presented detailed serologic studies demonstrating serotype-specific IgM and IgG antibodies in serum, IgG and IgA in tears (174) and the correlation of the serum IgM with active infection (176). Antibodies to the type-specific antigen were also found to be neutralising (175). The presence of tear antibodies was more closely correlated with clinical disease than serum antibodies (178). Subsequent work by Harlan Caldwell showed these antibodies were directed against the major outer membrane protein (MOMP) (179).

By 1973 the WHO recommended the microF assay (102,105,153). Although this was a very useful test, it was still susceptible to minor changes and required considerable expertise to perform reliably. Variability was reduced with the generation of much "cleaner" and more specific monoclonal antibodies in the 1980s (180). Many laboratories depended on slides prepared by Dr Wang in Seattle instead of preparing their own reagents (167).

MicroF serology was quite widely used in animal studies, various trachoma vaccine trials and field studies (105,181). Although tear anti-chlamydial IgG and IgA titres correlated with the presence of active disease were serovar specific, the correlation was not strong and less specific than immunofluorescent cytology (167). However, serology was much more widely used for diagnosing sexually transmitted diseases than trachoma (171). As distinct from ocular infection, genital tract infection was not amenable to ready clinical diagnosis or Giemsa cytology, and culture was problematic. Over time, as better diagnostic tests were developed, serology has gradually been abandoned.

Direct immunofluorescent cytology

The ability to culture chlamydia provided a supply of purified elementary bodies that could be used to immunise animals to produce specific antibodies. This allowed the development of fluorescent antibody cytology that used polyclonal antibodies to detect infection (182). Immunofluorescent cytology was found to be more sensitive than normal Giemsa stain, and twice as sensitive and much more convenient than egg culture (183).

Fluorescent cytology was also much easier and quicker to read than Giemsa cytology.

Nichols and collaborators from Harvard used quantitative immunofluorescent cytology for detailed studies of the community load of chlamydia infection in Saudi Arabia (92). They demonstrated a very high level of positivity in children under the age of four years. The highest number of inclusions were seen in children aged between three and nine months, although age specific prevalence rates of positive cytology continued to increase up to 36 months. Young children under the age of one year, were the most prolific shedders of chlamydia, a finding reconfirmed 40 years later with quantitative PCR (122,168). Fluorescent cytology was an exciting advance. For the first time it allowed meaningful quantification of the infectious bacterial load of individuals.

Not all polyclonal preparations were sufficiently specific and cross-reactivity was a problem. One study in American Indian children demonstrated that 35% with either no trachoma or Trachoma Stage IV tested positive with fluorescent cytology (184). The authors concluded that "beyond doubt TRIC agent antigen occurs in persons without evidence of inflammation and clinical activity in the conjunctiva" and postulated at length about subclinical or latent infections. However, they were unable to culture chlamydia from these eyes and many had persistently positive fluorescent cytology, even after topical tetracycline treatment. These aberrant findings were more likely to have been due to cross-reactive antibodies with a poor specificity that gave false positive results, rather than a new, transiently observed, biological phenomenon. These antibodies could adhere non-specifically to bacteria in the smear, for example. With time, better, more specific polyvalent sera were developed, and fluorescent cytology became the method of choice for the laboratory diagnosis of trachoma (105,152,185).

The identification and subsequent purification of MOMP (186) and the development of monoclonal antibody technology led to the next advance in chlamydial diagnosis. Direct fluorescent antibody (DFA) cytology using fluoroscein-conjugated monoclonal antibodies revolutionised the diagnosis of chlamydia (187). Monoclonal antibodies gave a significant improvement in specificity and when produced commercially, the MicroTrak test (Syva) gained rapid and widespread adoption (188) (see Figure 4.6).

Although specificity could still be a problem with genital specimens due to non-specific staining of genital discharge, bacteria and other debris in genital specimens, the specificity with ocular specimens was usually very high. The sensitivity was superior to Giemsa cytology and tissue culture, both in longitudinal studies in infected animals (189) and in human ocular infection including trachoma, ophthalmia neonatorum and inclusion conjunctivitis (190,191,192,193,194).

An adequate DFA cytology specimen required 100 to 200 epithelial cells. An advantage of a cytology specimen over a swab for culture or other tests was that one could assess the adequacy of each cytology specimen. A study in Tanzania showed that 11% of specimens collected in the field had an inadequate number of cells, although some of the slides with small numbers of cells still had EB identified and could be graded positive (167). However, compared to tissue culture, for trachoma, DFA had a sensitivity of 88% and a specificity of 87%. This relatively low specificity may have been a reflection of the lower sensitivity of the putative "gold standard" of culture, which was to become more of an issue in the assessment

of the even more sensitive, new DNA-based tests to be discussed in the next section. Although much quicker to read than Giemsa cytology, a DFA slide could still take up to one hour to read carefully (195). Five EB was found to be the optimal cut point for a positive test for trachoma specimens (167).

Lavelle Hanna and co-workers reported a marked increase in positivity of fluorescent antibody cytology following rescraping (151). The inclusion count increased on rescraping in 66%, compared to a decrease in the inclusion count seen in 6% of individuals. The positivity rate more than doubled when people were rescraped one to seven days later. This was attributed to the trauma of the scraping leading to an increase in the rate of positivity, although it could equally have been due to increased non-specific staining in inflamed, previously scraped eyes as relatively non-specific polyclonal antibodies were used. An effect of this magnitude has not been reported by other authors.

Using DFA, the discordant rate of specimens taken five minutes apart was 10% and 25% for those taken two days or more apart (195). Specimen adequacy could be determined in each case by identifying epithelial cells. This inconsistency in positive specimens was attributed

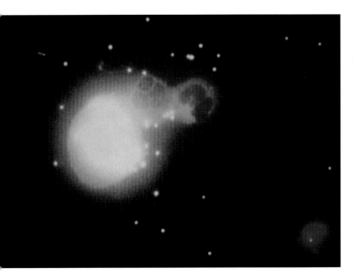 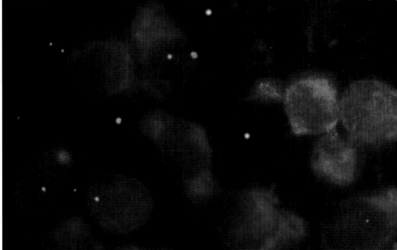

Figure 4.6 Direct fluorescent antibody cytology (DFA) showing
LEFT brilliantly staining cytoplasmic inclusion in an epithelial cell and multiple single extracellular elementary bodies. Inflammatory cells can also be seen
RIGHT scattered extracellular EB.

to both sampling variation and biologic variation in shedding. Both problems have continued to haunt the laboratory diagnosis of trachoma (196). Another study reported the detection of human DNA in only 70% of samples when tested by PCR (124). A more recent study found levels of human DNA confirmed that more than 100 cells had been collected in each specimen (197).

Advances in diagnostic technology also led to the development of a direct antigen detection by enzyme immunoassay (EIA). This technique initially was called enzyme linked immunosorbent assay (ELISA) and detected antigen extracted from collection swabs. Enzyme immunoassay involves the binding of antichlamydial antibodies to a specific chlamydial antigen. Bound antibodies are then labelled with horseradish peroxidase anti-IgG that allows detection of chlamydia (198,199) and a number of commercial EIA kits became available. Probably the most widely used was Chlamydiazyme (Abbott) that used a polyclonal antibody to identify a number of antigens including LPS and MOMP (200) (see Figure 4.7). Another popular test was the IDEIA (Boots CellTECH) that used a mouse monoclonal antibody against chlamydial lipopolysaccharide.

EIA were easy to perform, large batches of specimens could be processed at one time and EIA specimens did not require refrigeration. The enzyme induced colour change that indicated a positive test was machine-read and commercial kits contained all the reagents required. However, EIA tests were also susceptible to false positives from cross reaction with contaminating bacteria. This was observed in some trachoma specimens, but was more of a problem in genital tract specimens where the bacterial contamination was more frequent and of a much higher load (201).

With trachoma field specimens EIA performed slightly less well than DFA cytology, but were less dependent on laboratory technical experience (195). EIA were not used widely in trachoma research with the exception of the London group working in The Gambia (126,202,203) but these tests were extensively used in STD clinics for diagnosing genital infection (200). Overall, the sensitivity of the EIA for eye specimens was of the order of 80% to 95%. The lack of specificity really precluded the use of EIA tests for rectal or pharyngeal specimens. Further improvement and refinement led to second generation EIA with increased sensitivity. The use of confirmatory or blocking assays may have increased their specificity to around 99% (204).

However, commenting on EIA, Julius Schachter (1936–), Professor of Laboratory Medicine at the University of California, San Francisco, and a leader in chlamydial diagnostics and research, stated:

> All positive results seem to be accepted as valid. The same holds true, in a sense, with amplified DNA probes, where researchers often accept positive results as the truth without the adequate verification systems. Such an uncritical approach of accepting laboratory results is liable to cause considerable misunderstanding about the distribution of chlamydial infection and their clinical spectrum (204).

It is still worth reflecting on Schachter's words today.

EIA tests were eventually replaced as the detection of DNA became possible with nuclear acid amplification (NAAT) tests. However in 2006, a new EIA test specifically developed for detecting trachoma was reported (205). This rapid test or "point of care assay" was developed as a "dip stick" to detect chlamydial lipopolysaccharide. It has a sensitivity threshold of about 2500 EB per test and is thought not to cross react with the commonly found human ocular pathogenic bacteria. The initial study compared the new test to a PCR test and found that the dip stick test had a sensitivity of 84% and a specificity of 99.5% (205). It was easy and rapid to perform and four novice operators had very high inter- and intra-agreement. It will be interesting to follow the future development of this relatively cheap, quick and deceptively "low technology" test, to see if it replaces the clinical grading of trachoma to monitor trachoma rates in prevention programs (206) (see Figure 4.8).

Nuclear Acid Amplification Tests (NAAT)

Nucleic acid detection is the newest and most sensitive test and relies on the identification of unique chlamydial DNA or RNA sequences using

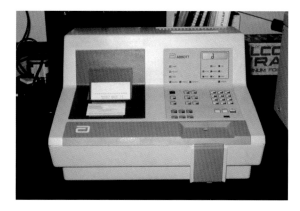

ABOVE **Figure 4.7** The self-contained instrument provided for reading the Chlamidiazyme EIA assay.

RIGHT **Figure 4.8** Field assessment of the new point-of-care EIA test (courtesy, Claude Michel).

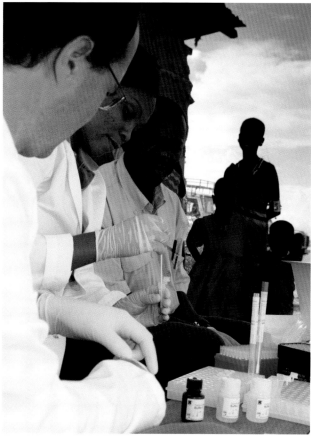

either probing or amplification techniques. The rapid developments in DNA biology and techniques in the 1980s were also applied to develop tests to detect chlamydial infection. The first generation of nucleic acid detection tests used a radio labelled DNA probe to bind to the target DNA. The first DNA hybridisation detection of chlamydia was reported in 1985 (207). Later a non radioactive DNA probe (GenProbe Pace II) became commercially available (204,208,209). These assays used a DNA probe directed to the DNA in the cryptic plasmid contained in all serovars of *C. trachomatis* not present in the other chlamydial species. This assay gave a sensitivity of 93% with a disappointing specificity of 83%. DNA probe tests were not widely used in trachoma (see Figure 4.9). Several probe assays to detect ribosomal RNA were also developed, although they had limited use (200,210).

The development of the polymerase chain reaction (PCR) lifted the detection of chlamydia to a higher plane by using nucleic acid amplification.

By cleverly using the ability of DNA to replicate, PCR essentially provided a "photocopier" that allowed minute amounts of specific sequences of chlamydial DNA to be multiplied to give sufficient quantities of DNA for easy detection. This involved a significant increase in complexity and cost (see Figure 4.10).

In 1989, Deborah Dean and colleagues from San Francisco reported the first use of PCR amplified DNA probes to assess trachoma (211). They used a probe to the 7.0-KB cryptic plasmid and compared PCR to tissue culture with repeated blind passage and to DFA. On replicate specimens collected from children with trachoma in Nepal, PCR had a sensitivity of more than 96% compared to tissue culture and was 100% specific.

Three studies using PCR to detect *C. trachomatis* were presented back to back at the 1990 International Chlamydial Meeting in Harrison Hot Springs (212,213,214). Two of these studies related to sexually transmitted diseases, but the third discussed patients presenting with chlamydial

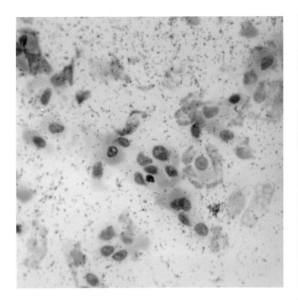

Figure 4.9 DNA probe indicates the presence of chlamydia in a conjunctival smear.

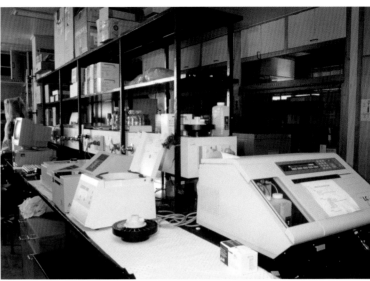

Figure 4.10 A laboratory set-up for LCR or PCR.

conjunctivitis. Each study reported sensitivities of the order of 98.5% and specificities also in the range of 98.5%. The new PCR technology also permitted the genotyping of chlamydia and the first report was also presented at this meeting (215).

Linda Bobo and co-workers from Johns Hopkins used PCR based on the detection of the MOMP gene in a study in Tanzania and compared their data to DFA and the clinical status assessed with simplified trachoma grading (216). Each of the PCR assays at this stage was in-house and their data are quite confusing. In humans who did not have active trachoma, only 1% tested positive for DFA cytology, but 24% were positive for PCR. For those with TF, 8% were positive for DFA, but 54% were positive for PCR testing. For TI, the percentages were 60 and 95 respectively. Inhibitors were subsequently identified in 75% of specimens that were positive for DFA but negative for PCR testing. These data were interpreted as indicating that PCR was more sensitive than clinical grading. Commenting on the finding of positive PCR results in humans who did not have TF, the authors said "clinical grading is subject to error and it is possible that less obvious clinical disease may have been present in these subjects". As the WHO simplified grading was used this is possible but the possibility of specimen contamination during collection does not seem to have been considered.

NAAT testing, specimen contamination and other issues

In a clinic setting one patient is seen at a time, and usually the medical staff will have washed their hands and possibly seen many patients between the collection of one swab and the next. In a STD clinic, it is also very likely that examiners will be gloved, and use at least a semi-sterile technique. However, trachoma fieldwork is conducted under very different circumstances.

With Giemsa cytology, there is almost no chance of having inadvertent contamination, as cells would have to be carried over from one patient to another. It has been a long-standing practice to flame the platinum spatula between cases or at least wipe with alcohol. Similarly, there is little likelihood of contamination of other cytology specimens such as DFA or with the collection of tears for serology. There is a theoretical risk of contamination of chlamydial culture specimens but given their relatively low sensitivity, this issue does not seem to have been raised or seriously explored.

However, with modern PCR, it is a very different story. The importance of even minor specimen contamination is greatly changed with the ability to detect 100, 10 or possibly even one elementary body—dead or alive. The potential for specimen contamination is a particular problem for ocular specimens in trachoma studies (see Figure 4.11). Eversion of the upper lid is required and a series of specimens are collected from one person after another. All schoolchildren in a class or all members of a family or community are likely to be placed in line and examined one after the other. In other settings, such as in an STD clinic, specimen contamination may be much less important.

Specimen contamination can occur in multiple ways. The most obvious is the specimen collectors who may have chlamydial EB or DNA on their fingers and contaminate a specimen. During either examination or cytology specimen collection, most trachoma field staff were not accustomed to scrupulously scrubbing their hands to remove all traces of foreign DNA between cases. In some areas, such as Tunisia or Egypt, the provision of alcohol swabs for wiping the fingers after each examination was supposed to be part of a long-standing ritual, but more often than not, they sat on the shelf unused. Only recently have those collecting PCR swabs started to glove and specifically wash their hands between handling each case (197,217).

Another very potent source of contamination can be an assistant who holds the child's head and may evert or "flip" the lid to facilitate specimen collection. These staff may well carry EB or chlamydial DNA from one eye to the next. To date, I am not aware of any instances in large field studies that have collected specimens for PCR where individuals have separately gloved and washed their hands between each case. Inadvertently, they could easily carry over infection from one individual to the next so that EB or chlamydial DNA is placed in or around the eye of the next child before the specimen is collected. A similar increased risk of contamination would follow for anybody else, such as a clinical grader or a photographer, who had examined or handled the child before specimens were collected. Studies have shown an occasional positive swab that is just open and closed in the field (an "air swab") (217). Others have used duplicate swabs (218), but positive PCR swabs have been reported from field staff fingers, chairs and tables (219).

Without being absolutely certain there is no chance of inadvertent contamination of the specimen, the explanation of unusual results from fieldwork is fraught with difficulty because of the

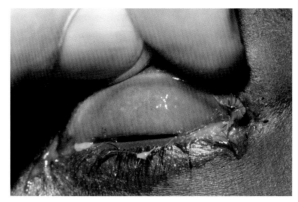
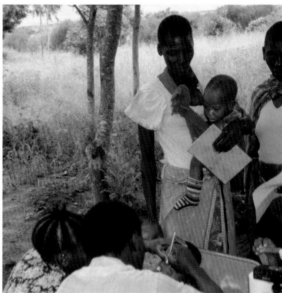
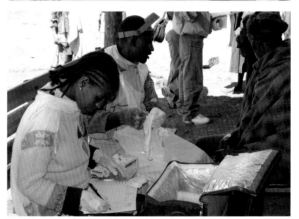

Figure 4.11 Specimen collection in the field
TOP an eye with marked discharge and active trachoma (TF and TI) that could easily act as a source of specimen contamination
CENTRE collecting a specimen for DFA. Bare hands may or may not be cleaned between subjects. Similar methods were used for the initial PCR studies
BOTTOM precautions now taken to prevent contamination of PCR specimens (courtesy, Tom Lietman).

potential risk of artefact. It is the exquisite sensitivity of PCR techniques in detecting such small trace amounts of DNA that makes this such an important issue.

Robin Bailey, then a student at the London School of Hygiene and Tropical Medicine, and co-workers compared an in-house PCR assay with an EIA (IDEIA) and clinical grading in The Gambia (220). The percentage of positive results with PCR was higher than EIA in each severity of disease category. Overall, they reported a sensitivity of PCR to clinical grading of 72% with 93% specificity; the sensitivity of EIA was 62% with 94% specificity. At the six month follow-up, the majority who had been clinical disease negative but PCR positive had not developed any clinical signs, although 17% developed TF, compared to only 8% of those who had been PCR negative at baseline and developed TF at six months.

Across the full range of chlamydial infection, PCR is a much more sensitive test than previous tests with a sensitivity generally in the range of 90% to 95% and a specificity of 99.5% (204). The commercially available system Amplicor (Roche) became widely used. Another commonly used test was the Ligase Chain Reaction (LCR, Abbott) in which after the Ligase enzyme ligated the DNA strands, an additional enzyme, polymerase was used to close a gap of two nucleotides between two incomplete ends of the ligated strands. The LCR test was particularly favoured by the San Francisco group and used in most early azithromycin field studies (221).

A problem that arose in the assessment of NAAT tests was that they appeared to be much more sensitive than chlamydial culture. If chlamydial culture was used as the "gold standard", NAAT testing would identify positive specimens that were negative on the "gold standard" test. This would show a lack of specificity. There was much discussion in the literature about the appropriate gold standard and the need to stop using culture as the standard. For example, while assessing an early DNA probe, Schacter and co-workers (135) "defined a true positive as a child who yielded a positive tissue culture, a positive Giemsa specimen or a specimen that was positive in two of the other three non-culture methods." Using this new definition, they found the sensitivity of culture to

be of the order of 75% to 90% (204).

Much has been written about the reliability of in-house NAAT assays for the detection of chlamydia (222,223). Apfalter and co-workers also give a comprehensive review of the difficulties of NAAT testing for chlamydia (222). They list four major areas of error in specimen collection, although they overlook specimen contamination. Presumably this oversight is because the authors deal predominantly with STD patients in a clinical setting. They also list eight major sources of laboratory error, four major sources for test design error and two major areas for interpretation error.

NAAT testing can also be affected by the presence of inhibitors (201). It is unclear whether inhibitors may have played a role in the somewhat unusual LCR results published from Nepal in 1999 (224). Although working in a relatively low prevalence area, the prevalence of active trachoma was less than 6% and none of the LCR specimens were positive. The interpretation of these results was that a "low prevalence of clinically active trachoma is not necessarily evidence of the presence of chlamydial infection". This suggests that trachoma may occur as some unique event without the need for chlamydia. Other experimentation might include the possibility that the test did not work for a variety of reasons. Amplification tests are susceptible to a number of inhibitors, many of which are unknown, but some like phosphate have been identified (225). Manufacturers will provide advice on further manipulation or "confirmation" tests to help resolve this issue. In addition, there may have been misclassification in the clinical grading or chlamydia may have been present intermittently to stimulate disease, but were not detectable at the time of testing. The latter has increased relevance when one considers the cycles of reinfection and the immunopathology of trachoma where delayed-type hypersensitivity is thought to be important.

One of the first trachoma studies to use LCR was the Azithromycin in the Control of Trachoma (ACT) in Egypt (221). Overall, 31% of those with active trachoma (TF or TI) were positive with LCR, as were 31% who did not have active trachoma. The age-specific prevalence of clinical disease dropped markedly with increasing age, from over 60% in four year olds to less than 10% in 16 year olds. There was almost no change with age with LCR positivity (infection); infection rates of 30% or higher were maintained in those over the age of 10. The authors concluded that "clinically active trachoma is not always a reliable marker of infection." This could well have been rewritten as "PCR positivity is not always a reliable marker of clinically active trachoma." And the authors did not consider the possibility of cross contamination from one individual to another during specimen collection. The LCR test was later withdrawn from the market because of reproducibility problems (226). Further developments in PCR technology led to the development of quantitative PCR that in theory allowed the quantification of the number of copies of the *C. trachomatis* omp1 gene in samples.

Quantitative testing initially gave somewhat confusing data, with many people having low levels of detectable organism irrespective of clinical status, possibly due to low level contamination (168) (see Figure 4.12). The distribution of these low levels varied from one site to another and may be linked to the different field teams and protocols followed. Nevertheless, there was a clear picture for young children and those with more severe disease to have higher levels of organism detected. This was an exciting advance and added greatly to the armamentarium available to study the amount of chlamydia present or shed. These data confirmed the findings from previous laborious studies which had used fluorescent cytology techniques (92). Quantitative PCR has also been useful for monitoring levels of infection after community antibiotic treatment.

NAAT testing of trachoma specimens used DNA assays of one sort or another, apart from one early report that detected RNA (210). However in 2006, Burton and co-workers used a 16S ribosomal RNA reverse transcriptase PCR assay (228). They compared an in-house assay against an in-house quantitative PCR assay for the omp1 gene. The RNA results were strongly correlated with increasing disease severity but in general, there was a relatively poor correlation between the DNA and RNA results. This suggested at least some of the DNA may have come from small numbers of non-viable chlamydia. In particular, of the 34 tests that had less than 100 DNA copies per swab, only two tests were positive for RNA. Some have argued this

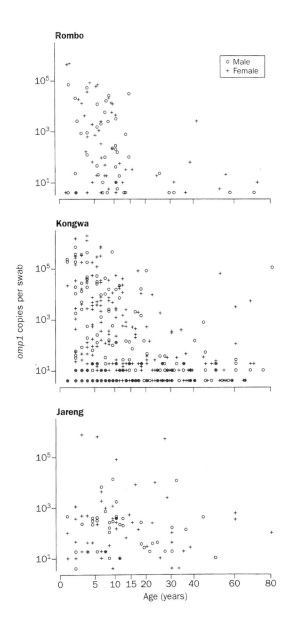

Figure 4.12 Results of quantitative PCR showing estimated number of copies of omp1 gene per swab by age. Rombo and Kongwa are in Tanzania and Jareng is in The Gambia. A logarithmic scale has been used for the y axis and a non-linear scale for the x axis (Solomon et al 2003 (168). Reprinted from The Lancet, Vol 362, Solomon AW, Holland MJ, Burton MJ, West SK, Alexander NDE, Aguirre A, Massae PA, Mkocha H, Mounoz B, Johnson GJ, Peeling RW, Bailey RL, Foster A, Mabey DCW. Strategies for control of trachoma: observational study with quantitative PCR, 198–204, © 2003, with permission from Elsevier).

assay showed a lack of sensitivity. Alternatively, the low levels of organism detected by the DNA PCR could reflect spurious contamination and could in reality be false positives. A second study used a commercially available 16S rRNA-based APTIMA *C. trachomatis* (ACT) assay (Gen-Probe) and compared it to DNA PCR (218). This study found that the RNA assay was more often positive and was more sensitive than the DNA assay. They speculated that rRNA is more abundant than DNA and may therefore contribute to increased sensitivity. This issue cannot be resolved with the current data and further studies comparing RNA and DNA testing will be of interest.

Current status of NAAT testing

Ribosomal RNA is of particular interest, as there is some debate as to whether 16S rRNA is present in elementary bodies, but we know that reticular bodies have about twice as many copies of rRNA as gene copies of DNA (228). This may make rRNA assays a better indicator of the presence of actual chlamydial infection. Other studies have shown that chlamydial DNA may persist for up to a week (204). In addition, residual killed EB may be detected in the conjunctival scrapings up to a week after ocular installation (229).

Both PCR and LCR became widely used. They provided convenient and automated assessment of a large number of specimens and did not require a cool chain for specimens. For STDs they performed well on non-invasive urine specimens and this was a significant advance. Best of all, these tests were highly sensitive. Their major downside was expense relative to other tests available (230), although pooling specimens was widely recommended to reduce costs (225,231).

Schachter has recently reviewed the current commercially available diagnostic kits (223). He dismissed in-house assays (or "home-brew" tests) because of problems of reproducibility. In 2006 there were three commercially available NAAT tests for DNA: Amplicor (PCR-based and manufactured by Roche); ProbeTEC, a strand displacement assay (Becton Dickinson); and the APTIMA Combo 2 (AC2) assay (GenPROBE), a second generation test using a transcription mediated amplification assay targeting a 23S RNA sequence. GenPROBE also has a 16S RNA assay recommended as a "confirmation test", APTIMA CT (ACT). The second generation tests include a target capture step that reduces their susceptibility to inhibitors.

The sensitivity of these assays is about 92% to 96%, and the specificity in excess of 99%. Specimen pooling for STD testing when the prevalence is less than 5% can reduce the cost of testing by half. Schachter speculated that further improvement in NAAT testing would come with improvements in specimen processing, methods for nucleic acid extraction and the use of international standards for quality control. This would in turn reduce the variation in test sensitivity. He previously stated "we are now approaching the level where false positives are more likely due to labelling errors and mistakes in specimen collection or processing than problems with technology" (225).

Correlation of clinical grading and laboratory tests

Despite modern, highly sensitive NAAT, many have reported a poor correlation between clinical examination and laboratory tests (196,232,233,234), particularly in areas with low prevalence of trachoma. A study in The Gambia identified 7% of the population with infection based on PCR, but only a quarter of these PCR positive individuals showed clinical signs of trachoma (227). In Nepal, where 6% of children had clinical trachoma, none had LCR evidence of infection (224). Similar reports with LCR testing also came from China (235). Some have suggested that nucleic acid tests should replace clinical grading for control activities and antibiotic distribution (196,236,237).

As detectable chlamydial infection rapidly declines after mass antibiotic treatment, it has been suggested that a reliance on clinical examination might lead to unnecessary antibiotic treatment in communities with clinically active trachoma, but with no or low levels of demonstrable infection (196,205). Anthony Solomon, a young Australian infectious disease doctor working in London, has written a useful review that includes the correlation of laboratory tests and clinical signs in which he considers factors that influence the accuracy of the

Figure 4.13 Prevalence of infection in active trachoma in children. Data were classified as being from hypoendemic (<10%), mesoendemic (10% to 20%), or hyperendemic (>20%) regions. Circles represent the mean percentage of positive laboratory testing from clinically positive individuals; error bars denote standard deviation. Each has been plotted as a separate data point with the reference provided in italics (Wright & Taylor 2005 (234). Reprinted from The Lancet Infectious Diseases, Vol 5, Wright HR, Taylor HR. Clinical examination and laboratory tests for estimation of trachoma prevalence in a remote setting: what are they really telling us?, 313–320, © 2005, with permission from Elsevier).

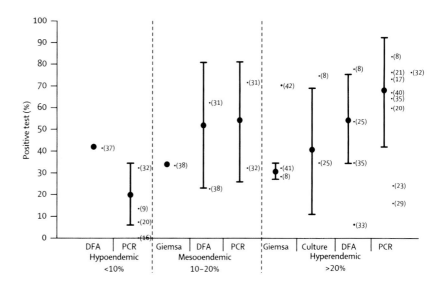

Figure 4.14 Results of laboratory tests on children with severe trachoma and intense inflammation. Circles represent the mean percentage of positive test results in children with follicular trachomatous inflammation (TF) but not intense trachomatous inflammation (TI), and in children with TI; error bars denote standard deviation. Each study is shown as a separate data point with the reference given in parentheses (Wright & Taylor 2005 (234). Reprinted from The Lancet Infectious Diseases, Vol 5, Wright HR, Taylor HR. Clinical examination and laboratory tests for estimation of trachoma prevalence in a remote setting: what are they really telling us?, 313–320, © 2005, with permission from Elsevier).

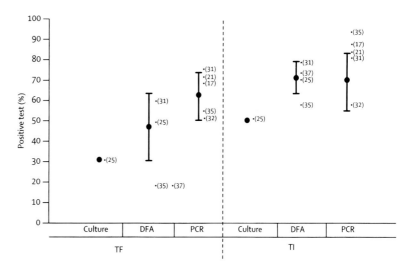

Figure 4.15 Rate of positive laboratory tests in individuals without active disease. Data are presented from published studies that provide the results of laboratory tests in people without signs of active disease and also for people without active disease who had signs of scarring. Circles represent the mean percentage of positive test results; error bars denote the standard deviation. The results for PCR are stratified by endemicity (Wright & Taylor 2005 (234). Reprinted from The Lancet Infectious Diseases, Vol 5, Wright HR, Taylor HR. Clinical examination and laboratory tests for estimation of trachoma prevalence in a remote setting: what are they really telling us?, 313–320, © 2005, with permission from Elsevier).

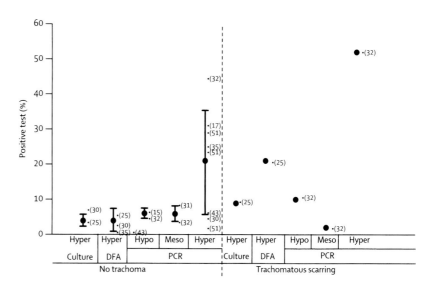

test, the accuracy of clinical diagnosis and those that relate to the natural history of infection (196).

The increasing sensitivity of laboratory tests is reflected in their ability to identify chlamydia in higher proportions of individuals with active trachoma (234). In areas hyperendemic for trachoma (>20% prevalence), swabs taken from children with active trachoma have reported positive 31% of the time for Giemsa, 39% for culture, 55% for DFA and 65% for PCR (see Figure 4.13). The sensitivity of laboratory tests also increases with the prevalence of clinical disease. In this case PCR was positive in 19% of children with active trachoma in hypoendemic areas (<10% prevalence), 59% in endemic areas (10% to 20% prevalence) and 65% in hyperendemic regions (>20% prevalence).

The intensity of the clinical disease is an important determinant of test sensitivity (see Figure 4.14). Children with intense inflammation (TI), for example, are more likely to have organism identified from a swab than those with active trachoma (TT) without TI (234). Quantitative PCR has confirmed this finding by demonstrating higher levels of organism in those with TI with or without TF than those with TF alone (122,168).

Chlamydia can be identified in people who do not have signs of current active trachoma (see Figure 4.15). However, the frequency with which this occurs is vastly different with PCR than with other tests, and the possibility of specimen contamination needs to be remembered. However, it is quite clear that a small percentage of people who are not graded as having TF do have demonstrable chlamydia.

This is an instance where the WHO simplified grading system does not give enough discrimination and a finer clinical grading scale is required. Some have used the 1981 WHO trachoma grading system (238) and others have used customised systems for grading milder disease. In a study of 1671 people in Tanzania, we subdivided follicular or active trachoma further into definitely normal, equivocal, definite but mild disease and TF or TI (239). Of the 47 who tested positive on culture or DFA and who did not have TF or TI, ("normal"), six (13%) were normal on fine grading, 15 (32%) had equivocal disease and 26 (55%) had a mild form of the disease. Thus only 1% who were truly

clinically normal tested positive on DFA. The six who were clinically normal included one girl and five mothers, four of whom had children with active trachoma in their families.

Of equal importance are cases misdiagnosed as having trachoma when the clinical disease is related to another cause. These clinical "false positives" for follicles could include other types of follicular conjunctivitis, or even the misdiagnosis of a papillary reaction and a severe allergic or vernal conjunctivitis. Some have suggested that infection with other organisms such as staphylococci may cause the re-expression of follicles from previous episodes of trachoma (224,232). Of course, severe acute conjunctivitis from a number of causes can cause the changes associated with correctly diagnosed TI (extensive thickening) and many factors can cause the misdiagnosis of TI (the simple obscuration of tarsal vessels). A more complete discussion of the differential diagnosis of trachoma is discussed in the final section of the previous chapter.

From this one concludes that chlamydia can be identified in the eyes of some people who are clinically normal at that time. Without close follow-up, one cannot separate those who may be incubating an infection and will shortly produce signs. In human volunteer and monkey studies, the incubation period for clinical disease is usually five to 10 days. Alternatively, it may represent the transient carriage of chlamydia in immune or non-immune people or possibly low levels of specimen contamination, although the latter is unlikely without NAAT tests. Whatever the ultimate explanation, this seems to be a relatively rare event.

Equally, it is clear that a large proportion of people with active trachoma, including some of those with intense inflammation (TI), do not have demonstrable organism. As discussed in detail in chapter seven, this is a reflection of the pathogenesis of trachoma as an immune mediated disease.

Community assessment of trachoma

The only way to establish the prevalence of trachoma is to conduct a prevalence survey, although population-based prevalence surveys can be difficult, time consuming and expensive (see Figure 4.16).

A good estimate of prevalence is deemed by many to be desirable, if not essential, for monitoring when one needs to establish baseline prevalence and then repeat prevalence surveys periodically (240). The suggested criteria for the certification of the elimination of blinding trachoma is to mandate multiple prevalence surveys. These surveys are seen as an essential part of the azithromycin donation program. Conceptually, large prevalence surveys are fairly straightforward. They can keep a lot of people busy for a long time, but often become an end in themselves rather than the means to an end. In programmatic activities, as distinct from research activities, careful consideration needs to be given to whether a detailed population-based prevalence survey is required, or whether some other sampling or indicator methodology can suffice.

The WHO has published extensive guidelines on the methodology of prevalence surveys including the selection of random sampling and data analysis. The 2006 *Trachoma Control, A Guide for Managers* (127) is a useful update of many previous versions (102). There are many good published examples of prevalence surveys (125,241,242,243,244,245). However, population-based prevalence surveys are relatively weak at

distinguishing between low level trachoma and its absence, unless they use a large sample size. This is particularly important when a disease like trachoma has a lumpy distribution and classically occurs in pockets. The focal nature of trachoma becomes especially marked as prevalence levels fall.

In an attempt to give some flexibility to programs in determining whether trachoma still exists in certain areas and in making some first order assessments for prioritising intervention, the WHO developed the Trachoma Rapid Assessment Methodology (TRA) (246). A further refinement of this has been suggested with the use of Lot Quality Assurance Sampling, a methodology developed for monitoring manufacturing processes. This technique became known as Asymmetric Sampling Trachoma Rapid Assessment (ASTRA) (247). It is another attempt to estimate the prevalence in the community without a full population-based study.

In 1997 at the start of the WHO program "The Global Elimination of Trachoma by the Year 2020" (GET 2020) (248), there were some 55 countries listed as being either known to have or thought to have endemic trachoma. In some of these countries trachoma had been a serious problem in the past, but no further data were available from the last 10 or 20 years. In these countries, one had the option of doing a population-based prevalence survey to ascertain whether trachoma still existed anywhere

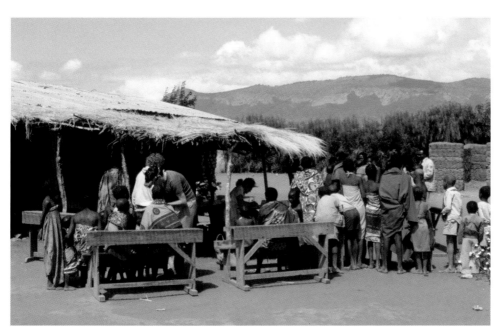

Figure 4.16 Examining villagers at a central site during a population-based prevalence survey in the Kongwa district of Tanzania (1986).

in the country. This would have been an almost impossible task that certainly would be expensive and utilise valuable resources better spent on various specific health intervention programs. Alternatively, one could use a more targeted approach by seeking out and visiting areas most likely to still have trachoma, and examine the children who were most at risk. If these children did not have trachoma, then it would be highly unlikely that trachoma would exist elsewhere.

The methodology for rapid assessment has also been set out in some detail (246), using a two phase technique to obtain "optimally biased" samples in the "worst places" within those communities most likely to have trachoma. At risk communities are selected within a region using available information from past records of trachoma and current socio-economic and hygiene conditions. Within these communities, the children from the families with the poorest hygiene and highest risk are examined (see Figure 4.17).

It is important to emphasise that TRA does not indicate a prevalence, although it is likely to set the upper bound of a possible prevalence, that is, if 10 of the 50 children examined during TRA have

trachoma (20%), it is unlikely that the true prevalence of trachoma would be any greater than this percentage. If the highest risk children were truly examined, other children would be at lower risk and have a lower rate of trachoma, if they had trachoma at all. This could only reduce its overall prevalence. Thus TRA can indicate the presence of trachoma and maximum prevalence, although it gives no lower bound of prevalence (249,250,251).

The ASTRA assessment uses the trade-off of a rapid survey using a random sampling method against a relative lack of precision in prevalence estimates. It applies a "stopping rule" so that examinations continue until a predetermined number of children with trachoma have been identified. At that point, there is no need to examine the rest of the sample as the true prevalence will lie within preset bounds. For example, if the threshold is set at four of 50 children with trachoma, there is no need to identify or examine the remaining 46. With ASTRA one can determine whether the true prevalence of trachoma in a community lies within a range defined by a preselected upper and lower prevalence boundary (247,252). A further hybrid

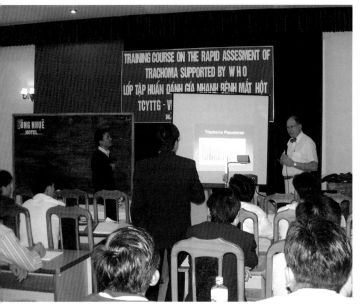
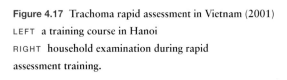
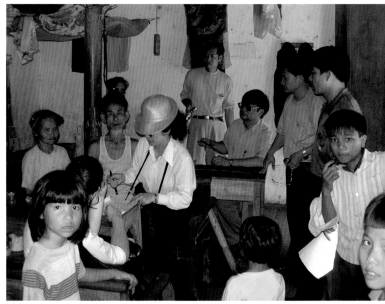

Figure 4.17 Trachoma rapid assessment in Vietnam (2001)
LEFT a training course in Hanoi
RIGHT household examination during rapid
assessment training.

method has been used that selects a random sample of children using the method suggested for ASTRA but does not apply the stopping rule (253). This is a variation of a population-based survey and gives a true prevalence of trachoma in the age group examined.

Many of these surveys have used a technique that randomly selects the starting household and systematically moves to either the next closest household or the next house in a given direction known as the "Random Walk" (254). These sampling techniques are still susceptible to a certain degree of subjectivity in the selection of households, particularly when village guides are used. The "helpful" village guides may bias the sample by steering enumerating teams towards particular households (255).

All these assessments of trachoma are based on clinical grading. Others have suggested that laboratory tests for the presence of chlamydia infection use either NAAT tests, or the new dip stick could be used instead (205). Another suggestion was to use quantitative PCR to develop a community ocular chlamydia trachomatous load (COCTL) (256). The use of these new laboratory tests to assess trachoma has not been fully evaluated and begs the question of the relative importance of clinical and laboratory indicators of trachoma, and which method is the better indicator of the need for intervention to prevent the ultimate development of trachomatous blindness.

Efforts to control trachoma are undertaken to prevent vision loss from trachoma or eliminate trachomatous blindness (257). It is well established that the development of trachoma blindness is strongly correlated to the preceding presence and severity of clinical disease. Active clinical disease generally correlates with infection load, but there are clear exceptions (122,168,258). Those with more severe "active trachoma" are more likely to test positive for chlamydia, but it has not been established that they have a higher infection load. The frequency of positive laboratory tests (prevalence of demonstrable organism) increases markedly with more severe active disease, that is, TI compared to TF (234). However, the highest levels of infection (the number of organisms shed) are usually seen in young children, whether this be determined by cytology or NAAT testing (92,122,168).

Cost is another factor to consider in comparing clinical and laboratory diagnosis. Laboratory tests will always cost more than field examination. The logistic costs of putting a team into the field and identifying a sample of children will be the same whatever test was used, but once a team is in place and the children identified, there are essentially no additional costs for clinical examination. However, even if the total costs including labour were only one dollar per child, it would add a very significant cost to any large-scale assessment.

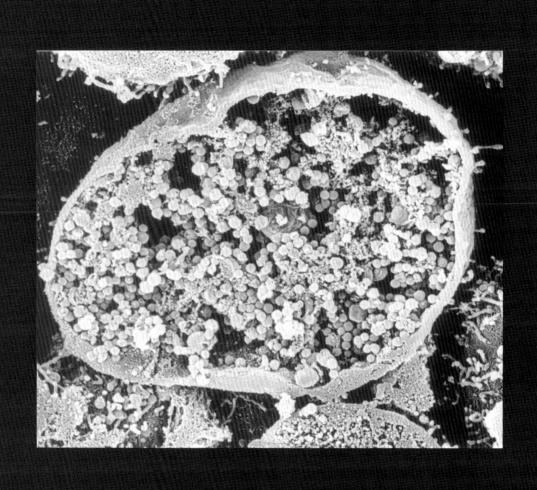

CHAPTER FIVE

Biology of chlamydia

We therefore propose grouping them between both classes (bacteria and protozoa) under the name Chlamydozoa χλαμύς *cloak, mantle;* ζώον *animal*

LUDWIG HALBERSTAEDTER & STANISLAV VON PROWAZEK, 1907

The classification of chlamydia

MUCH HAS BEEN learnt about chlamydia and the recent advances in molecular cloning, PCR technology and mass spectroscopy, and other tools of cellular and molecular biology have greatly expanded our understanding of these unique intracellular parasites.

The name *Chlamydozoa* ("cloak" or "mantle", and "animal") was first proposed by Halberstaedter and von Prowazek to reflect the way elementary bodies appear to be cloaked within the intracellular inclusion (142). However, over the years, a number of other names were used. The similarity between the trachoma organism and organisms associated with psittacosis and lymphogranuloma venereum led to the transient use of the terms Bedsonia, Miyagawanella, TRIC (Trachoma and Inclusion Conjunctivitis) agents and PLT (Psittacosis Lymphogranuloma and Trachoma) agents. For a while they were considered to be *Ricketssia* (162). The most recent classification was proposed by Karin Everett and colleagues in 1999 from the National Animal Disease Center, US Department of Agriculture (259). This classification has not been universally adopted and, in fact, has generated much discussion. Most workers in the field continued to use the term chlamydia for the two genera, *Chlamydia* and *Chlamydophila* (5) (see Table 5.1).

Chlamydiae are characterised by their unique development cycle with the extracellular infectious form (elementary body) and the intracellular replicative form (reticulate body). They are Gram-negative bacteria, but they are smaller than many viruses and were initially classified as viruses because of their small size. They could pass through the Berkefeld V

Table 5.1: Scientific classification of Chlamydiae (259)

Kingdom:	*Bacteria*
Phylum:	*Chlamydiae*
Order:	*Chlamydiales*
Family:	*Chlamydiaceae**
	Simkaniaceae
	Parachlamydiaceae
	Waddliaceae
	Rhabodochlamydiaceae
*Genus:	*Chlamydia***
	Chlamydophila⁺
**Species:	*C. trachomatis*
	Ocular serovars A, B, Ba, C
	Genital serovars D to K
	LGV serovars 1, 2, 3
	C. muridarum
	C. suis
⁺Species:	*C. pneumoniae*
	C. psittaci
	C. pecorum
	C. abortus
	C. felis
	C. caviae

filter (143), for example, but when it was possible to study their growth in culture, they were reclassified as bacteria. The EB is typically 0.2μ to 0.6μ in diameter, with an RB up to 1.5μ. The RB divide by binary division and after consolidation to form new EB, the inclusion ruptures or is extruded to release the infectious but metabolically inactive EB. Members of the family Chlamydiaceae share a family- or genus-specific lipopolysaccharide epitope and 90% RNA sequence identity (260). The two genera *Chlamydia* and *Chlamydophila* differ in that the former produce glycogen and have two ribosomal operons whereas the latter do not produce detectable glycogen and only have a single ribosome operon.

The genus *Chlamydia* contains three species. *C. trachomatis* only naturally infects humans and the four ocular serovars A, B, Ba and C are universally responsible for blinding endemic

trachoma. *C. muridarum* was originally called the mouse pneumonitis agent (MoPn) which only infects mice. It was initially thought to be similar to *C. trachomatis*. Recently a second strain of *C. muridarum* has been identified in hamsters. *C. suis* is endemic in pigs where it causes conjunctivitis, enteritis and pneumonia. It has a number of diverse strains.

The genus *Chlamydophila* is still often referred to as chlamydia. Many of these species were formerly lumped together as strains of *C. psittaci*. *C. pneumoniae*, formerly known as TWAR, is an important cause of pneumonia in humans and has also been associated with arteriosclerosis, asthma and even age-related macular degeneration. *C. pneumoniae* also causes infection in a wide range of animals and reptiles including koalas, snakes, iguanas, chameleons, frogs and turtles. The DNA of *C. pneumoniae* is about 20% larger than that of *C. trachomatis*. *C. psittaci* is predominantly an avian infection. Although persistent inapparent infection is very common, *C. psittaci* is associated with epidemics in birds and causes respiratory infection psittacosis in humans and contains at least five serovars. *C. pecorum* predominantly affects mammals including cattle, sheep, goats and pigs, and also koalas. *C. abortus* is common amongst ruminants but also occurs in horses, rabbits, guinea pigs, mice, pigs and humans. Infection is frequently associated with abortion. *C. felis* is endemic amongst cats and causes feline conjunctivitis, rhinitis and respiratory infection. Finally, *C. caviae* occurs in guinea pigs and was formerly known as guinea pig inclusion conjunctivitis.

Chlamydial infection is highly prevalent in animals and as such, over 70% of domestic cattle and pigs and nearly 60% of feral pigs will be PCR positive (260). Most calves are infected within two weeks of birth and the prevalence and intensity of infection increases exponentially with crowding. Twelve per cent of cats carry *C. felis*. In many cases animal infection is endemic and asymptomatic, although as mentioned, epidemics of infection will occur, particularly in birds, if the animals are stressed or crowded together. More typically, the asymptomatic infection makes the animal more susceptible to other infections and less able to resist other pathogens. Chronic latent or persistent infection may also have important implications in animals raised for food production, decreasing growth rates, fertility and milk production.

Australian marsupials are unique animals and have been geographically isolated from the rest of the world for millennia. It is interesting to note that in these animals not only have *C. pneumoniae* and *C. pecorum* been identified, but multiple new strains are still to be classified (261). One study found *C. psittaci* present in 70% of koalas, with only 9% showing symptoms (262).

Analysis of sequence changes in 16S rRNA provide a molecular clock which can be used to monitor the early evolution of bacteria (5). (See also Figure 1.1). *Chlamydia* appear to have separated from the *Parachlamydiaceae acanthamoeba* some 350 to 830 million years ago. *Chlamydia* separated from *Chlamydophila* between the Cretaecous and Jurassic era 50 to 200 million years ago. *C. suis* diverged from the other *Chlamydia* 31 to 74 million years ago as the mammalian species started to differentiate and *C. muridarum* about 19 to 46 million years ago. Primates first appeared about 20 to 30 million years ago and Homo sapiens some 500,000 years ago. LGV diverged from the other strains of *C. trachomatis* four to 13 million years ago and the genital and ocular strains were differentiated about two to five million years ago. The trachoma biovar differentiation started about 0.8 to 1.8 million years ago. Richard Stephens at the Proctor

Foundation in San Francisco points out that this suggests ocular infection occurred surprisingly early in human evolution.

The chlamydial developmental cycle

The unique developmental cycle of chlamydia was first documented by Lindner by 1913 (147). When Bedson isolated the psittacosis agent in the 1930s it was possible to study this developmental cycle in more detail (263). The ability to culture chlamydia, especially in tissue culture, greatly facilitated these studies.

The length of the chlamydial developmental cycle varies considerably with different species and strains of chlamydia and host cells. Typically in the laboratory, *C. trachomatis* will take 24 to 48 hours to complete a developmental cycle, although in *in vivo* studies *C. trachomatis* may take more than twice that long (264) (see Figure 5.1). The host response or the presence of interferon-γ *in vitro* may arrest development and lead to "persistent" infection (265). Much has been learnt about detailed mechanisms involved in the chlamydial life cycle and these have recently been reviewed and summarised by Hackstadt (266), Hatch (267) and Clarke (268).

Chlamydia use "parasite-specific" phagocytosis (269) to initiate an active process of phagocytosis.

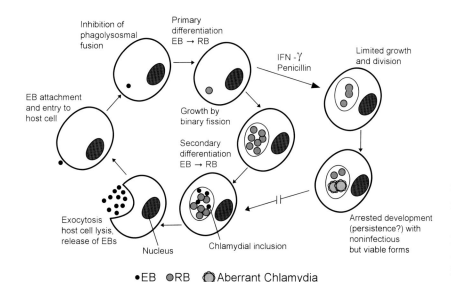

Inhibition of phagolysosmal fusion

Primary differentiation EB → RB

EB attachment and entry to host cell

IFN -γ Penicillin

Limited growth and division

Growth by binary fission

Secondary differentiation EB → RB

Exocytosis host cell lysis, release of EBs

Nucleus

Chlamydial inclusion

Arrested development (persistence?) with noninfectious but viable forms

•EB ●RB ◯ Aberrant Chlamydia

Figure 5.1 Simple schematic representation of the *C. trachomatis* developmental cycle *in vitro*. EB attachment to RB formation may take eight hours; RB to EB about 24 hours and release 48 hours. The normal cycle may take 48 to 72 hours (redrawn from Beatty WL, Morrison RP, Byrne GI. Persistent chlamydiae: from cell culture to a paradigm for chlamydial pathogenesis. Microbiol Rev. 1994; 58:686–99. Reproduced with permission from the American Society for Microbiology and Gerald Byrne).

The complete process is still not understood, but there is a multi-faceted interaction between chlamydial and host signalling pathways. Multiple attachment mechanisms have been identified and they may be used by different species with different cell lines or under different conditions. Initially, a reversible electrostatic adhesion is noted. This seems to be mediated by glycosaminoglycans, although it is unclear whether these are chlamydially derived or originate from the host cell. An irreversible attachment develops. The role of Type III Secretion (TTS) and tyrosine phosphorylation of Tarp is not yet known, although these mechanisms are activated. In addition, plasma membrane proteins (PMPs) may also be important. Changes are noted in actin filaments within the cells and a number of GTPases are activated along with cascades of other enzymes.

Once inside the cell, the chlamydia replicate in a unique niche, the intra-cellular vacuole. There are a variety of mechanisms that are still not clearly elucidated by which the vacuole containing chlamydia is able to avoid or delay liposomal fusion, and still interact with host cell microtubules and metabolic processes. Chlamydia is dependent on the host cell ATPase, energy generation and also lipids, such as sphingomyelin and cholesterol. Chlamydia release recently identified inclusion-modifying proteins (Incs) that modulate host cell response in unknown ways.

Elementary bodies have a number of surface exposed proteins. The major outer membrane protein (MOMP) is the predominant protein, which is also immuno-dominant. It has four variable domains and domain variation provides the basis for serotyping and serovar classification of *C. trachomatis*. MOMP is a porin with a molecular weight of 39 kDa. Other surface proteins include the PMPs of which there are between nine to 20 species. They are autotransporters and cleaved on the surface to give a final molecular weight of about 70 kDa. PMPs are also thought to be important in attachment and may form a target for future vaccine development. The surface also contains chlamydial lipopolysaccharide. Unexplained hemispherical domes can also be seen on the surface of EB by electron microscopy.

Elementary bodies are characterised by their small size, about 0.5μ, compared to the RB of about 1.5μ (see Figures 5.2, 5.3). The compact shape of the EB seems to be maintained by disulphide bonds that tightly crosslink the surface proteins and compress the EB, almost like a tight net. The chlamydia DNA is also tightly packed and histone-like proteins prevent transcription and hold the DNA tightly together. Once the EB has entered an intracellular vacuole, the disulphide bonds break and EB expands again to form RB. The histone-like proteins are removed and their production is stopped. The chlamydia becomes metabolically active and transcription starts within 30 minutes of entering the cell.

Some beautiful studies have been undertaken with micro arrays to identify chlamydial genes that

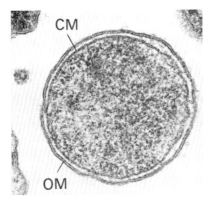
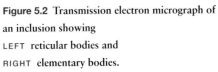

Figure 5.2 Transmission electron micrograph of an inclusion showing
LEFT reticular bodies and
RIGHT elementary bodies.

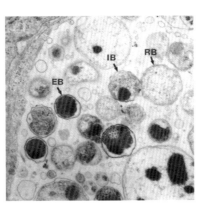

Figure 5.3 Scanning electron micrograph of an inclusion showing reticular bodies and elementary bodies, (courtesy, Michael Ward).

are "up regulated" during the development cycle (270) (see Figure 5.4). Twenty-nine genes are up regulated within the first hour and have been called "immediate early genes". By mid cycle (eight to 16 hours) nearly all genes are expressed and 26 genes are expressed late in development (24 to 40 hours). Nicholson has grouped these genes into seven temporally cohesive clusters (271). Much is still to be learnt about the fine control of these mechanisms, but a picture is now emerging of the ways in which chlamydia control gene expression and use sigma factors to regulate the transcription of specific genes.

The sequencing of C. *trachomatis* serovar D by Rick Stephens of San Francisco was a major

achievement (272). Since then, the complete sequences of C. *trachomatis* serovar A, C. *muridarum*, two isolates of C. *pneumoniae*, C. *caviae*, C. *abortus* and C. *felis* have become available (273).

The chlamydial genome is small with approximately 1.04Mbp and codes for 894 proteins (272). Some 28% of these proteins are unique to chlamydia. There is a strong "core genome" of conserved genes that are common amongst all chlamydia, but there is also an area of greater variability near the replication terminus labelled the "plasticity zone". This particular part of the genome codes tryptophan synthetase, the chlamydial toxin and the Tarp gene. Variation is

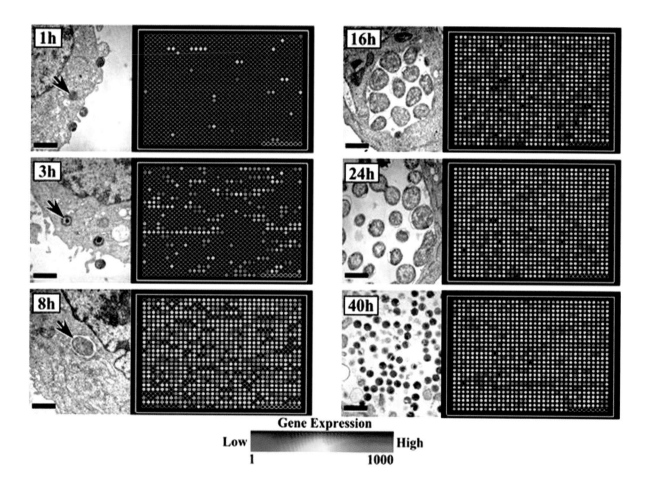

Figure 5.4 Transcriptional profiling of the developmental cycle of C. *trachomatis* serovar D in HeLa 229 cells with accompanying transmission electron microscopy of bacterial inclusions at 1, 3, 8, 16, 24, and 48 h PI (Belland et al 2003 (270) Belland RJ, Zhong G, Crane DD, Hogan D, Sturdevant D, Sharma J, et al. Genomic transcriptional profiling of the developmental cycle of Chlamydia trachomatis. Proc Nat Acad Sci USA 2003;100:8478–83 © (2003) National Academy of Sciences, USA, courtesy Robert Belland).

also found in the incA locus and in the ompA gene that codes for MOMP, although ompA shows clonal stability.

More detailed studies of the ompA gene have shown diversity within a given serovar. A study in Egypt showed five variations of genovar A and six variations in genovar Ba, but only a single genovar for serovar C (274) (see Table 5.2). The overwhelming majority of isolates had the common genetic sequence, but a small number of isolates had one or two point mutations in either variable segment 1 or 2 of the ompA gene. These minor genovar variations could be used to track household clustering and were also used to monitor the re-emergence of infection after treatment.

Another study in Nepal had similar findings, but three genotypes of Ba and six genotypes of C were found (275). Again the vast majority shared a common genotype with small numbers of isolates with single point mutations.

Another study examined multiple loci dispersed through the chromosome to determine the occurrence of recombination amongst 19 laboratory reference strains of chlamydia and 10 recent isolates (276). They found that recombination was widespread, although point substitution was relatively infrequent. Hot spots for recombination were identified downstream from the ompA gene. These findings suggest there may be more divergent clones of chlamydia than

Table 5.2: Location and encoding outcomes of point mutations distinguishing genovars from the prototype A, Ba and C sequences (274)

Genovar A	56 (VS1)	93	125	256 (VS2)
A1 (138)				
A2 (7)		C→A None		
A3 (3)	C→T			G→A Gly→Ser
A4 (4)	Ala→Val			
A5 (1)			C'T Ala→Val	

Genovar Ba	18 (VS1)	35 (VS1)	262 (VS2)	328	413
Ba1 (45)			A→G Ser'Gly	G→T Ala→Ser	
Ba2 (9)			A→G Ser'Gly		
Ba3 (2)			A→G Ser'Gly	G→T Ala→Ser	C→A Pro→His
Ba4 (1)		A→G Thr→Ala	A→G Ser→Gly	G→T Ala→Ser	
Ba5 (2)			A→G Ser→Gly		C→T Pro→Leu
Ba6 (1)	C→T Ala→Val		A→G Ser→Gly	G→T Ala→Ser	

Genovar C	56 (VS1)	165
C1 (25)	T→C Ile→Thr	C→T None

Numbers in parentheses indicate genovar frequency and VS indicates variable sequence.

previously identified from studies of the ompA gene alone. The significance of these findings is yet to be established. The toxin expressed by some chlamydia (*C. muridarum*, *C. caviae* and *C. pecorum*) is similar to the large clostridial cytotoxins that block the GTPases activated by interferon-γ (266).

In addition to their own DNA, all chlamydia contain four to eight copies of a highly conserved plasmid whose function is unknown (268). The plasmid, known as a chlamydiaphage, is 7.5 Kb and features eight major open reading frames (see Figure 5.5). Many chlamydia are also infected with a bacteriophage. These microviridae constitute the smallest known DNA virus (22nm). Six different but related phages have been identified. They contain a single strand circular DNA of 4.5 Kbp with eight open reading frames. The function of the phages is also unknown.

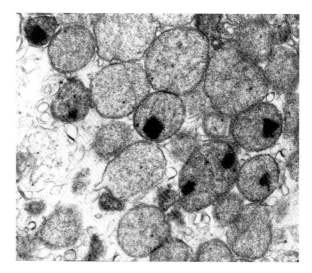

Figure 5.5 Thin section EM of *C. abortus* A22 RBs infected by chlamydiaphage Chp2 at a high multiplicity of infection (Clarke 2006 (268); courtesy, Ian Clarke).

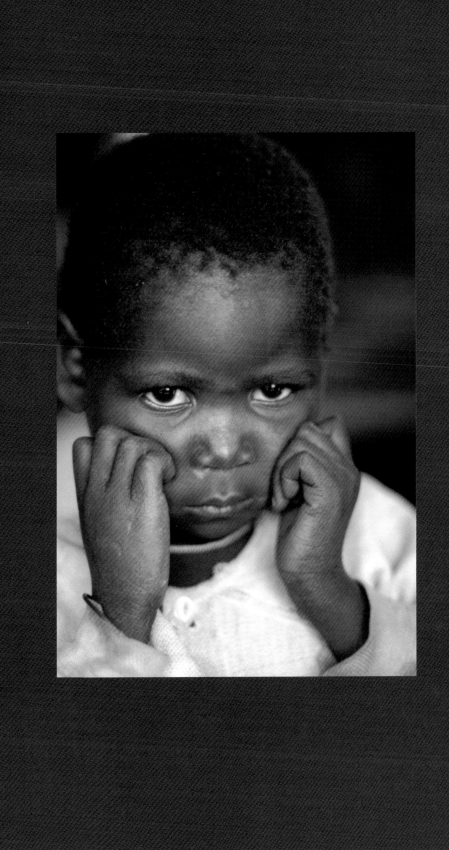

CHAPTER SIX

The epidemiology of trachoma and reinfection

The best predictor of trachoma in a child is trachoma in his or her siblings.
So trachoma is a disease of the home, especially when the home is also the crèche

FRED HOLLOWS, 1989

TRACHOMA IS A disease of the crèche and clusters in large or small pockets. These pockets may be countries (currently 54 of 200), districts or regions, villages or household clusters within villages, but ultimately trachoma is a disease of individual families. Epidemiology can describe where trachoma occurs but more importantly, why some are affected and others not. It can also explain the patchiness of these pockets of infection and the basis of family clustering.

Although there was much confusion in the 19th century about definitions of trachoma (its cause, its course and complications), by the 1900s, the clustering of trachoma within the family was well known and described. Boldt firmly stated "The chief seat of infection is the family, especially the poor with their small dwellings" (15). Thygeson later said "Since trachoma is known to spread chiefly in the home, the characteristics of the home environment are important … One can almost pick out on sight the homes where trachoma will be found rampant" (69). Similar observations came from Kentucky (75), Indian reservations in the USA (76) and Egypt (26) (see Figure 6.1).

There are copious reports from around the world confirming family clustering of trachoma. These include studies from the USA (77), Japan (83), Tunisia (277), Jordan (278), Saudi Arabia (92), Iran (279), Egypt (280), Samoa (281), South Africa (282), Tanzania (241,283), The Gambia (284) and Brazil (285). About the only study to specifically look for family clustering and not find any evidence was undertaken at a time in Taiwan when trachoma was rapidly disappearing (286). That study found marked regional variation and clustering by socioeconomic stratification, although many families had just a single person

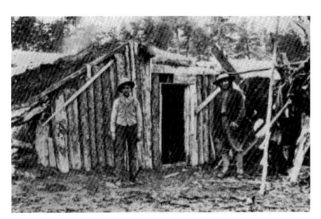

Figure 6.1 American Indian home in 1915. "It provides a splendid place for trachoma..." reads the caption in Berry GL. Trachoma in the United States. Mod Hosp,1915;5: 368–71 (reproduced by Allen & Semba, 2002 (74). Reprinted from Survey of Ophthalmology, 47, Allen SK, Semba RD, The Trachoma "Menace" in the United States, 1897–1960, 500-9 © (2002), with permission from Elsevier).

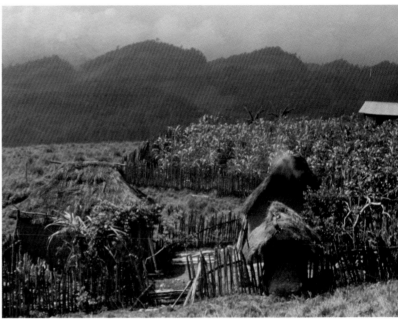

Figure 6.2 A Mayan village in Chiapas, Mexico, where family clustering was noted (1982).

RIGHT Figure 6.3 Age of acquisition of trachoma demonstrating the importance of infection in very young children (Nichols et al 1967 (92). This article was published in the American Journal of Ophthalmology, 63, Nichols RL, Bobb AA, Haddad NA, McComb DE. Immuno-flourescent Studies of the microbiologic epidemiology of trachoma in Saudi Arabia, 1372–1408, © Elsevier (1967)).

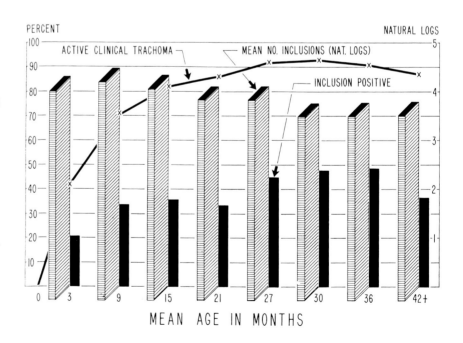

with residual disease. However, other studies in Taiwan did show family transmission (287,288). Our study in Mexico found family clustering in one village with a lower prevalence of trachoma, but not in the other village with a higher prevalence, where most families were affected (110) (see Figure 6.2).

Many of these studies, particularly the earlier ones, were not very detailed; they used the MacCallan Classification and often used only rudimentary analytic techniques. Other studies have looked more specifically at the particular factors within the family that are associated with the family clustering of trachoma.

Carl Taylor (later Head of International Health at Johns Hopkins) and his colleagues in the Punjab in India undertook one of the first trachoma studies that used the tools of "modern epidemiology" (289). They found the principal place of infection was in the home, and if the mother was affected— irrespective of the status of the father—the children were at higher risk. Taylor described the possibility of both the direct transfer of infection and indirect contact with "reciprocating infection" between mothers and children, through the use of the mother's dopatta (or shawl) to wipe children's eyes and faces and the use of suoormi (a Kohl-like substance placed around the eyes). He believed that children who suffered a relapse after being treated at school would have been almost certainly reinfected at home.

In the Samoan Islands, Ostler attributed the family clustering of trachoma to the custom of families eating together and sharing a common bowl, and to using a common towel to wash their hands and faces before and after meals (281). This was culturally important and meals were eaten by hand.

Nichols and the group from Harvard studied the intrafamily spread of trachoma infection in Saudi Arabia and concluded the "reservoir infection lies somewhere in the household environment" (92,290). Their extensive cytology studies used quantitative fluorescent antibody cytology and showed the vast bulk of infection was in children under five years of age (see Figure 6.3). They also demonstrated that a child was much more likely to have trachoma if they had one or more siblings with active trachoma. Similar findings were

reported from Lebanon (291) and have been rediscovered in more recent studies.

Bailey and colleagues from London showed trachoma clustered in family compounds in The Gambia and furthermore, it clustered by bedroom (292). They postulated that trachoma spread was facilitated by prolonged intimate contact in the bedroom. This concept was consistent with the notion of ocular promiscuity and the sharing and swapping of ocular secretions put forward by Barrie Jones (see below) (91). Bailey could find no other explanation for the spatial clustering and there was no direct link with water supply (284).

Further analysis from The Gambia showed that children who shared a bedroom with an active case had a twofold risk increase of having trachoma (293). As the number of children with active trachoma in a bedroom increased, there was also a trend for an increased risk of more severe active disease. A more sophisticated study used a geographical information system (GIS) to map villages in The Gambia. It also confirmed significant clustering of trachoma in bedrooms after adjusting the study for age, room size and distance to water (283).

A detailed study we undertook in Malawi quantified the very strong clustering of trachoma (294) (see Figure 6.4). This statistical analysis compared the clustering of trachoma and xerophthalmia. Trachoma was found to be strongly clustered in villages and even more so in families. For children, there was a 12-fold clustering effect for trachoma. When one child was found to have trachoma, it was more likely that other children in the same family would have trachoma too. This has important consequences for sample size estimates for trachoma prevalence surveys that would need to be increased ninefold. A recent report from Senegal assessed this design effect to be about sixfold (253).

Our large population-based study in Tanzania of 8409 also demonstrated strong family clustering apparent even with controls for distance to water, religion and facial cleanliness (295) (see Figure 6.5). Similar findings came from a smaller study in Egypt of 1107, where both hygiene and crowding within the family were considered to be important determinants for family clustering (280). In addition, pre-schoolchildren had a significant increased risk if they had either another sibling of

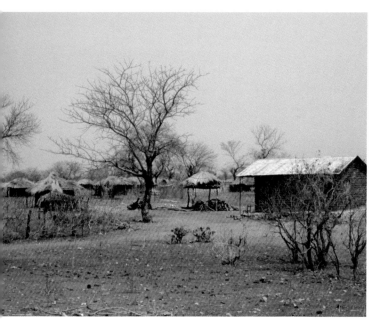

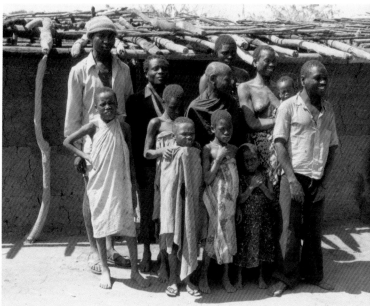

Figure 6.4 A village in the Lower Shire Valley, Malawi, where family clustering of trachoma was strong (1983).

Figure 6.5 A Tanzanian family (1986).

similar age, or an older sibling with trachoma. However, the Egyptian data suggested that trachoma was transmitted between younger children rather than from school-age youths to their younger siblings. This notion was strongly supported by earlier reports from Tunisia, Algeria and Japan (46).

Several studies have used serotyping of chlamydia to study family clustering. Those from Saudi Arabia were amongst the first studies to show the consistency of serovar specificity of serologic response of family members (177). Similar findings came from Taiwan (288) and serotyping of isolates in southern Iran over five years "clearly confirms transmission on an interpersonal basis mainly within the confines of the family" (279,296). Studies in Tanzania showed stable serovar specificity of tear antibodies over a 12 month longitudinal study of nine families (297). The use of PCR technology to look at genetic variation in chlamydia in The Gambia also confirmed strong household clustering (220), as did the Tanzanian studies (124).

As technology has developed, so has the sophistication of various studies. Genovar studies,

for example, show frequent single point mutations in the variable segments (VS1 and VS2) of MOMP, and this allows the "finger printing" of individual strains of chlamydia. In Egypt, relatively rare genovars are confined to a single family and recurrent infection after treatment is usually from the genovar prior to treatment (274). (See also chapter five, Table 5.2). At the same time, it was not uncommon to find mixed infections with two genovars present in the same family. Similar studies in Nepal show that even though half the samples were of a single genovar, the number of genovar variants increases as prevalence increases; presumably as more families are involved, more will have their own genovar (275).

Studies of the re-emergence of chlamydial infection after community-wide treatment with azithromycin strongly support intra-family spread. Baseline analysis showed strong household clustering after controlling for other known risk factors (298). After azithromycin treatment, the risk of new infection in a household member was increased 3.5 times if another member of the family was also PCR positive. The occurrence of new infection was not related to travel outside the

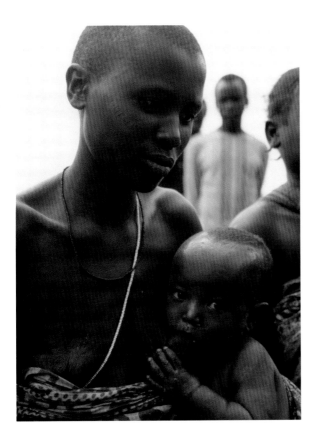

Figure 6.6 Examining small children can be quite difficult. Note the nasal discharge, scabies and the flies around the face in this Tanzanian baby (1986).

village or to visitors staying in the village. A further analysis showed the risk of an individual having infection demonstrated by PCR at two months was related to their own status at baseline. Those infected at baseline were more likely to be still infected at two months. The risk of infection at six months was related to the presence of other infected individuals in their household (299). By 12 months, households with recrudescent infection clustered within 1.2 kilometres. This analysis suggested infection finally may spread between households with children, and that nearby households will also share the same risk factors. Nearby houses are often interlinked by family ties, and there was a high level of interchange of infection between extended family members (283). To my mind, these observations firmly establish the notion that trachoma is a family-based disease and transmission occurs within this living unit.

The age of first infection

Active trachoma is a disease of early childhood, or as Fred Hollows succinctly put it: "Trachoma is a disease of the crèche"— the child-care group. However, little information exists about the dynamics and acquisition of chlamydial infection and the development of clinical trachoma in the first years of life.

Very young children are often difficult to examine (see Figure 6.6). They are small, not co-operative and physically hard to hold. Trying to evert the eyelid of a crying infant is distressing to everybody, especially the mother, and other mothers quickly become reluctant to have their young children examined. For these reasons, many trachoma studies have not examined children under the age of one, in fact, some studies even confine themselves inappropriately to schoolchildren.

Rowland Wilson (who became Director of the Giza Laboratory after MacCallan's retirement) studied 40 newborn Egyptian children (300). Giemsa cytology was collected every two weeks and all developed inclusions within the first few months of life. The number of inclusions decreased rapidly after the first three months from their first appearance.

Sowa and co-workers studied the age of acquisition of trachoma in The Gambia (301). They followed 79 newborn children, five of whom developed chlamydial conjunctivitis in the first three weeks of life. This was presumed to be genitally-acquired ophthalmia neonatorum, although two mothers also had active trachoma with positive ocular chlamydial cultures. Two babies resolved the infection without sequelae. Two of the babies were twins; one of the twins and two of the other three babies had ongoing chlamydial infection and developed signs consistent with trachoma including pannus. It is unclear if those with ongoing disease had persistence of their initial infection or whether they were exposed to further infection within their family environment. The discordance of disease in the twins was not discussed further. Eleven of the remaining 74 babies also acquired chlamydial infection with positive ocular cultures and signs consistent with trachoma, starting from three months. By three or four months, the immune system is sufficiently mature to be able to form follicles and germinal centres, so trachoma can be clinically distinguished from conjunctivitis.

Detailed studies in Saudi Arabia show the bulk of chlamydial infection occurred in children under five years, and infants between three to nine months shed the highest number of organisms (demonstrated by fluorescence cytology) (290). This was a striking finding as the prevalence of infection occurred well before the peak of clinical infection at 30 to 36 months. Clinical trachoma has been commonly reported in children about four months (123,162,300,302,303,304,305,306,307). In Egypt and Morocco almost all children were reported to have clinical signs within the first few months of life (139,300).

In the Sudan, 48% of children under the age of one year had already acquired trachoma with a peak prevalence of 71% in those aged one to four years (308). In Egypt, the highest age-specific rate of active trachoma was found in children under the age of one who had the most intense disease (304). Recent data from southern Sudan continue to confirm the high prevalence of active trachoma in the first two or three years of life (254). In fact, in this hyperendemic area 56% of infants between two weeks and 11 months showed signs of active trachoma.

Schachter and Dawson followed 88 infants from birth for one year and infection was defined by cytology and tear antibodies. They calculated the incidence of infection in the first year to be 6% per month (309). These children form a huge pool of infection and the need to call on a genital reservoir of infection in their words was "moot". When trachoma was still endemic in Japan an incidence of clinical disease in infants of 2.1% per month was reported and 26% had trachoma by their first birthday (83). The difference between these two studies may reflect real differences in the force of infection and transmission potential between hyper and mesoendemic areas, or they may reflect differences in ascertainment.

There are multiple reports in the literature describing the age-specific rates of trachoma. Earlier studies that used the MacCallan Classification tend to be confusing because the progression from one stage to another does not correlate with current concepts of disease, and active trachoma can exist in the first three

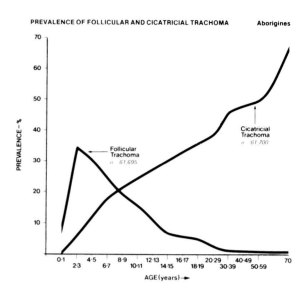

Figure 6.7 Age-specific prevalence of trachoma in Australian Aborigines 1976–78 (NTEHP 1980 (103); courtesy, Royal Australian and New Zealand College of Ophthalmologists).

MacCallan stages. The data become even more confusing when various composite indices of gravity and severity were used, as they bear almost no relation to our current understanding of the disease (286). The simplified grading gives probably the clearest indication of the community distribution of trachoma (121).

Studies show that peak prevalence of active trachoma is almost invariably in children, usually aged between two to five depending on the overall level of endemicity, and show a rapid decline in the prevalence of active trachoma after seven to 10 years (see Figure 6.7).

Interestingly, studies in Australian Aborigines also show a maximum age-specific infection in pre-schoolchildren, but there are also considerable rates of active trachoma into the teenage years (103,310,311).

The infectious pool

Probably the single, biggest unresolved question with trachoma is the relative importance of episodes of reinfection versus the presence of persistent or latent infection. This issue has been intensely debated for the last 100 years, ever since trachoma was finally confirmed to be an infectious disease, rather than a disease from the myasm, or an "endogenous" condition such as gout or rheumatoid arthritis. This debate has been further fuelled by the apparent similarity of the chlamydia that cause such different ocular outcomes in trachoma and inclusion conjunctivitis. Initially, most authors assumed that trachoma was a chronic disease that resulted from a single chronic infection; once acquired, trachoma would progress relentlessly like syphilis, tuberculosis or leprosy (148). This assumption was explicit in the MacCallan grading and it was based on the understanding of the evolution of other chronic infectious diseases.

Observations from the field suggest reinfection was in conflict with the notion of ongoing chronic infection. These inconsistencies were frequently seen, but were glossed over or somehow tucked into the general theory of chronic persisting disease. At present, this issue is still unresolved and it is possible that both mechanisms may operate to some extent. However, I believe that most of the features of the disease including its epidemiology and pathogenesis can be explained by the notion of repeated episodes of reinfection.

Further field observations suggesting reinfection include the rapid recurrence of active trachoma in Indian children, who had been treated at school with topical tetracycline in some of the early treatment studies (289). This was attributed to reinfection at home. Trachoma was seen to become "periodic" in Taiwan, where living conditions were dramatically improving (312). First grade children showed "conversions" from active disease with demonstrable organism to apparently normal conjunctiva without organism, and then they became reinfected and had active trachoma again. This could occur three or four times over a period of five years. Similar observations that trachoma was a disease that "waxes and wanes" were made in Saudi Arabia (92). Nichols observed that "the duration of infection is thought to be primarily determined by the living conditions of the subject". The occurrence of disabling sequelae was determined by the duration of infection rather than climate, geography, race, virulence or susceptibility to the "force of infection", a term introduced by Assaad (94).

Barrie Jones in London promoted the concept of ocular promiscuity (*pro* in favour of; *miscere* to mix) (91). He related the duration and severity of trachoma to both the magnitude of the source of shedding of infection and the level of ocular promiscuity within a family, that is, the interaction of the individual with the family "pool of infection".

Suggestions that trachoma was not a simple chronic infection also came from a study of Indians in the Punjab and those who migrated to British Columbia (313,314). Those who migrated to Canada as adults had as high rates of trachoma sequelae (scarring and trichiasis) as those who had lived all their life in the Punjab. However, if individuals had migrated to Canada before the age of 20, they had less disease and were less likely to have severe complications. The chance of "relapse" in British Columbia was assessed to be very small, the prevalence of trachoma was reduced, the disease was less "active" and milder and did not spread to young children. The authors pointed out that as the children in Canada were not affected there was little chance of infection or reinfection occurring within these families after migration. This meant the only way the disease could progress in the migrant adults would be through "endogenous relapse". However, as the adults showed little progression, the authors concluded that endogenous relapse was not occurring and therefore did not play an important role in the disease. This formalised the observation previously made anecdotally many times in areas where trachoma has disappeared.

Probably Tom Grayston (1924–) in Seattle was one of the first to advocate the importance of reinfection (287,288,315,316). A leader in chlamydial research for 50 years, Grayston started work on trachoma in Taiwan before moving to Seattle, where he later became Dean of Public Health. He has made many major contributions to the field and is a friend and mentor to many. Grayston's evidence for reinfection came from two areas. First, his experimental infections in monkeys showed that a single primary inoculation with chlamydia would eventually resolve the infection without cicatricial sequelae. However, with secondary infection, or challenge infection of previously immunised animals, a proportion (about 12%) developed more severe disease with pannus or scarring. He concluded that the cicatricial sequelae were only seen with reinfection. His second line of evidence came from his family-based studies. These studies were hampered as trachoma was disappearing with rapid socioeconomic development in Taiwan. However, he undertook detailed, longitudinal studies of families that used tear and serum serology, chlamydial culture and clinical grading. They demonstrated the recovery from infection in children, followed by relapse or reinfection. As in the animal studies, reinfection in children was associated with a more severe response and the development of cicatricial changes, whereas initial or primary infection could be resolved without sequelae (178,316). As early as 1963, Grayston clearly and emphatically stated that inclusion conjunctivitis was seen with single ocular chlamydial infection and that trachoma occurred with repeated infection (315).

An interesting discussion is recorded during the fourth International Chlamydial Meeting that assessed the status on this debate in 1976 (317). Roger Nichols was one of those who spoke of the importance of persisting infection and stressed that a small number developed long-term severe disease apparently from a single infection. Others including Grayston, Dawson and Jones spoke of the importance of reinfection. Dawson explained the decrease in active infection in children after the age of six as being due to "increasing social distance and better hygiene", both of which would decrease the likelihood of reinfection.

The importance of reinfection

While this meeting was going on, I was having my first experience of trachoma fieldwork with the National Trachoma and Eye Health Program (NTEHP) in Australia, and was totally oblivious to these erudite discussions. A year or so later at the Wilmer Institute, the possibility of establishing an animal model of trachoma was raised in discussion with Art Silverstein, one of the first immunologists to work full-time on ophthalmic issues, who had a very enquiring mind.

My own field experience convinced me of the importance of reinfection for three reasons. The first came to me in the first few months of trachoma fieldwork. I had examined many hundreds of Aboriginal children and a hundred or

so European children living in the same communities and was struck by the different rates of trachoma. Whereas trachoma prevalence in Aboriginal children ranged between 40% to 70%, in those few non-Aboriginals it was only about 1%. All lived in the same communities, shared the same desks at school, played football together and shared the same flies. However, they went home to different families where they had vastly different standards of personal and family hygiene (see Figure 6.8). This illustrates the importance of close or continuous exposure to infection within the family. Much later, I learnt of similar observations previously made in different areas in North Africa (46).

The second observation was the vastly different levels of personal and community hygiene one saw in trachoma areas. Thygeson had noted that you could usually recognise people and families with trachoma from a distance (69). Poor hygiene, copious ocular discharge and dirty faces gave ample opportunity for the sharing of ocular secretions by ocular promiscuity, as Jones had suggested (91) (see Figure 6.9). Frequent exposure to infected ocular secretions could occur easily and often with the poor hygiene present in these trachoma areas.

The third observation was that none of our field staff developed trachoma or even inclusion conjunctivitis (318). Although we did not wash our hands between every child we examined, the field teams did practise reasonable levels of personal hygiene in the clinic and during field activities (see Figure 6.10). This suggested that chlamydia was not "highly contagious" and one needed fairly close contact to pick up infection. Jones related the close interpersonal contact needed to exchange ocular chlamydial infection to that required for the exchange of genital tract infection and coined the term "ocular promiscuity" (91).

In my naïvety, I replied to Silverstein that it would be easy to establish an animal model of trachoma, and that all one needed to do was to repeatedly reinfect the animals. I had no knowledge of previous controversies and the many "failed" monkey experiments. As detailed in the following chapter, we were able to induce chronic disease resembling trachoma in monkeys with repeated reinoculation. The monkey experiments reinforced the importance of repeated reinfection and my

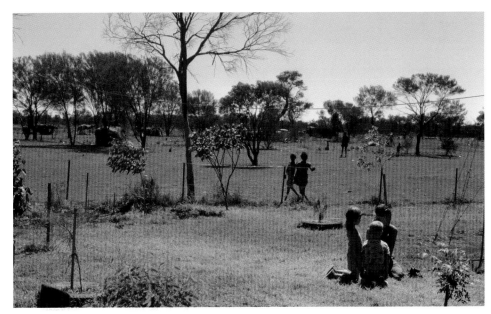

LEFT **Figure 6.8**
The strikingly different
environment of white
children living in a
remote Aboriginal
settlement (foreground)
compared to Aboriginal
children in the
background (1977).

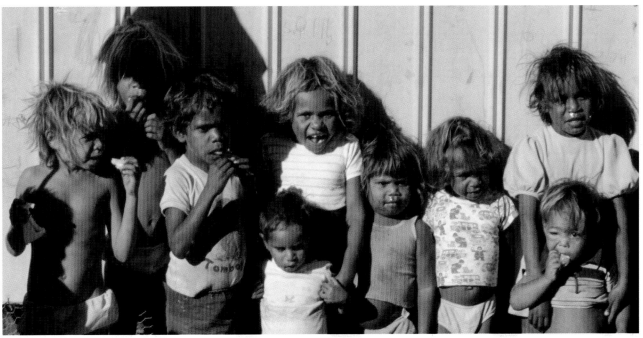

ABOVE **Figure 6.9** A group of Australian
Aboriginal children with a high prevalence of
active trachoma. Many also show nasal
discharge and dirty faces (1977).

RIGHT **Figure 6.10** NTEHP field
examinations in a schoolroom in Central
Australia (1976).

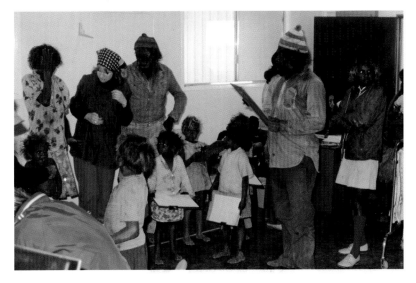

subsequent field studies were built on this premise.

The next step was to return to the field to look at factors that favoured frequent transmission and episodes of reinfection. The first attempt was a study of face washing we undertook in Mexico. This line of research led to further epidemiologic studies into facial cleanliness in Tanzania, Malawi and elsewhere, the clinical trial of facial cleanliness in Tanzania and the inclusion of facial cleanliness as a component of the SAFE Strategy.

Reinfection or persistence

With all this information, one can make a very convincing argument about the importance of repeated episodes of reinfection. However, there are some anomalies and outlying observations that do not entirely fit with this concept and these could be explained by the occurrence of persistent infection.

To properly evaluate "anomalous" results suggestive of persistent infection, one must ensure that the possibility of repeated episodes of reinfection are either totally excluded, or have been measured and quantified. Without knowing the status of exposure to further infection, one cannot interpret the finding of apparent presence of ongoing or persistent infection. One also has to be confident of the validity of both the assessment of clinical status and the detection of infection. A more comprehensive clinical assessment is needed than the WHO simplified grading system. There are always issues of test sensitivity and specificity, and with the supreme sensitivity of modern tests, the possibility of specimen contamination needs to be confidently excluded.

The occasional occurrence of individuals with apparent persistent severe infection needs more understanding. Mabey found in The Gambia that a child with moderate severe disease at one visit was 15 times more likely to have moderate or severe disease at the next visit, some eight or 13 months later (293). He observed that "host factors may be more important determinants of severity than the frequency of episodes of reinfection". This led to a series of studies that suggested that major histocompatibility antigens may explain a difference in the immune response in some individuals, and subsequent work has shown individual variations in inflammatory mediators

that modify the risk of infection or sequelae (319,320).

Longitudinal studies in Tanzania also have identified children with apparent persistent severe infection. One such study of families we performed used culture, DFA and EIA and showed that young age was a more important indication of the likelihood of severe persistent disease three months later, rather than high inclusion counts on DFA and high antigen loads determined by EIA (297). In another study, we looked at environmental factors that may facilitate reinfection and the maintenance of constant severe disease in three of four examinations over a 12 month period (321) . The children with severe persistent TI were almost three times as likely to have a sibling with TF; twice as likely to have a dirty face, live in a house more than two hours from water, or keep cattle nearby. The study was confined to children aged one to seven, but girls were more likely to have persistent disease in this age range than boys.

West extended these observations and showed that children who had constant severe disease incurred a five times increased risk of developing conjunctival scarring at the seven-year follow-up, and were also more likely to still have intensive inflammation at the seven-year examination (322). She also speculates that in addition to the role played by reinfection, there might also be a subgroup of children who responded more strongly to exposure to chlamydia, and developed more severe diseases that they were unable to resolve. These children therefore would be at higher risk of scarring. West noted that about 10% of children showed constant severe inflammation over a 12 month period, and the seven-year incidence of scarring (TS) was 11%. She calculated the attributable risk of TI for conjunctival scarring to be 28%. The remaining 72% of TS would come from children who were not in the group with constant severe disease. This is an important observation to keep in mind when assessing the relative importance of these mechanisms and indications for continuing programmatic interventions.

Another study from Tanzania examined a group of women who had positive PCR in two examinations three years apart; 73% were infected with the same genovar (323). Given half these women were not living in households with

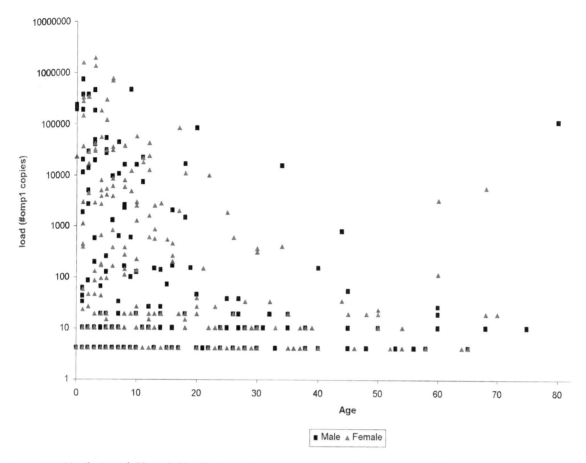

Figure 6.11 Distribution of chlamydial load in the total population by age and gender in Central Tanzania (West et al 2005 (122). Reprinted with permission from the Association for Research in Vision and Ophthalmology, © 2005).

children, this was taken as evidence for "persistence of infection". Those with persistent infection were more likely to have scarring and trichiasis. However, none of these studies were able to quantify the ongoing exposure to chlamydia and transmission.

The source of infection

What is the source of chlamydial infection that gets recycled? Reinhards strongly stated that children below the age of four are the prime source for infection within the family (324). Not only did they have the highest prevalence of trachoma and bacterial conjunctivitis, they also have the most severe disease and attract the most flies to their face. The more sophisticated quantitative laboratory studies, especially those using NAAT

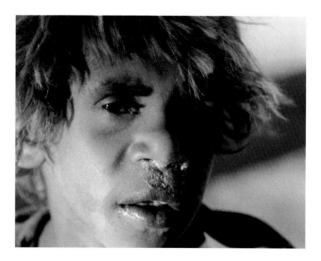

Figure 6.12 Nasal discharge can be an important source of chlamydial infection.

testing, have confirmed earlier cytology findings that the vast majority of infection is in young children, particularly pre-schoolchildren (92,301,324).

In a longitudinal study in nine Tanzanian families, we used elementary body counts in DFA to give a measure of infectious load (297). Most infection was found in young children and in those with severe disease (TI) (297). Studies using semi-quantitative EIA in The Gambia showed a predominance of infection in children under 10. Bailey undertook a longitudinal study using EIA in which he examined some 250 people in 20 households each week for six months (126). The incidence of new infection decreased threefold with age. The highest infectious loads as determined by EIA were seen in younger children. He also noted an apparent reduction in the duration of episodes of infection with age; in 0 to 3 year olds infection lasted some 13 weeks and in those 15 and above, infection lasted only 1.7 weeks. This notion of decreasing duration of infection with age is consistent with field observations previously made by Grayston, but in neither case was there a measure of the exposure to potential episodes of reinfection (126,316). Studies in Tanzania

suggested TF would resolve in three to nine months after a child ceased to be DFA positive (297).

However, the advent of quantitative PCR gave a very compelling picture of the distribution of infectious load. Both in north and central Tanzania, studies showed the overwhelming predominance of demonstrable DNA was in young children (122,168). More than 90% of the community load of infection was in children under the age of seven in Rombo, a mesoendemic area, and two individuals with the highest loads were aged five and eight months. Over 50% was found in children under the age of two in the hyperendemic area of Kongwa (122) (see Figure 6.11).

However, young children in endemic areas not only have ocular infection with chlamydia, but chlamydia can also be cultured from other sites. In Egyptian villages 34% had extraocular infection (325). Positive cultures came from the eyes of 28% of children, and one-third with ocular infection also had extraocular infection. Nasopharyngeal infection was also examined in Tanzania where 27% of children aged one to seven had chlamydia in nasopharyngeal swabs demonstrated by PCR (326) (see Figure 6.12). The presence of nasopharyngeal chlamydia was correlated with the

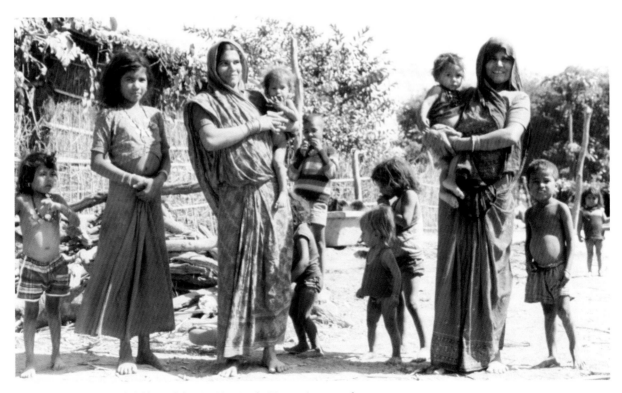

Figure 6.13 Women and children of the Terai in Nepal. Here, as in many places, women are more severely affected by trachoma than men (1989)

presence of trachoma, both clinically and by PCR. West examined the effect of topical tetracycline treatment and concluded that nasal infection was not the source of ocular reinfection following topical treatment. A further study using quantitative PCR showed nasal carriage was higher in children with higher ocular loads or with TI (327). More recently, Gower has shown that nasal discharge tested positive for chlamydia by PCR in one-third of Tanzanian children with trachoma who have nasal discharge, and this strongly correlates with a positive ocular PCR test (328). The presence of a positive nasal discharge was more likely in those with TI, and increased the likelihood of the presence of infection two months after treatment. Of course, chlamydia-infected nasal discharge could easily transfer infection from one child to another by direct contact or via handkerchiefs, sheets or other means.

Chlamydial genital tract infection in adults has not been studied frequently in trachoma endemic areas. Some early studies in The Gambia (301) and South Africa (282) found it occurred relatively infrequently. More recent studies in Somalia using EIA antigen tests demonstrated chlamydia in 6% of men, but 18% of women (329). Brunham and colleagues examined families with trachoma in Central Kenya (330). Although a range of serotypes were cultured from the eyes of children (serovars A, A/L$_2$, B, Ba, D, E and F) only 4% of their mothers had positive cervical cultures and these were a genital strain (serovar E).

It is worth re-emphasising the potential importance of children in the first year of life as a source of infection in their families, especially when considering the efficacy of family or community-based distribution of azithromycin or other antibiotic treatment. These young children may have very high infectious loads. Most treatment programs have only treated children aged one year or more and in some cases, six months or more. This leaves this most potent reservoir of infection in the family untreated with the youngest children being the family-based, infantile fountains of infection. The few existing studies suggest that these infants alone may account for 25% or even 50% of the entire infectious load or pool of infection in the community!

Trachoma in women

It has become widely recognised that in general women are particularly affected by trachoma. There are several good logistic and political reasons to continue to emphasise this ongoing trend. The potential linkage of trachoma control activities with maternal and child health programs offers great advantages, as does the alignment with goals to improve health, literacy and social standing of women specifically re-enunciated in the Millennium Development Goals. The recognition that women are disproportionately subject to trachoma is implicit in the aphorism that trachoma is a disease of the crèche, based on observations that in many areas women have a significantly higher rate of scarring and trichiasis than men (see Figure 6.13).

Schereschewsky reported American Indian women were more affected than men (76). In India, the prevalence of complications was similar for men and women in hyperendemic areas, but as prevalence decreased, scarring trichiasis and blindness decreased more rapidly in men (289). Overall, Indian women had twice the rate of cicatricial complications of trachoma compared to men (302). In China, women were reported to have higher rates of trichiasis and entropion (159) and similar observations were made in Poland (46), Morocco (331), Burma (332), Mexico (110) and Vietnam (333,334).

In South Africa, trichiasis was eight times and blindness four times more common in women (284). In Tanzania, trichiasis rates were four times higher in women with corneal opacity and vision loss was twice as common (295). In The Gambia scarring was 50% more common in women than men (293) and blindness from trachoma 3.5 times higher (335).

Kupka and co-authors comment that in Morocco young girls are usually less well cared for than boys, and females usually have constant and close association with young children throughout their lives (331). They speculated that:

> Although the mother may at first be the source of infection for very young children, with the prevalence of active cases among children close to 100 per cent, one can easily speculate on the possibility of the

mutual intensification of infection between mother and child reaching a vicious cycle. Higher rates of reinfection amongst females and thus a prolonged course of the disease, increase the risk of severe lesions such as conjunctival or corneal complications and an early age of onset of trichiasis (331).

A Moroccan woman who as a child spent more than 15 years living with other children (brothers and sisters) incurred a 50% increased risk of having grave trachoma (trichiasis or corneal scarring) (331). However, the risk was even greater for women who as adults had looked after children. Those adults who cared for children for more than 15 years incurred a threefold risk of grave lesions. Women who had not looked after children incurred the same risk as men. The higher exposure of women to (potentially infected) children is shown in The Gambia, where 95% shared a room with a child, but only 10% of men did the same (293).

Our population-based study in Tanzania confirmed the higher rate of cicatricial sequelae in women and increased rates of active disease in women who cared for children compared to those

who did not (295). In another Tanzanian study, the risk of active trachoma in women was directly related to caring for children with active trachoma, irrespective of facial cleanliness (336) (see Figure 6.14). Compared to women living without children with trachoma, the risk of active trachoma for women living with children with active trachoma was 1.6 times for non-caretakers and 2.4 times for caretakers. A subsequent case control study of the risk of trichiasis in Tanzanian women identified a number of indicators of poverty and poor hygiene including having a mother with trichiasis (337). The latter finding is tantalising and begs the following questions. Is it nature or nurture, a genetic risk or a shared environment?

The increased risk of trachoma for women starts from childhood. Girls tend to have more severe trachoma than boys. In Mexico most TI was found in girls and active disease was also seen in older girls and young women. The rate of TF was twice that in girls compared to boys (110). In this area of Mexico, girls aged five or more had a major responsibility in caring for their youngest siblings (120). Similar findings come from Tanzania, where girls incur higher rates of active disease which continued for longer periods in girls than boys (338) (see Figure 6.15). Many studies have now

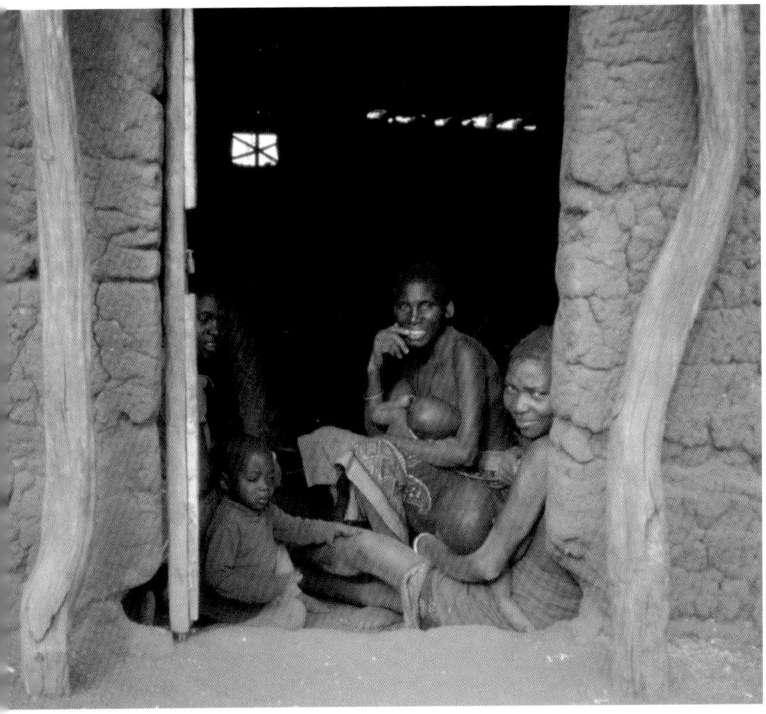

Figure 6.14 Trachoma is a disease of the crèche. Women and children in Central Tanzania (1986).

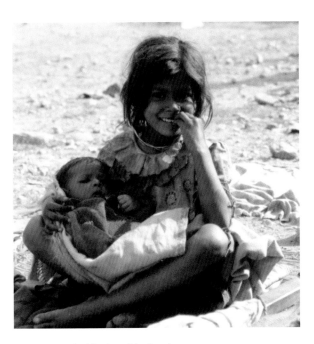

Figure 6.15 A "big sister" looks after a baby sister in Nepal.

confirmed the slower age-related reduction of active trachoma rates in girls.

In addition to contributing to the ocular pool of infection, mothers may interact with children in other ways. Reinhards postulated that trachoma was worse in women because they contracted bacterial conjunctivitis from children (324). Schachter and Dawson examined the role of transmission of genital infection in women, and concluded the genital tract was not an important reservoir for transmission of trachoma (309). This is consistent with the findings of Brunham and co-workers in Kenya, although they identified occasional episodes of genital to ocular infection (330). A related study in Nairobi found 7% of babies had chlamydial ophthalmia neonatorum and the overall prevalence of genital tract infection with chlamydia in women was 21% (339). Although this was a hospital-based study, many women came from rural trachoma areas.

However, the predominance of trachoma in women is not universal. As was the case in India, the gender difference was more marked in areas of lower prevalence (289). In areas of high prevalence, the rates between men and women may be more equal. In Egypt where trichiasis rates were very high (75% for women and 57% for men), the gender difference was quite small, although rates of blindness and corneal opacity were still twofold

higher in women (304). In Egypt, it was interesting to note that the rate of active trachoma in boys was higher than girls, even though women had higher rates of scarring. No gender difference in active trachoma rates was reported from the large study in Mali (242). A recent study in Ethiopia also reported no significant differences in rates of active trachoma, scarring or trichiasis between men and women (243).

There are some areas in which the rates of scarring, trichiasis and blindness are reported to be marginally higher in men than women—for example, Aboriginal people in Australia (103,340) (see Figure 6.16). Aboriginal boys and girls also have similar rates of active disease (311,341). In some other areas, more severe disease is reported in boys, although these reports may be biased. In Samoa, this was attributed to boys tending fires and smoke irritation (281). In Okinawa, schoolboys had more trachoma than schoolgirls, but of course girls from poorer families would be more likely to have trachoma and less likely to attend school (342). In Qatar it was noted that more males than females had scarring (118), but this was a hospital-based study and may reflect the differential utilisation of health care services.

If the explanation for the generally higher rates of trachoma in women was due to their prolonged exposure to children and the attendant risk of

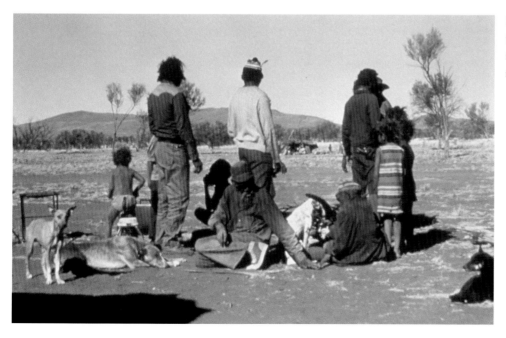

Figure 6.16 The rates of trichiasis and blindness are marginally higher in Aboriginal men than women.

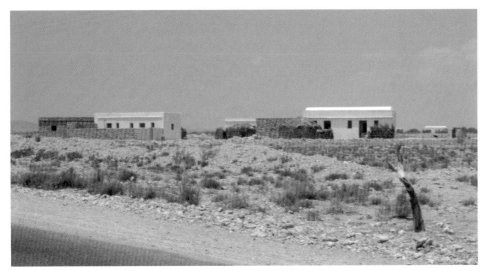

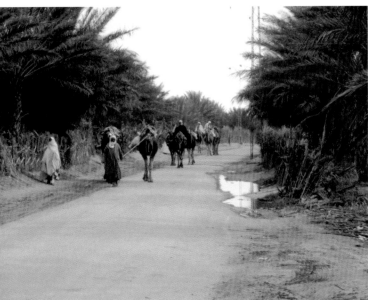

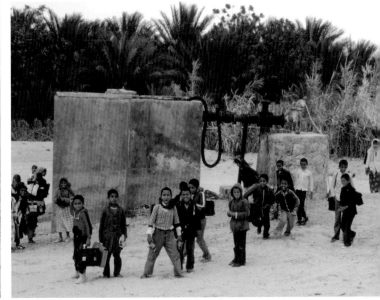

Figure 6.17 By the early 1980s, trachoma had essentially disappeared from Tunisia, with concomitant socioeconomic development that included

TOP new houses

CENTRE LEFT made roads and electricity

CENTRE RIGHT more secure water supplies, and

BOTTOM in one case, the building of a chemical factory.

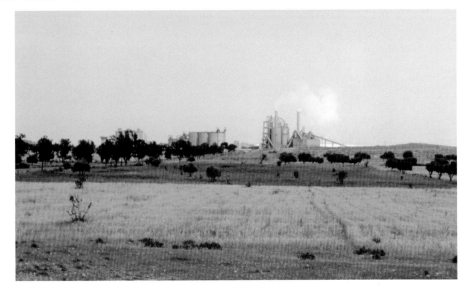

repeated episodes of reinfection, what was different in areas where women and men were equally affected? Why were men still exposed to the infectious pool? It is my impression that in subsistence farming settlements in Africa or Asia young children aged five to seven are more likely to move away from the "childcare group". If they are lucky they may go to school, but if they are boys, they may well start farm work or tend animals. On the other hand, girls are more likely to stay at home and care for younger children and assist their mothers. This division of activities by gender is far less clear-cut in Australian Aboriginal communities for example, with little commercial activity or subsistence farming and intermittent school attendance.

Natural experiments and the impact of socioeconomic development

As discussed earlier, trachoma progressively decreased in Western Europe over the last century as living conditions improved. Over the last 60 years, many have commented on the progressive decrease in trachoma with concomitant socioeconomic development and subsequent improvement in living standards (162). For example, a decrease in trachoma was noted in the Punjab with decreased crowding, improved sanitation and drainage, and increased provision of open space (289). In Jordan socioeconomic development led to a lower prevalence of trachoma in towns than in surrounding villages (278). The decreased amount of trachoma in Indians who migrated to Canada was ascribed to better personal and community hygiene with decreased crowding, dust and flies and cases of mucopurulent conjunctivitis (314). Jones related a specific decrease in trachoma rates in southern Iran with the development of oil pipelines and pumping stations (91).

Trachoma had declined in Malta by 1960 after it was made a notifiable disease in schoolchildren, overcrowded housing was addressed, piped water was provided, and sanitation and fly control were introduced (343). However, making trachoma a notifiable disease was not always an effective measure in other areas. For example, Mackenzie

notes it had little effect in France in the 1920s (46). The general improvement in the standard of living in Saudi Arabian villages in the 1960s led to falling rates of trachoma, although no specific factors were identified (344). Thirty years later active trachoma had essentially disappeared from Saudi Arabia and the amount of blindness from trachoma had decreased dramatically (345). Trachoma decreased with the improved socioeconomic conditions in a Tunisian village after the opening of a power station and chemical factory (138) (see Figure 6.17). There was a dramatic decrease in the overall prevalence and severity of trachoma in The Gambia over a 37 year period that paralleled improvements in sanitation, water, education and health care (346). A similar decrease was also noted in Kenya (347). Economic analyses also quantify the link of less trachoma in areas of greater prosperity (348).

None of these reports identified any specific intervention that led to a reduction in trachoma. Several explicitly state that "no single factor" could be identified (138,344). They share the common theme of non-specific socioeconomic improvements leading to a decrease in trachoma. However, several have noted that these general improvements first led to a lowering in the intensity of active trachoma. This was followed by a reduction in the levels of infection and the incidence of active trachoma that was followed in turn by a gradual decrease in prevalence and ultimately a decrease in the cicatricial complications (91,139,288,313,349). This sequence should have considerable significance when one considers the selection of indicators used in the assessment of the impact of trachoma control programs, where the emphasis has been on the prevalence of active trachoma (TF), almost the last measure to decline.

Specific risk factors for trachoma

The previous section broadly discussed some general environmental factors that impact on the prevalence of trachoma. No doubt, if one sat and waited for general socioeconomic development to occur in every household in every village around the world, trachoma would ultimately disappear. After all, it has disappeared from the whole of

Table 6.1: WHO Expert Committee on Trachoma, 1962 (49)

Factors favouring transmission of infection

Race, climate, including temperature, rainfall, altitude and amount of exposure to ultra-violet light

Transmission by insect vectors (especially *M. sorbens*)

Density of population (crowding and institutions)

Diet and nutrition

Cultural and social customs, including organisation of the household; nomadic or stationary habits; religious practices; use of cosmetics; occupation (especially as a possible influence on varying sex or age distribution of cases); and availability and use of water

General economic level of the area

History, from the point of view of extrinsic contents (migration, invasion and trade routes)

Status of education in the community

Presence of other ocular or general diseases

Information on as many as possible of the above points should be obtained in preliminary surveys of an area. This will require, in many cases, the co-operation of an epidemiologist and a sociologist or anthropologist; it is evident that any or all of these factors may have importance in explaining the incidence and characteristics of trachoma in a particular population.

In heavily infected areas of low social and economic level, treatment campaigns alone have not been entirely effective, but education and sanitation, with emphasis on water supply, must also be improved concurrently.

Europe and North America and many other parts of the world over the last 50 to 100 years with progressive improvements in the standard of living.

One hundred years ago, Boldt was quite clear: "There is no doubt that a *low state of civilisation, want of cleanliness and overcrowding* play an important part in spreading infection"(15). Even more specific, MacCallan in 1908 listed a range of "uncleanly habits of the lower classes" that included poor water availability, crowded huts, sleeping together and with their cattle, dust from unpaved and unwatered streets, daily gales and sandstorms and for the rich, the presence of infected servants (89). In addition, of course, MacCallan also listed the epidemics of bacterial conjunctivitis in the early and late summer months. He also went on to state that "trachoma is a purely local disease" and maintained that "the severity of the disease depends on ... the personal habits of the individual and the conditions under which he lives" (89). The beautiful back-to-back papers by Stucky and Schereschewsky paint a strikingly similar picture in Kentucky and American Indian reservations (75,76).

The challenge for those of us who follow is to identify the specific personal habits and particular conditions that expose an individual to increased risk of trachoma, and then develop specific strategies to address them. We cannot, with good conscience, sit and wait for gradual improvement in socioeconomic status to reach the last family with trachoma sometime in the next 100 or 200 years.

The second WHO Expert Committee listed the risk factors for trachoma that included "poverty, dirt, crowding and ignorance" and associated bacterial infection (33). The third WHO Expert Group expanded this list considerably (see Table 6.1) (49). Although somewhat more specific, this was still a very broad umbrella and covered almost every conceivable aspect of life, and did not materially advance our understanding, or foster the development of specific intervention strategies.

Individual workers had identified various specific risk factors. Mann specifically identified the importance of the introduction of textiles, clothes and blankets, in the absence of good personal hygiene in outback Australia, Papua New Guinea

TABLE 6.2: Odds ratios for the range of community, family and individual risk factors for active trachoma (TF or TF/TI) examined by population-based epidemiologic surveys (significant associations are shown in bold)

Author	Taylor 1985 (110)	Tielsch 1988 (361)	Taylor 1989 (241)	Courtright 1991 (280)	Luna 1992 (285)	Katz 1996 (123)	Sahlu 1992 (360)	Schemann 2002 (242)	Schemann 2003 (372)	Cumberland 2005 (306)	Faye 2006 (253)	Mesfin 2006 (243)	Abdou 2007 (394)
Population	Mexico n=1097	Malawi n=5436	Tanzania n=8409	Egypt n=1107	Brazil n=2939	Nepal n=836	Ethiopia n=1222	Mali n=15,187	Burkina Faso, n=1960	Ethiopia n=1960	Senegal n=1648	Ethiopia n=3900	Niger n=651
Environmental risk factor	all ages	< 6	all ages	all ages	all ages	2 to 6.5	all ages	<10	3 to 9	3 to 9	2 to 5	all ages	1 to 5
Community													
Development services ‡		n*	n			n		1.2					n
Tube well						1.3							
Altitude							4.2						
Family													
Socioeconomic status		n			2.0	n		1.1					
Servants						n							
Size/number of children	n	n	n	1.3	1.5			n		3.4			n
Crowding		n				1.5	2.9	n			n	n	
Migration		n		n	n								
Distance from school	n												
Construction roof	n		n		n			n					
Construction walls	n			n	n	n		n					
Construction floor	n			n	n	n							
Number of rooms	n			n	n								
Separate kitchen	n						2.7					n	
Family possessions †			n	n		n		n					
Source of water	n	n	n		3.7	1.9		n		n		n	
Distance to water	n	2.6	1.3			n		1.3 / 1.4		n	n	n	n
Volume of water/household			n										
Volume of water/person					2.8			n			2.2		
Household flies			1.5 / 1.6						5.8	n			
Latrine absent	n	1.7	n / 1.4	3.3	n	n		1.9	n	2.0	n	n	n
Rubbish disposal	n				2.3		2.7	n	1.7	n	n	n	n
Religion			1.4 / 1.7			n							
Paternal education	n	1.3		n	2.9	n	n	n				1.4	
Maternal education	n	1.6		n	n	n		n					
Maternal age						n							
Maternal reproductive history							n						
Knowledge of trachoma										n			
Father's occupation	n	1.3		n	n	n							
Animals owned	n		n	n		n	2.3				n		
Cows/kept by house			1.4				1.5	n	1.2	1.8	3.1	n	n
Farm ownership/size				n		n							
Individual													
Frequency bathing	n						n	1.1	1.7 / 1.8	2.4			
Frequency clothes washing					n								
Frequency face washing	3.7	n	n		n		n	1.25	n		2.5	1.4	
Clean face			1.3 / 1.7					3.8 / 3.3	15.1 / 15.6	3.0#	4.1		3.1
Clean hair										1.7			
Use of soap	n							1.1 / 1.4			1.9	1.5	
Use of towel/drying	n		1.3		n					n			
Use of used water	n												
Nose cleaning method	n	1.6	1.6 / 2.3										
Clothes washed frequently	n												
Clothes washing site	n												
Washing bed linen	n												
Facial flies		n						1.9/1.5		3.4#	1.9		2.4
Sleeping with cooking fire			1.2										
Number in bedroom		n			3.9¶			n		n			
Siblings with trachoma		4.2			4.4								
Preschool siblings			n	n									

* examined but no significant association found

‡ urban/rural, size, presence of store, market, mill, health centre/pharmacy, church/mosque, school, bus route

† family ownership of bicycle, car, watch, radio, television, iron, refrigerator, farm equipment

¶ sleeping with other children

ocular discharge plus flies Odds ratio = **8.3**

and various Pacific Islands (90,350). Others had drawn specific attention to the use of mothers' clothes, a saree, dohti or shawl, to blow children's noses and clean and dry their faces (289,302). This was potentially a potent way of spreading chlamydia, as chlamydia had been shown to withstand drying on cloth for several hours from the earliest studies (143,351,352). And, of course, face washing with clean running water and not sharing towels was enshrined in military practice since the Egyptian campaign (15,16).

Others produced encyclopaedic lists of problems such as poverty-stricken homes, lack of water for washing, cultural and religious traditions, education, dust and flies (69), or smoke, dust, UV, sand grains, lack of water, poverty, overcrowding and heat (332), or lack of water, humidity, mechanical trauma from sandstorms, dust, frequent hand shaking, flies and poor hygiene (308), direct or indirect contact with infected material (hands, clothing, towels, etc.) and environmental and behavioural features including the presence of young children, crowding and lack of safe water, inadequate disposal of human and animal waste and increased flies (353). To advance, specific epidemiologic studies of risk factors were required. The list of potential factors that have been examined in rigorous studies is enormous and included community, family and individual factors (see Table 6.2).

In examining these studies and the data they generated, it is just as important to look at those factors that were not included in particular surveys, for example, the work in Nepal did not collect individual data other than the presence or absence of trachoma in the child (123). This study could therefore not assess facial hygiene, although other factors that were indirectly linked (proxies) might appear to be linked to trachoma. If the more proximate factor—a clean face—had been included, the proxy probably would no longer appear to be important. In the final analysis, it is the individual's status and behaviour that is most important. Without individual information, the family and community level data can only provide proxies or indicators of individual behaviour. Although these broad studies can give leads, without the ultimate or most proximate factor(s) they can only be indicative.

The more consistent risk factors identified by these studies will be discussed in more detail in the following sections. Many other studies have looked at one or two risk factors, but have not had a broad enough scope to assess the impact of potentially confounding factors. They have also been limited by their small sample size. A few have examined the link between nutrition and trachoma but consistent associations have not been demonstrated (300,354,355,354). At the Dana Center, we examined in detail a potential link between xerophthalmia and trachoma in multiple studies in Malawi, Zambia, Tanzania and Nepal but failed to find an association, and these negative findings were not published in detail. Before moving on to studies of specific risk factors, I want to review the work undertaken by the National Trachoma and Eye Health Program (NTEHP) in Australia.

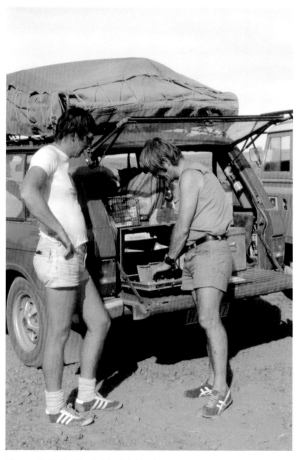

Figure 6.18 In the field with Fred Hollows during the NTEHP (1977).

The National Trachoma and Eye Health Program

My first experience of working with trachoma was in the NTEHP, directed by Fred Hollows, funded by the Australian Government and run by the Royal Australian College of Ophthalmologists. The College conducted fieldwork across Australia from 1976 to 1978. In total, 62,116 Aboriginal people and 38,616 non-Aboriginal people were examined in 426 communities and towns (103). I spent a year or so in the field as Assistant Director and learnt a tremendous amount from Fred Hollows and experience in the field (see Figure 6.18). As previously mentioned, an overwhelming impression was the difference in hygiene in those individuals or communities with trachoma compared to those without.

The NTEHP examined Aboriginal people living over the entire continent with the exception of major cities. Because of the broad geographic area covered, the program was able to look at environmental factors such as latitude, daily hours of sunshine, evaporation, rainfall, humidity and UV radiation. These analyses confirmed that trachoma was more common in the hot, dry desert areas of Australia than along the more humid or temperate coastal regions (103) (see Figure 6.19).

A high level assessment was made of six hygiene parameters: water access, nutritional status, food storage facilities, waste disposal systems, sewerage systems and housing (103,357). These were collected at the community level, with a grading of "worse half" and "better half" of the community (see Figure 6.20). An aggregate index was constructed known as the Waterford Index. Each parameter had four grades (except food storage and waste disposal, which were only given three grades). An extensive analysis was undertaken, but it was limited to the presentation of stratified univariant analyses as multivariant analysis was not generally in use at that time. As these factors are inevitably linked in various ways it would have been interesting to see the results of a more sophisticated analysis. Follicular trachoma, cicatricial trachoma and blindness were each strongly and significantly related to poor rankings in each of the above hygiene parameters (see Figure 6.21).

In reviewing these findings, Hollows stressed that good home hygiene required the use of certain "health hardware" and pointed out that:

> During the last 35 years, home hygiene for white persons in Australia has undergone significant but unsung improvement. For white Australians, reticulated and heated washing-water, showers, clothes-washing facilities, the single occupancy of beds and no overcrowding in rooms have become universal; not so for most inland Aboriginal Australians.

Hollows set out some basic housing requirements he considered everyone should have:

> All houses should have reticulated water supplied to them at a rate of 100 litres per person per day; one shower for every 10 persons; a means of heating water; a means of washing clothes and bed linen (this almost always requires electricity in Central Australia); elevated, separated and ventilated beds; no more than two persons per three metre square bedroom; all exterior openings with fly screens; washable floor surfaces; all inside areas free of animals; and one toilet per 10 occupants.

Having worked with Fred in the field as a mentor, and having developed a strong personal friendship taught me that if one disagreed with Fred, one was usually wrong. Although I agree with his broad range of requirements for healthy living, I hope these subsequent sections dealing with some specific epidemiologic studies of trachoma will show why I believe a much more focused approach to facial cleanliness is the key to understanding trachoma epidemiology and hence its control. Facial cleanliness seems to be the final common pathway through which all the other health and environmental parameters impact on the one hand; and on the other, it is the pathway by which infection is spread from one eye to another.

Crowding

Many have suggested that crowding is an important risk factor for trachoma and as an infectious disease, this would not necessarily be surprising. Although attention to crowds was drawn by earlier observers, it was not until the

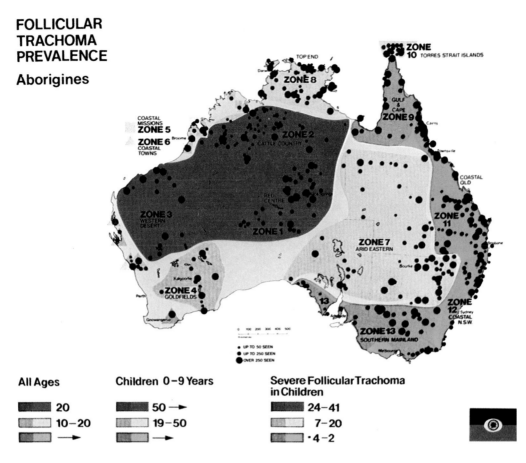

FOLLICULAR TRACHOMA PREVALENCE

Aborigines

All Ages	Children 0–9 Years	Severe Follicular Trachoma in Children
20	50 →	24–41
10–20	19–50	7–20
→	→	·4–2

Figure 6.19 Prevalence of follicular trachoma in Australian Aborigines (NTEHP, 1980 (103); courtesy, Royal Australian and New Zealand College of Ophthalmologists).

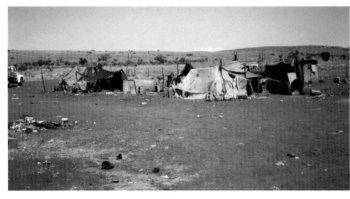

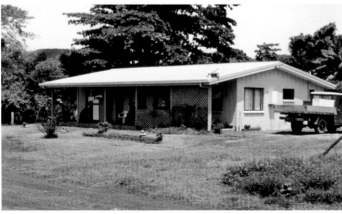

Figure 6.20 Aboriginal housing in the 1970s
TOP some of the worst BOTTOM among the best.

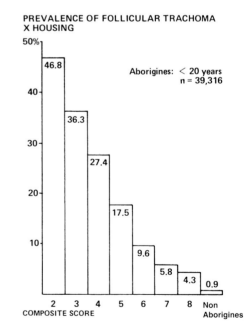

PREVALENCE OF FOLLICULAR TRACHOMA X HOUSING

Aborigines: < 20 years
n = 39,316

Figure 6.21 Prevalence of follicular trachoma by housing quality in Aboriginal communities (NTEHP, 1980 (103); courtesy, Royal Australian and New Zealand College of Ophthalmologists).

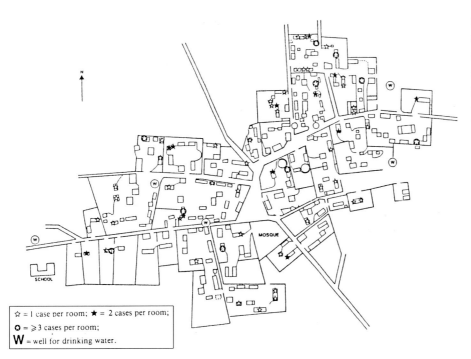

Figure 6.22 Map showing the distribution of cases of active trachoma by room and compound in Jali (Bailey et al 1989 (284) with permission of Oxford University Press).

1960s that its impact was quantified.

Detailed studies in Taiwan showed that the number of people per ping (the Taiwanese unit of area approximately 3.3 metres square) was a significant risk factor for trachoma after stratifying for water supply, parental occupation and socioeconomic status (349,358). In areas of low endemicity people with a lower socioeconomic status had increased risk of trachoma, but in areas with a higher level of endemicity, even those with a high socioeconomic status were at risk. The increased rate of trachoma amongst the war-time cohort of infants and children was attributed to increased crowding during the war.

Other indicators and proxies have been used to assess the effect of crowding, such as family size or the number of children in the family (282). More refined measures have ascertained the number of people sleeping together in one bedroom (123,280, 283,285,359,360,361).

An even better indicator of the risk of acquiring trachoma attributable to "crowding" or sleeping close together is the presence of another child with trachoma who shares the same bedroom (see Figure 6.22). This has been found to be a significant risk factor in multiple studies in The Gambia (284), Malawi (361), Egypt (280) and Tanzania (283),

although it was not significant in Mali (242) or Senegal (253).

These studies have shown that by increasing precision in the measurement of "crowding", the key effect turns out to be the close proximity of children with other children with active disease, especially if this occurs during prolonged contact through the night when children sleep together, usually on the same cot or mattress or under the same blanket or animal skin.

Water

It can be difficult to measure the availability of water. Should access to the water source be measured in time or distance, is an estimate acceptable or does access change with the season? Can other surrogates be used? These issues plague the assessment of water supply, let alone the actual utilisation of household water. Punjab villages with hand pumps or a well had less evidence of trachoma than villages without (289). However, the real difference was attributed to the quality rather than quantity of water.

No link between active trachoma and distance to the water source was found in a study in Morocco that examined distances from less than 50 metres to those over 2.5 kilometres (331). Nor was a link

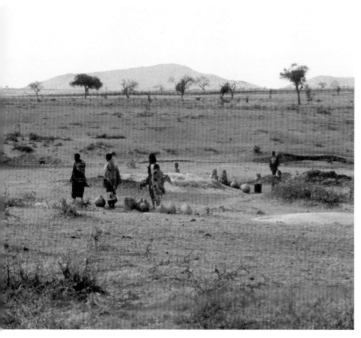
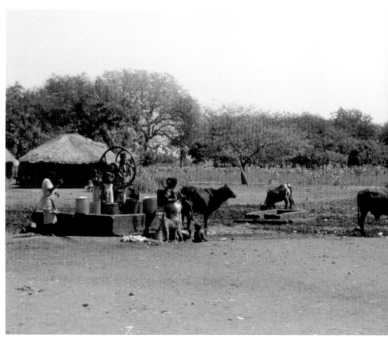

Figure 6.23 Water sources

ABOVE LEFT Tanzanian women collecting water from a well (1986)

ABOVE RIGHT a bore hole in a Malawian village—this water source is shared by cows, goats, pigs and dogs (1983).

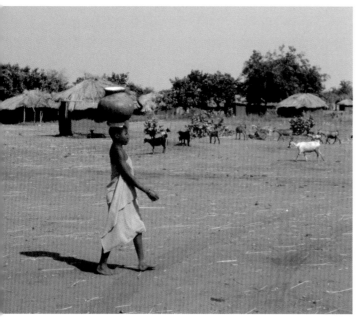
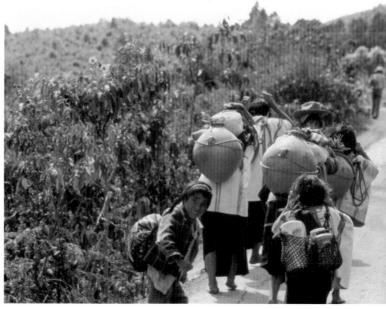

Figure 6.24 Almost invariably it is the women who carry the water

ABOVE Malawi

ABOVE RIGHT Mexico

RIGHT Tanzania (courtesy, Sheila West).

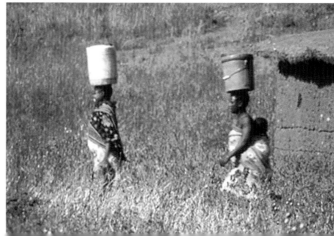

found between the quantity of water used and the distance to the water source. However, families that used more water used the extra water for hygiene purposes, particularly for washing their children, and there were lower rates of active trachoma. Thus the quantity of water used was important. These findings have been repeated in a recent study in Tanzania (362).

In Okinawa and the Ryukuyu Islands, the provision of piped water changed patterns of water use from "water scarce" to "water rich", and this was associated with a decrease in trachoma prevalence (342). As water became more readily available more was used for personal hygiene. The volume of water was considered more important than its purity, the opposite conclusion to the Punjab study (289). A rather perverse occurrence was noted in a school that had had piped water installed. A long trough with multiple washing taps had been installed. Each child was required to wash their face and hands before eating and each was expected to bring their own clean towel. Many children forgot their towels and Marshall comments: "I observed the same towel used to dry the hands and faces of more than a dozen children". He was concerned that this would lead to an increase in trachoma.

Others have widely reported a variable association between water availability and trachoma (110,120,284,332,358,361,363,364, 365). Prost and Negrel undertook a thorough review of available studies of water and trachoma in 1989 and concluded there was a general reduction in trachoma rates as water access improved (366).

Our population-based study in Tanzania looked at water availability in some detail (241,367). There was a significant linkage, for example, between water distance and the risk of trachoma (see Figure 6.23). Although definable, the increased risk was quite small; for those whose water sources were more than 30 minutes distance, the risk increased by about 40% (odds ratio 1.45 for 0.5 to two hours to the water source; 1.37 for greater than two hours). The total volume of household water was also assessed, although not adjusted for family size. Household quantities were grouped as using less than 15 litres per household per day, between 15 and 45 litres or greater. Household

water quantity was not linked to the risk of trachoma.

We also examined the relationship between clean faces and both the distance to water (time) and quantity of water used (367). Again, time was an important factor with approximately 40% increase in trachoma risk with an unclean face in children whose family lived more than 30 minutes from their water source (0.5 to two hours, odds ratio 1.14; greater than two hours, odds ratio 1.55) (see Figure 6.24). We concluded that distance to the water source was not the prime determinant for the presence of trachoma, but rather distance influenced the value placed on water, and therefore its priority. When water was seen as a scarce resource, it was not used for personal hygiene and the children's faces were not clean. This would point to the importance of facial cleanliness. However, this not only showed the need to improve access to water but also the need to address utilisation behaviour. Further work would show the complexity of this behaviour (368). Along with the notion of health hardware learnt from Fred Hollows came the additional component of "health software" to make the hardware effective (2).

Evidence to support this notion was also seen in studies in Brazil, where those with either an isolated tap outside the house or no piped water had lower monthly water consumption than those with piped water inside the house and the latter population had higher rates of trachoma (285) (see Table 6.3). Frequency of face washing could not be analysed because almost every mother said their children's faces were washed every day. An analysis of water use in The Gambia showed on average that children without trachoma used more water (6.4 litres/child/day) than children with trachoma (4.2 litres/child/day) (364). In northern Tanzania, only a weak association was found between GPS-determined distance to the water source and trachoma after adjustments were made for the family clustering of trachoma (62). Other studies have shown that household consumption of water does not vary much when water is obtained from sources between five and 30 minutes away (369). In general, water use increases when the source is closer and decreases with distance, although extreme (greater than five hours) water use is much more restricted (370).

TABLE 6.3: Significant risk factors for trachoma (TF/TI) in Bebedouro, Brazil (logistic regression) (290)

Variable	Odds ratio
Water source (inside pipe versus other)	3.69
Water consumption per person (<5000L/month versus ≥5000L/month)	2.77
Frequency of garbage collection (daily versus other)	2.27
School level of head of household (some versus none)	2.86
Number of children (1–2 versus ≥3)	1.50
Number of children sharing beds	
0	1.00
1	2.33
≥2	3.88
Socioeconomic stratum	2.03

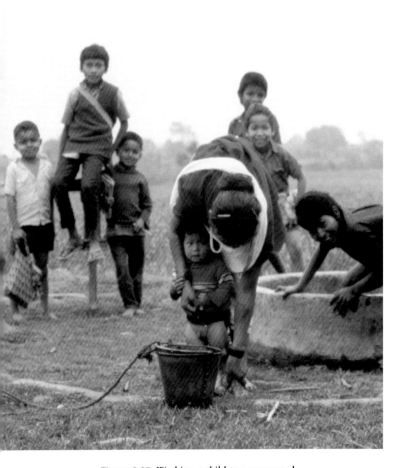

Figure 6.25 Washing a child at a communal well in Nepal (1990).

As we have seen, the actual utilisation of water and priority given to washing children varies from family to family, and water availability seems to be linked to trachoma indirectly through facial cleanliness (see Figure 6.25). The family needs enough water to keep a child's face clean and also needs to prioritise water use for this purpose. In Tanzania, we found as little as 30mls of water was sufficient to wash one face.

Faye in Senegal found the risk of trachoma doubled if less than 10 litres of water were used to bathe a child (253). Trachoma was not related to the distance to water. In Mali, Schemann found that the presence of a well inside the compound reduced the risk of active trachoma (TF/I) and also TI, but the volume of water used for washing was not significant in a multivariate analysis (242). One wonders what the outcome may have been if the volume of water used was substituted for distance in his final analysis. Possibly the presence of a well in the compound is a better surrogate for the actual use of water than the self-reported estimate of volume. Mesfin found an association between water source or distance in Ethiopia (243).

The use of water was studied in more detail in Northern Tanzania (362). Although those who lived closer to water (less than 85 minutes) had less trachoma and used more water, there was not a significant correlation between quantity of

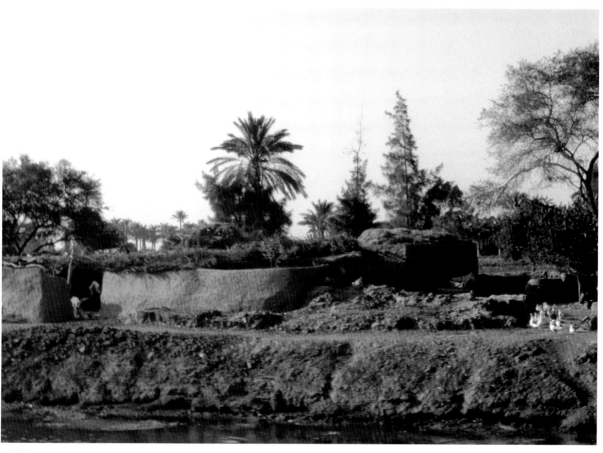

ABOVE **Figure 6.26** A village in the Nile Delta where there is often a mixture of animal and human faeces that accumulate in large piles (1981).

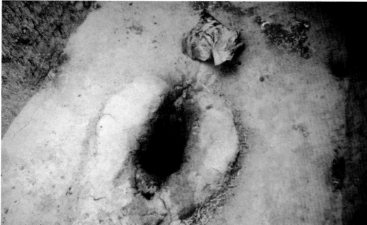

LEFT **Figure 6.27** Tanzanian latrine (1986).

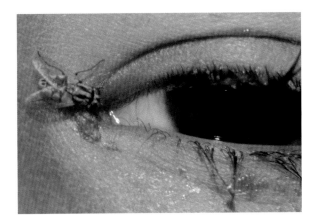

Figure 6.28 Flies drink from the tear film.

household water used and active trachoma in children. Further analysis showed the important factor was the proportion of water prioritised for personal hygiene. Households closer to their water source used more water for bathing and face washing. The mean daily volume used for personal hygiene was 4.25 litres per person or 24% of household water. This study emphasises the importance of behaviour and attitudes around water use over the absolute availability of water.

The role of latrines

Some have seen the presence of a nice clean, but used latrine as the answer to trachoma, even a ventilated improved pit (VIP) latrine. Certainly many have observed that the absence of latrines, or other more advanced methods of human faeces disposal, is an important indicator of inadequate family hygiene.

In Egypt, the absence of a latrine increased the risks of trachoma about threefold (odds ratio 3.3) (280). For comparison, the odds ratio associated with trachoma in a school-age sibling was 4.4, and for other preschool siblings 1.3. However, a more recent study in Egypt found the association with latrines to be inconsistent (371). Attention was drawn to the linkage between human and animal faecal matter around the house and increased fly density (see Figure 6.26). This issue was also examined in some detail in central Tanzania (241). We found no significant association with the presence of active trachoma (TF) and the method of household faecal disposal, although the

likelihood of severe inflammation (TI) was reduced with a latrine. Studies in Malawi (242), Mali (361) and Ethiopia (306) also found less trachoma in houses with a latrine, whereas other studies in Mexico (110), Brazil (285), Burkina Faso (372), Ethiopia (243) and Senegal (253) did not. GPS mapping in a mesoendemic area in northern Tanzania also found no association between trachoma and the presence of a latrine or its distance from the house (62) (see Figure 6.27).

The installation of improved household pit latrines in Gambian villages significantly decreased the numbers of eye-seeking fly *Musca sorbens*, although the domestic fly (*M. domestica*) and a large green fly (*Chrysomya albiceps*) were still present in unabated numbers (373). As discussed below, eye-seeking *M. sorbens* has been implicated in transferring trachoma infection from one child to another or from one eye to another. This study showed *M. sorbens* can be controlled, at least in part, by improved human faecal disposal, although this intervention did not significantly reduce the prevalence of trachoma (374).

It is hard to determine a direct link between pit latrines and trachoma, although a reduction in eye-seeking flies could provide an indirect linkage in some areas. The presence of a nice new latrine, of course, can be a proxy indicator of general family hygiene. It is linked to the readiness to adopt new ways and behaviours and also is an indicator of socioeconomic development and family attitudes to personal hygiene. To my mind, as we will see, the key is faces, not faeces.

Flies

References to flies around children's faces and trachoma in Egypt date to the late 1500s and Baron Harant of Poljitz (4) (see Figure 6.28). Equally there are claims and examples that flies were not important that date back almost a century. Stucky commented that there were not many flies in the mountains in Kentucky. Trachoma persisted in these small communities not because of flies, but because everybody used one towel: "It is a filth disease. They are ignorant; they are unlettered. They know nothing of hygiene, nothing of sanitation" (77)—strong words.

MacCallan also quotes many other commentators on the importance of flies (4).

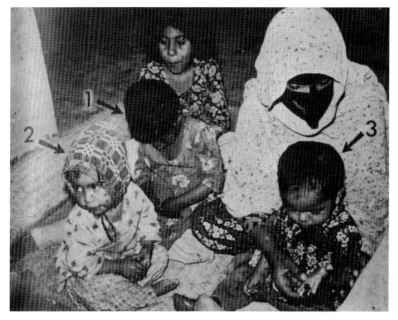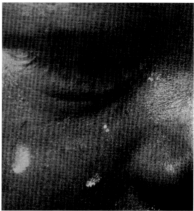

Figure 6.29 Fly-borne transmission of ocular discharges within a pool of ocular promiscuity (Jones 1975 (91) © 1975 Eye, reproduced with permission).
LEFT fluorescein placed in the eye of child 1 transmitted by fly vomits to the eyes of child 2 and child 3 within 20 and 40 minutes
RIGHT child 2 – fluorescing spots of fly vomit photographed in blue light through a yellow filter, indicating fly-borne transmission of conjunctival discharge from child 1 within a period of 20 minutes.

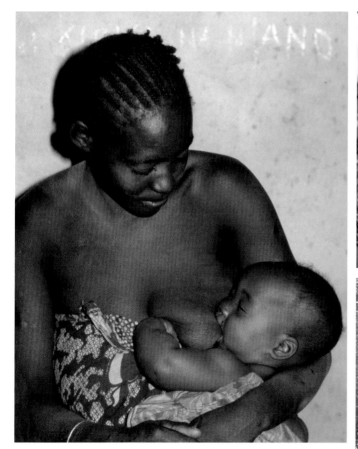

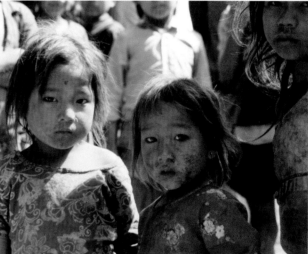

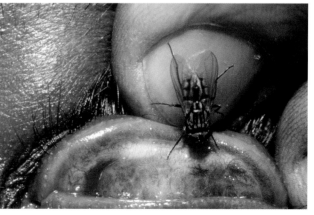

Figure 6.30 Flies may aid the spread of trachoma
ABOVE a Tanzanian mother and her breast feeding baby share flies around their eyes
ABOVE RIGHT Nepalese girls with *M. sorbens* on their face
BELOW RIGHT an inquisitive *M. sorbens* in Tanzania.

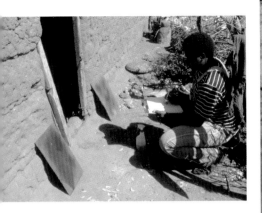

Figure 6.31 "Mirinda" boards used to quantify household flies in Tanzania (1986).

RIGHT Figure 6.32 An aerial view of a Tanzanian village showing the circular cattle briars partially enclosed by the flat-roofed rectangular houses (1986).

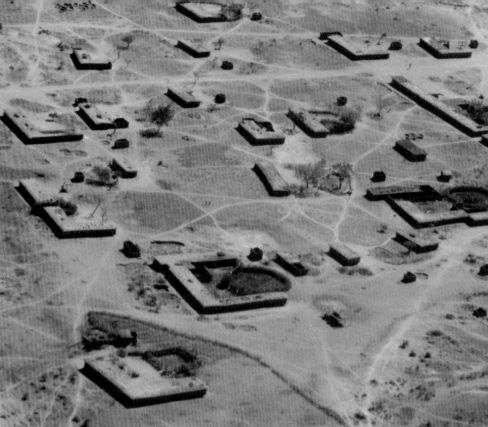

Wilson and Meyerhof drew attention to seasonal epidemics of flies in Egypt and associated epidemics of bacterial conjunctivitis that in turn were also linked to the transmission of trachoma (26,32).

In 1911 Nataf showed that flies could transmit experimental trachoma infection from an infected human to a monkey and from the eyes of one monkey to another (4). Darougar showed flies could transmit viable and infectious chlamydia (*C. caevi*) from one guinea pig to another (375). Emerson found chlamydia DNA by PCR in 0.5% of flies caught on children's faces and documented frequent fly-eye contact (376). In Ethiopia Lietman's group identified chlamydia by PCR in between 15% and 23% of *M. sorbens* caught on the faces of children (377,378).

Barrie Jones performed some beautiful experiments in southern Iran with a group of women and children sitting together on a blanket (91) (see Figure 6.29). He placed a drop of fluorescein into the eye of a child and examined them with a blue light 20 and 40 minutes later. He was able to demonstrate the transfer of fluorescein from the child's eye to the eyes of the others in the group and also found "fly spots" around their faces and on their clothes. This elegant study indicated the ability of flies to easily transfer ocular secretions from one human eye to another.

The first WHO Expert Committee on Trachoma came out very strongly on the importance of flies and the control of vectors (20) stating "The Committee considers that fly control is really efficacious, at least in the prophylaxis of acute conjunctivitis". This was in the era when DDT was first widely used to control many vector-borne diseases and its long lasting environmental effects had not yet been appreciated. In the same year, a massive hygiene improving intervention in Egyptian delta villages was underway that included the control of flies with DDT (379). The impact that fly control had had on trachoma was unclear, although there was a marked reduction in gonococcal conjunctivitis and some reduction in conjunctivitis associated with Koch-Weeks bacillus (379,380).

Studies in India showed a marked seasonal variation in Koch-Weeks conjunctivitis with peaks in April and May and August and September attributed to increased numbers of *M. sorbens* (302). These were similar to those trends seen in Egypt (32). However, in India there was no seasonal change in active trachoma in children. Female *M. sorbens* were particularly attracted to the faces of children with trachoma and they were more likely to suffer from episodes of acute bacterial conjunctivitis (see Figure 6.30). This observation is both consistent with flies being attracted to ocular discharge and conveying bacterial secondary infection.

Reinhards considered flies to be the main vector

Table 6.4: Association between active trachoma (TF/I) and observed characteristics of children studied in Ethiopia, 2005 (n = 1960) (306)

Factor	Number and percentage	Multivariate odds ratio (95 per cent CI)*
Discharge from eyes and flies in eyes		
No discharge or flies	627 (47)	1
Discharge but no flies	103 (75)	3.0 (1.94–4.55)
Flies but no discharge	682 (79)	3.40 (2.37–4.88)
Discharge and flies	539 (92)	8.30 (4.94–13.90)
Clean hair		
Yes	1090 (64)	1
No	867 (82)	2.50 (1.66–3.76)

*Adjusted for *kebele*, age, clean hair, discharge from eye and flies in eyes

of trachoma in Morocco. He also stated that large numbers of flies were able to breed "because of complete lack of sanitary measures to dispose of human and animal excretia" (324). Flies contributed to the spread of bacterial conjunctivitis (381) that in turn facilitated the transmission of trachoma. However, although fly control with chlordane residual insecticides gave a temporary reduction in bacterial conjunctivitis, it had no effect on trachoma prevalence or trachoma resolution (139).

Flies were implicated in the transmission of trachoma in Malta (343) but not in Saudi Arabia (290) or in the Punjab studies (289). Sowa in The Gambia remarked "flies are often blamed as vectors, but trachoma is known to flourish in areas that are comparatively free of these insects" (301). Mann also pointed out there are no flies in many parts of the highlands of Papua New Guinea and various Pacific Islands, despite much evidence of trachoma (382). However, in the Australian outback Flynn commented on the incessant presence of the eye-seeking Australian bush fly, *M. vetustissima* (383). It occupies the ecologic niche occupied by *M. sorbens* elsewhere (384) and is ubiquitous in the Australian bush (385).

When preparing for our studies in the mountains of Chiapas, Mexico, my colleague Milan Trpis, Professor of Medical Entomology at Johns Hopkins, accompanied me to work out how we

could quantify flies in this area. It was too easy for him, for there were none. This was yet another area where trachoma occurred in the absence of flies and Milan spent the week collecting butterflies.

For our studies in Tanzania, we developed a simple method of assessing household fly densities (386). A wooden board was moistened with sugar water and set on either side of the door to the house (see Figure 6.31). These boards attracted *M. sorbens* and the number of flies that alighted on the board were counted. This method gave a reproducible household count. Fly densities were highest around the doorway to the house. Counts were fairly constant throughout the day and did not vary markedly with sun or shade. Higher counts were associated with the presence of food scraps and rubbish that attracted flies with their moisture, although this rubbish did not provide a breeding ground because *M. sorbens* breeds in human faeces (387). We found a significant correlation between household fly density and the presence of active and severe trachoma in children (241).

Our study in Malawi found a weak association between the presence of flies on the face and trachoma (388). This work was extended by Brechner and colleagues who found that the measure of the presence of flies on the face had a more consistent and stronger association with the

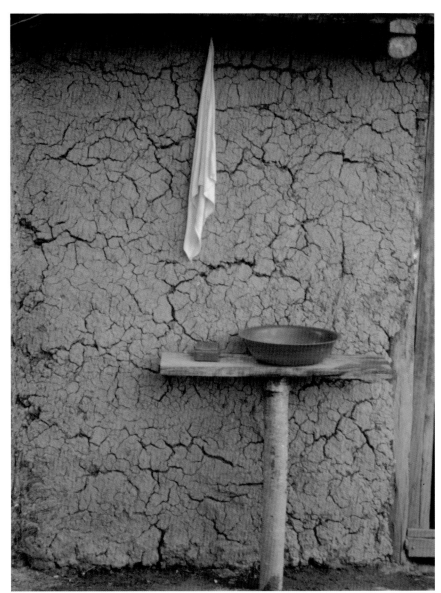

RIGHT **Figure 6.33** A towel, wash basin and soap outside a school in Mexico. It is unclear how often it was used (1982).

BELOW **Figure 6.34** Trachoma fieldwork in Chiapas, Mexico (1985).

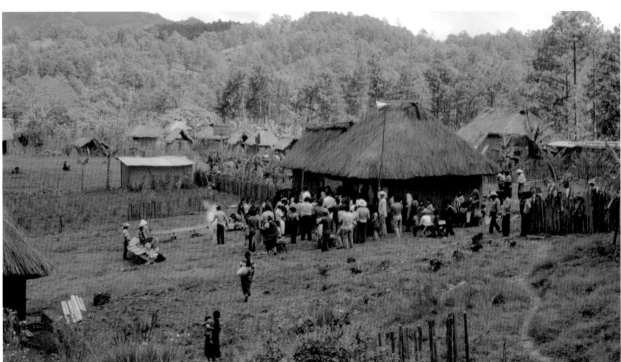

presence of active trachoma than the household fly score and was less susceptible to seasonal variation (389). A similar significant association between flies on the face and trachoma has been confirmed in a number of other studies in Mali (242), Ethiopia (306) (see Table 6.4) and Senegal (253). Flies are preferentially attracted to the faces of children with trachoma, especially those with dirty faces (376). In Burkina Faso, the presence of flies on the face increased the risk of active trachoma nearly 5.8 fold, a dirty face increased the risk of trachoma 15 fold, but a dirty face increased the risk of flies on the face 334 times (372). An earlier study in Ethiopia also found an association between trachoma and both the presence of flies on the face and cattle ownership (390). This study focused on the association with cows rather than flies and recommended the construction of corrals to reduce trachoma.

In a large and labour-intensive study Paul Emerson and colleagues used insecticide fogging to control *M. sorbens* in Gambian villages (374). They found they could reduce the number of flies for as long as they continued their fogging activities and subsequently trachoma rates were also reduced. Interestingly, a recent study from Tanzania has shown no added benefit to fly reduction in addition to the community-based treatment with azithromycin in a hyperendemic area (391). This large, thorough prospective clinical trial objectively graded clinical disease with photographs and assessed infection by PCR. It used the same fogging methods to control flies as the Gambian study, but complemented these with azithromycin distribution. However, a facial hygiene component was not included. In this context, fly control gave no benefit in addition to antibiotic treatment.

A number of studies have looked at the association between animal ownership and trachoma. In some studies, animal ownership is regarded as a measure of economic wealth and has a protective effect against trachoma (123,360). In Tanzania and some areas in Ethiopia animals, especially cattle, are kept close to the house (see Figure 6.32). This is usually associated with increased numbers of flies and an increased risk of trachoma (241,306,390) but not always (243,372).

The cows themselves will not directly influence the presence or severity of trachoma. As mentioned, *M. sorbens* breed almost exclusively in human faeces and so the presence of animal faeces will not contribute to breeding, although *M. domestica* and other flies will breed in animal faeces. However, animal faeces provide moisture and sheltered resting spots for flies. In this way, the housing of cows close to the household may increase the overall fly density including *M. sorbens*, and thus increase the likelihood of flies on the face.

As Miller points out, flies can be convincingly implicated as vectors of trachoma and they fulfil Barnett's criteria of (1) effective contact under natural conditions, (2) convincing temporal and geographic association of the presence of vector and infection, (3) the vector harbours the pathogen, and (4) experimental transmission can be demonstrated (377). However, although flies may play a contributory role as vectors, they are clearly not essential as blinding endemic trachoma can still occur in areas without flies.

Facial hygiene

In the Napoleonic Wars and in 19th century European barracks, there was an inverted U-shaped association between face washing and military ophthalmia or trachoma (16). Officers who washed their face in the privacy of their tents with their own water were protected from trachoma as were those soldiers who were dirty but never washed their face. The big risk factor for trachoma was the sharing of common washing water and common towels amongst ordinary soldiers who washed from time to time. This led to fastidious recommendations about face washing practices for soldiers and also laid the foundation for hygiene practices in trachoma schools that were established for children in England and North America.

New cases of trachoma amongst Indian children in the American south-west were attributed to the sharing of washing water and towels (76,359). The use of the mother's clothes or a common towel to wipe children's faces clean was noted in Kentucky (75) and India (289). In Morocco, children under the age of four had the highest frequency of trachoma and bacterial conjunctivitis (324). They also had the most severe ocular discharge and attracted the most flies because their faces were dirty, and "they are touched by their mothers or their sisters in a most unhygienic way" (324). As previously mentioned, Marshall was concerned about the sharing of towels when water was introduced to schools in Okinawa (342). However, when children in an Aboriginal community in Western Australia were showered and provided with clean clothes each day at school, trachoma decreased (365).

My opportunity to examine the role of facial hygiene and trachoma first came about unexpectedly. I was working in a lovely little town in the highlands of southern Mexico called San Christobal de las Casas. We were conducting drug studies on onchocerciasis and I was examining patients in a dark room. A young Mexican public health doctor, Francisco Millan-Velasco, came in looking for the ophthalmologist who was in town who knew something about trachoma. We subsequently did a quick survey and confirmed the presence of trachoma in the small Mayan Indian villages clustered along the mountain ridges of central Chiapas (109) (see Figures 6.33 and 6.34).

We then undertook a more formal study specifically looking at potential risk factors for trachoma, especially those that would favour frequent episodes of transmission and the possibility of reinfection (110). As shown, we selected a large range of possible indicators, one of which was the frequency with which children had their faces washed (Table 6.2). This study found a strong, consistent association between trachoma and children whose faces were washed less than seven times a week and those children whose faces were washed more often (see Table 6.5) (110). This association was independent of the use of soap or towels, although the use of a handkerchief to clean the child's nose was also protective (odds ratio 1.5; for face washing, odds ratio 3.5). The population attributable to risk of face washing was 57%.

We were fortunate in this study as we seemed to get reasonably reliable answers to our questions about face washing. In a follow-up study in the same area, we failed to demonstrate a statistically significant association as two-thirds of the children were reported to have their faces washed every day. In a separate study in Malawi, almost two-thirds of the children were reported as having their face washed twice a day! (361). A clean face reduced the risk of trachoma by 40% but this finding was not statistically significant. Similar reporting problems were encountered in Brazil (285) and Ethiopia (360).

Then the penny dropped and we recognised that it was not the process, or the frequency with which the face was washed, although this was important. It was the outcome. Did the child have a clean face? If the child's face was already clean it would not matter if it were washed or not. If the child's face was dirty and had been washed, but was still dirty or had become dirty again, it required further washing until it was clean. Another confounding factor may be the ascertainment bias related to the difference between an observed clean face and the report by the mother or child of the frequency of face washing.

In our next study in Tanzania, we documented both the frequency with which faces were washed (process) and whether faces were clean (outcome) (see Figure 6.35). Facial cleanliness was found to be strikingly important to protect against both active trachoma (TF/TI, odds ratio 1.30) and severe inflammatory trachoma (TI, odds ratio 1.72) (241). The frequency of washing was less strongly associated. A case control study in The Gambia supported the importance of outcome; an unclean face increased the risk of trachoma 2.96 times, but the association with washing a child's face less than twice a day was much less strong (odds ratio 1.14) (364).

Other recent studies have also looked at the question of face washing and facial cleanliness. Jean-Francoise Schemann and his team from IOTA in Mali undertook a major study of 15,187 children under the age of 10 (242). They found a high risk of active trachoma as their measure of personal hygiene became more specific; for those who bathed less than once a day, the odds ratio was 1.12, for those who usually used soap 1.14, washed their face less than once a day 1.32 and for those with a dirty face 3.80 (see Table 6.6) (242). A further large study in Burkina Faso reinforced the importance of facial cleanliness and found an odds ratio of 15.1 for active trachoma and 15.6 for TI (372). Similar data comes from Senegal where those whose faces were not washed daily incurred a 2.50 risk of active trachoma and those with a dirty face, 4.07 (253). In Ethiopia a correlation was found between the number of days since the child's face had been washed and the risk of trachoma; odds ratio 1.35 per day (243) and the study in Mali found a linear reduction with the number of times the face was washed in a day (242). Although these are interesting findings, these analyses address the process of washing and not the outcome of a clean face (see Figure 6.36).

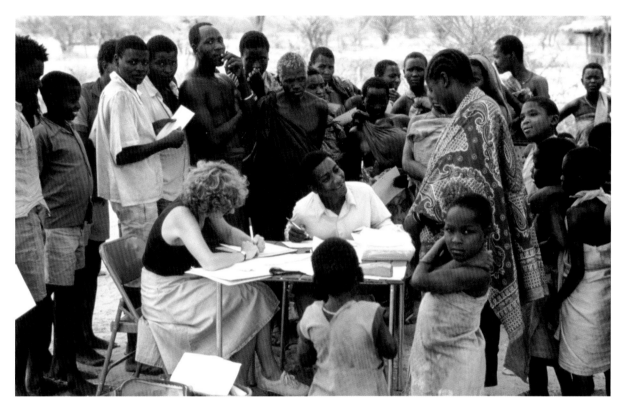

Figure 6.35 The Tanzanian trachoma risk factor study
ABOVE Sheila West co-ordinating fieldwork
BELOW a household interview (1986).

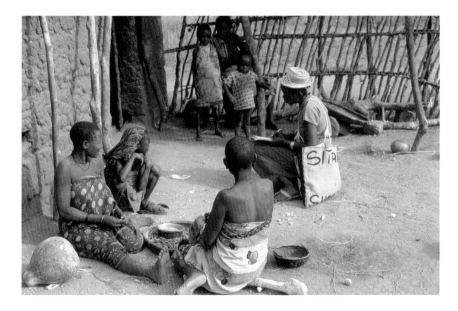

Table 6.5: Occurrence of trachoma in children aged 10 or less by the frequency with which their faces are washed in Mexico, 1985 (110)

Frequency of face washing (times per week)	Number of children			Percentage with trachoma
	Severity of trachoma			
Both communities*	None	Moderate	Severe	
0	11	8	2	48
1–2	77	36	7	36
3–6	207	35	5	27
≥7	154	17	1	10

*Comparison of the severity of trachoma between face washing 0–6 times per week and ≥7 times per week. Both communities $\chi^2_{2df} = 28.7$, $p < 0.001$; χ^2 trend = 27.8, $p < 0.001$

Table 6.6: Multivariate analysis of risk factors for active trachoma (TF/TI) in Mali, 2002 (242)

Explanatory factor for active trachoma	Odds ratio	95 per cent CI
≤ 500 inhabitants	1.14	1.02–1.28
Medical centre		
5–15km	1.19	1.08–1.38
>15km	1.37	1.30–1.63
Flies on the face	1.92	1.62–2.29
Dirty face	3.80	3.42–4.21
Well inside	0.76	0.68–0.86
Mother's education	0.85	0.72–1.00
≥1 bath a day	0.89	0.85–0.95
≥1 face washing a day	0.76	0.67–0.86
Use of soap	0.88	0.79–0.99
Latrine	1.20	1.09–1.32

The components of a dirty face were studied in more detail by Sheila West and her team in Tanzania (392). They demonstrated that the key component of a dirty face was the presence of nasal discharge (see Table 6.7) (392). Of even greater importance was the increase in risk associated with the combination of both flies and nasal discharge (odds ratio 1.74). In families with three or more pre-schoolchildren, the presence of flies and nasal

discharge increased the risk of trachoma 2.1 times, with a sibling with trachoma 4.3 times, and both having a sibling with trachoma and flies and nasal discharge increased the risk 6.8 times (see Figure 6.37). As mentioned earlier, chlamydia can be identified in nasal secretions (328).

To my mind, these studies in Tanzania really provide the key to unlock the critical components of the "trachoma friendly" environment characterised

Table 6.7: Facial cleanliness and risk of trachoma in children aged one to seven years in Tanzania (n=472) (392)

Facial sign	Percentage with facial sign	Age-adjusted odds ratio (95 per cent CI)
Food	40	0.91 (0.63–1.34)
"Sleep" in eyes	60	1.13 (0.77–1.64)
Nasal discharge	70	1.31 (0.87–1.97)
Dust	70	1.18 (0.79–1.76)
Flies on face		1.37 (0.93–2.00) [sic]
1–2	49	
>2	14	
Nasal discharge and flies	54	1.74 (1.19–2.55)

by Thygeson as "poverty-stricken homes, want of water for washing, culture and religious traditions, education, dust and flies" (69). The final common pathway for all these environmental factors is through ocular and nasal discharge that produces a dirty face in young children (see Figure 6.38). Adequate water is required to keep children's faces clean and in areas where water is in short supply, personal hygiene is given a low priority within the family. This is particularly true in hot, dry, dusty and dirty areas. In areas where water is not readily available, the provision of adequate water often comes at a relatively late stage in socioeconomic development. Families that are better off will be more likely to have better water supplies sooner. Thus trachoma can appear to be a disease of poverty. However, the volume of water itself is not critical; even in those families who used less than 15 litres of water per day, some children have clean faces and do not have trachoma.

A dirty face and ocular discharge increases the possibility of the direct spread of trachoma by direct face to face contact as children sleep together, or by indirect means through fingers with one child rubbing their face or eye and then playing with other children. Dirty fingers will contaminate clothes and other items. Mothers' fingers are also used at times to remove ocular nasal discharge. A dirty face is also more likely to attract the shawl or saree of the mother who will clean or wipe one of her children's faces and then the next. A dirty face is an attractant to flies which can pick up chlamydia with or without other bacterial

pathogens, fly to the next child's face, and regurgitate the previous meal with its bacterial load and ingest fresh ocular secretions. In this way, flies could convey both trachoma and bacterial pathogens.

Of course, the proof of the pudding is in the eating. In this day and age, one needs a prospective randomised clinical trial. With Sheila West and a large team we undertook specific intervention promoting facial cleanliness in central Tanzania (393). We were very careful to emphasise the outcome—clean faces, not the process—face washing. We studied 1417 children aged one to seven in six villages. At one year, children in intervention villages were 60% more likely to have consistently clean faces. As found in the observational studies of hygiene improvement, severe trachoma (TI) was the first sign to reduce, and odds in intervention villages were 0.62. Of equal importance was that a consistently clean face reduced the odds of active trachoma (TF/TI) to 0.58 and TI to 0.35, over and above the impact of community-wide antibiotic treatment (topical tetracycline).

In 1989, I wrote:

It seems likely that these two key factors, facial cleanliness and fly density, would both directly influence transmission. An unclean face would increase the likelihood of that child transmitting trachoma to others either by direct contact or by contact with fingers, flies, or with clothes or other fomites. Similarly, a child with an unclean face is more

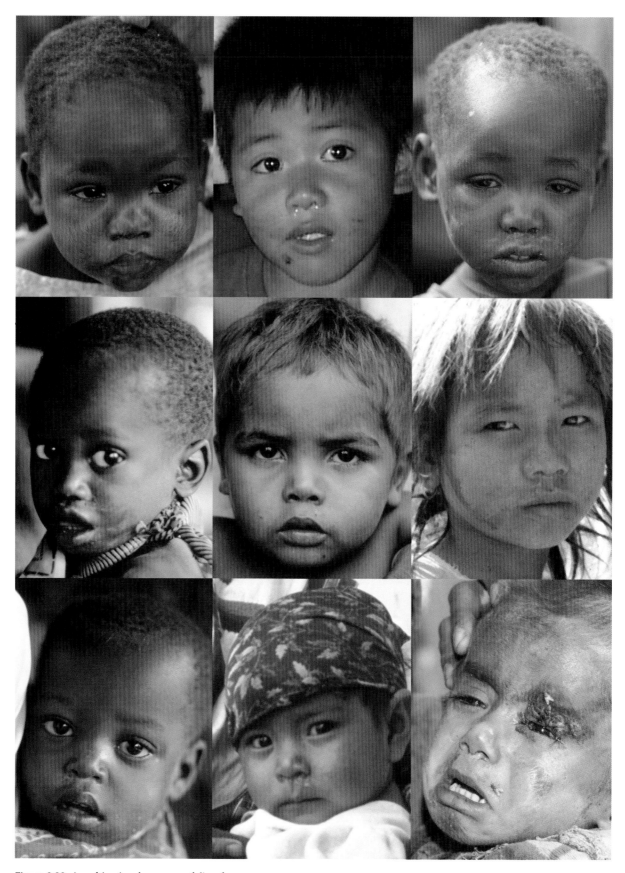

Figure 6.36 A multinational montage of dirty faces.

Figure 6.37 Estimated probability of active trachoma in 224 children in families with three or more preschool-aged children (West et al, 1991 (392), reproduced with permission © 1991, American Medical Association. All rights reserved).

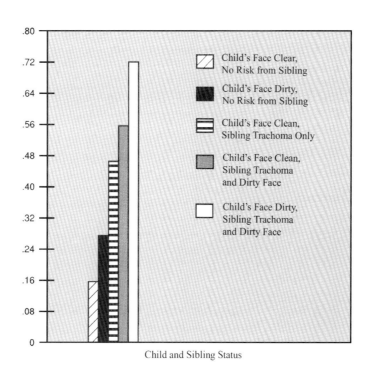

Child and Sibling Status

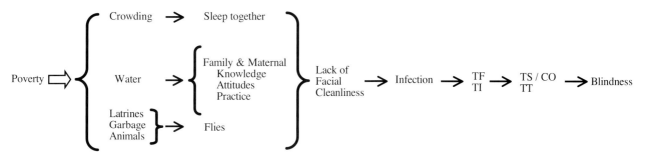

Note: Bacterial infection can hasten the progression of TF/TI to TS and TT to CO.
Genetic factors may influence the progression of TF/TI to TS

Figure 6.38 The interaction of trachoma risk factors.

likely to become infected, as it is more attractive to the mucus-seeking flies that can transfer chlamydia. Within a family, an increase in transmission by children being either "transmitters" or "receivers", together with facilitated transfer due to increased fly numbers, would lead to more frequent episodes of reinfection within that family. This would lead to a higher prevalence and severity of disease and an increased risk of eventual blindness (241).

Today, I would give much more weight to the dirty face.

As we will see, the recognition of facial cleanliness gives a clear focus and target for intervention strategies and means that we—those who are interested in eliminating blinding trachoma—do not need to wait for the broad improvement in personal and community hygiene that comes with socioeconomic development. We can hone in on facial cleanliness and immediate environmental barriers to achieve this in any given community.

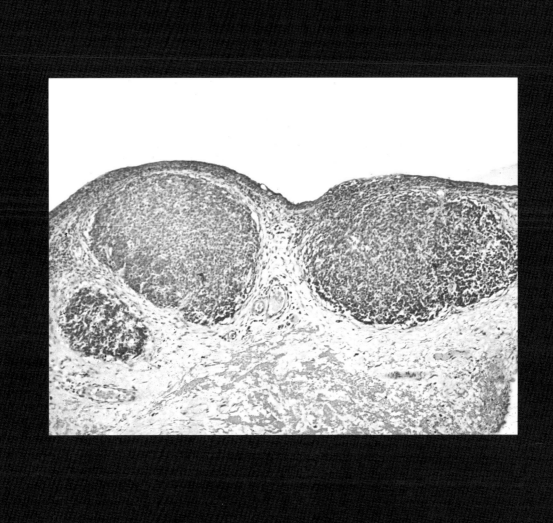

CHAPTER SEVEN

Pathogenesis

Trachoma is not a disease of poverty,
it is an immune disease—it is like chronic poison ivy
Hugh Taylor, 2005

ONE NEEDS TO explain why chlamydia persists in some people and not others. In part, this variation seems to be ecological as blinding trachoma occurs in certain environments, but disappears with improved living standards. Variation may be due to genetic factors in the host (or in the organism). What is the evidence for host genetic factors to play a major role in determining the severity of trachoma? Trachoma is not really a "disease of poverty" but a disease of immunopathology, characterised by a delayed-type hypersensitivity reaction maintained by the continuing presence of infection. Trachoma can thus be likened to "chronic poison ivy".

Most studies suggest the overwhelming importance of repeated episodes of reinfection in maintaining the presence of chlamydial antigens. However, the notion of persistent infection can be dismissed as merely unrecognised reinfection. There may be a few individuals in whom chlamydia truly persists for prolonged periods, but the interpretation of these findings is difficult and one needs to balance the general and the particular.

A tobacco industry analogy is instructive. If everyone smoked, lung cancer would be considered a genetic disease. In this scenario, even though everybody was exposed to cigarette smoke, only a proportion of people would develop lung cancer. Therefore one would falsely conclude that genetics played the major role, overlooking the overriding importance of exposure to cigarette smoke. In areas with hyperendemic trachoma, not everyone becomes blind; usually "only" 10% to 20% will end up with trichiasis and may become blind without further intervention, even though "everyone" will have been exposed or infected as children. Is this genetic or environmental? If environmental, is this due to a persistent single infection or repeated reinfection? In developed countries, blindness from chlamydial conjunctivitis (trachoma) is no longer seen, even though trachoma may have been a major problem in that population as recently as half a century or so earlier. Chlamydia infections are still prevalent and 15% or 20% of young adults may have chlamydial genital tract infection and therefore episodes of inclusion conjunctivitis are not uncommon (see Figure 7.1). Why do people become blind from trachoma in areas where reinfection can occur often, but do not become blind from chlamydial infection in areas where ocular reinfection is rare? The genetics of the population have not changed. Persistent infection could occur in either setting but the occurrence of reinfection seems to be the key (see also chapter six).

Clinically we have seen how trachoma can be characterised initially as a conjunctivitis (active or acute inflammatory trachoma) with follicles and papillae associated with inflammatory thickening. This is followed by the development of cicatricial changes with conjunctival scarring and distortion of the lid (cicatricial trachoma).

The pathologic changes in trachoma reflect the clinical picture. In active trachoma inflammation occurs in all layers of the conjunctiva with striking lymphoid infiltration, the development of characteristic germinal centres or follicles and associated papillary hyperplasia. Subsequently, in cicatricial trachoma there is the proliferation of subepithelial connective tissue resulting in scarring and distortion of the eyelid.

This chapter will first review the histopathologic changes and then explore the information that has come from animal and human studies on the disease mechanisms and processes involved. In some ways the studies on whole animals, whether human or experimental, look "outside the black box", studies of cellular and molecular events look "inside the black box".

Histopathology

The infection in trachoma occurs in the conjunctival epithelium; the disease in trachoma occurs in the subepithelial tissues. Chlamydia can be easily demonstrated growing in the epithelium in cytologic smears. However, intraepithelial inclusions can be surprisingly difficult to find in vertical histologic sections through the epithelium, although they exist (395,396) (see Figure 7.2). This difficulty is due in part to the multiplicity of sectioned nuclei and the difficulty in differentiating these from sectioned inclusions. Rarely has chlamydia been reported in the subepithelial tissue; probably they were ingested in macrophages that

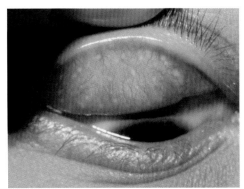

ABOVE **Figure 7.1** The lid changes in acute inclusion conjunctivitis in a young adult in Melbourne.

RIGHT **Figure 7.2** Intraepithelial infection with chlamydia in the monkey model shown by DNA probe.

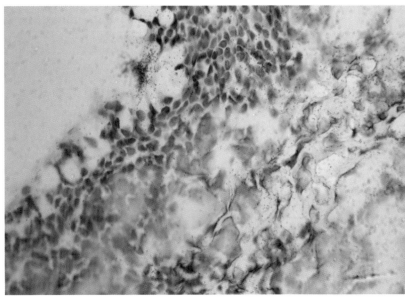

have travelled to deeper tissues (397). Alternatively they may represent an artefact with tissue distortion from scarring with epithelium seen in deeper sections. However, it seems to be universally accepted that chlamydial infection in trachoma is confined to the epithelium.

Universally serovars A, B, Ba and C of *C. trachomatis* are associated with trachoma, although usually one or two serovars will predominate in a given endemic region (5,296) and in fact, in a given family (274,275). Only occasionally are other serovars isolated and their significance is unclear (330,398) (see Table 7.1) (296).

Immediately following infection with chlamydia, a mild acute inflammatory response starts that is initially indistinguishable from that seen with other infectious causes of conjunctivitis. However, within days there is the increased accumulation of lymphocytes (32) which will go on to form the characteristic lymphoid follicles fully described first by Raehlmann (86). Between the follicles is a dense mantle of lymphocytes and an intense inflammatory infiltrate (see Figure 7.3). With time, this infiltrate is replaced with fibrous tissue and scarring.

The epithelium

The epithelium over the follicles is thinned and heavily infiltrated with polymorphs and mononuclear cells (395). The epithelial cells are activated to express both Class I major histocompatibility complex (MHC) antigens and Class II HLA-DR antigens on their surface (395,399). This activation can be induced by interferon-γ and allows the epithelial cells to present chlamydia surface antigens and react with Th-1 T-cells. In active trachoma, epithelial cells also express vascular endothelial growth factor (VEGF) (400). IL-1, a pro-inflammatory cytokine, can be found in the epithelium (401). In addition, the epithelium is infiltrated with macrophages in the superficial layers and dendritic cells in deeper layers. Many lymphocytes are present in the epithelium (mainly T-cells), with more CD8+ T-cells than CD4+ T helper cells, and a few B cells (395).

Studies of infected epithelial cells in culture show that when infected cells lyse and release the inclusion with new EB they also release IL-1α (402). IL-1α then stimulates other epithelial cells to release the pro-inflammatory chemokines and cytokines

Table 7.1: Distribution of *C. trachomatis* serovars found in hyperendemic trachoma (296)

Area	Serovars
Gambia	A, B [D]
Tunisia	A, B [C]
Egypt	A
Ethiopia	A, Ba
South Africa	A, B, [D, E]
Saudi Arabia	A, B, C
Iran	A, B, C, [D]
Afghanistan	B, C
India	B, C
Taiwan	B, C [D]
Australia	B, C
Guatemala	C
USA	Ba, C

[ ] less frequently found

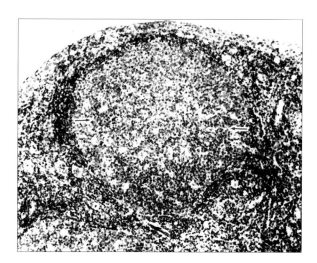

Figure 7.3 Conjunctiva obtained from a patient with trachoma stage 2a showing secondary lymphoid follicle containing a large pale follicular centre (arrows) surrounded by a thin lymphocytic mantle (arrowheads) (Abu El-Asrar 1989 (395) © (1989) BMJ Publishing Group Ltd, reproduced with permission).

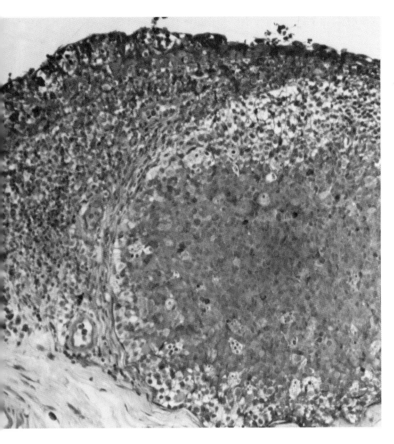

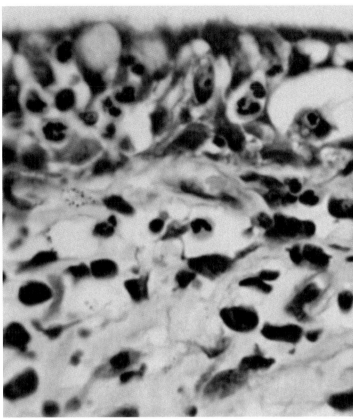

Figure 7.4 Conjunctival changes in the monkey model of trachoma
ABOVE LEFT a typical follicle with an intense surrounding inflammatory infiltrate and marked inflammatory infiltration in the abnormal and thinned overlying epithelium
ABOVE RIGHT intense intraepithelial infiltrate.

RIGHT **Figure 7.5** Scanning electron micrograph of surface topography of conjunctiva five weeks after inoculation in the monkey model. Note the typical rugae-like folds of the conjunctiva. Goblet cells (GC) are interspersed between the absorptive secretory cells (SC). Small lesions (arrows) are also apparent (x520).
(a) shows both the polygon shape of the secretory cells and the normal microvilli on the surface of the secretory cells
(b) shows the normal topography of a goblet cell. Note that the microvilli are larger and fewer in number (Patton & Taylor 1986 (396), reproduced with permission from the University of Chicago Press).

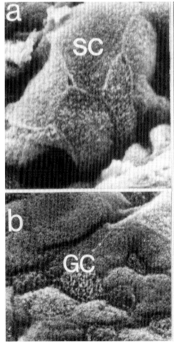

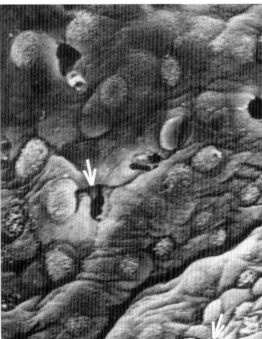

IL-8, GROα, GMCSF and IL-6, but not TGFβ1 or β-actin. These molecules attract inflammatory cells, especially macrophages, and initiate inflammatory cascade.

Findings in monkeys are strikingly similar to those in humans (396) (see Figure 7.4). Transmission electron microscopy (TEM) shows marked intercellular oedema and intracellular degeneration of the epithelium with decreased microvilli, vacuolation and fragmentation of the endoplasmic reticulum. Scanning electron microscopy (SEM) shows many patchy lesions with decreased microvilli and extruded lymphocytes can be seen on the surface (see Figure 7.5). These areas lay over follicles where the epithelium is thinned and infiltrated by plasma cells, eosinophiles and degranulating mast cells. Away from the follicles, the epithelium becomes hypertrophic beneath which large numbers of subepithelial plasma cells, T-cells and a few macrophages exist. Similar changes are seen in experimental animals and further studies confirmed the presence of anti-chlamydia specific IgM, IgG and IgA-producing B cells in and around the follicles (403). The plasma cells are prominent subepithelially and mainly IgA producing, with lower numbers of IgG and much fewer IgM or IgE expressing cells (395). In human tissue T-cells are mainly CD4+, although CD8+ cells predominate in "quieter" eyes (404). Interestingly, decreased bulbar conjunctival goblet cells were seen in children with PCR positive infection, but this did not correlate with clinical disease (355).

Trachoma follicles

Numerous well-formed follicles or germinal centres are the hallmark of trachoma. In humans these follicles have a pale centre containing lymphocytes, plasma cells and macrophages in the centre as a classical lymphoid germinal centre. Occasional giant cells may also be seen in the centre (395). These germinal centres are uncapsulated and are similar to Peyer's Patches in the intestine. They are surrounded by a mantle of small lymphocytes that are predominantly T-cells, but also include some plasma cells, macrophages and polymorphonuclear leukocytes. Some scattered mast cells and eosinophiles will also be seen (395). Again, the changes in monkeys are strikingly similar and show the majority of T-cells are T suppressor-cytotoxic

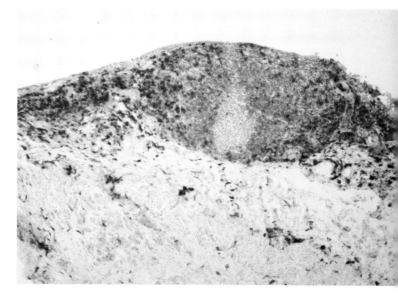

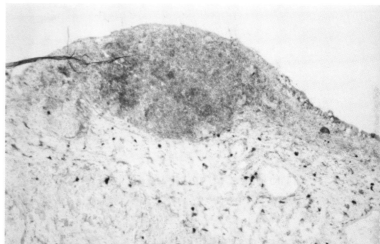

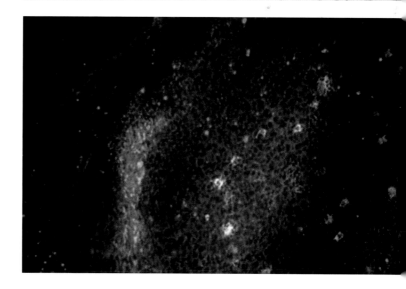

Figure 7.6 Immunohistochemical staining for lymphocytes in the monkey model
TOP CD8+ T cells predominate in monkey conjunctiva compared to
CENTRE CD4+ T cells
BOTTOM antigen specific IgA cells can be seen in follicles.

cells (CD8+) rather than T helper (CD4+) cells (396,405) (see Figure 7.6).

As the subepithelial tissues become more heavily infiltrated, the thickened conjunctiva shows an increasing papillary appearance that includes both the projection of papillae above the surface and the presence of downward projecting epithelial crypts (32). The papillae contain numerous dilated blood vessels with prominent vascular endothelium and surrounding inflammatory cells. There is a marked increase in the number of goblet cells and dense infiltration of plasma cells around the accessory lacrimal glands (395). At times, the crypts between the papillae become blocked with debris and form pseudo-cysts (32). Ultimately these may form calcareous deposits seen as small concretions.

Scarring

Although fibroblastic changes may be seen in the early stages of trachoma, these changes are much easier to see as intense inflammation decreases. This inflammatory process overlies a dense proliferation of connective tissue that eventually forms compact scar tissue covered by a thin flattened layer of epithelium (see Figure 7.7). The thickened, compact subepithelial fibrous membrane becomes adherent to the tarsal plate (406). The tarsus thickens and develops retention cysts, hyaline degeneration and focal replacement by adipose tissue (406,407). The deformed meibomium glands atrophy and show thickening of the acinar basement membrane with a loss of goblet cells (408). Similar cicatricial changes have been seen in the monkey model (108). Marked inflammation persists in some people with a large number of CD4+ T helper cells (404,407). In uninflamed biopsies CD8+ cells predominated. Although B cells are still present, germinal centres are not found and polymorphonuclear leukocytes are rare.

In the normal conjunctiva, Types I and III collagen are found in the substantium propria and Type IV collagen forms the basement membranes of the epithelium, endothelium and the lacrimal gland (409). Type V collagen is not normally seen. In active trachoma, an increased deposit of Types I, III and IV collagen is found (409,410). The increased deposition of Type IV collagen and the new

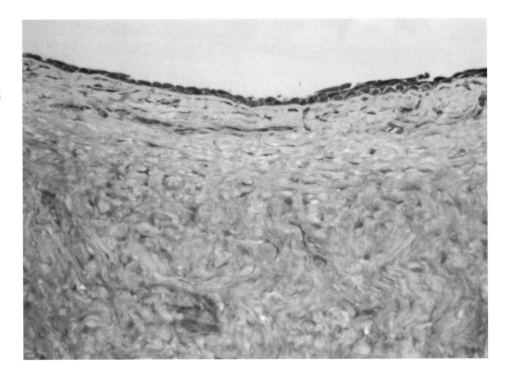

Figure 7.7 Tarsal conjunctival scarring with thinned epithelium over dense subconjunctival scarring that extends into the anterior tarsus (hematoxylin-eosin).

Table 7.2: Summary of collagen staining (410)

Collagen	Controls (n=9)				VKC (n=6)				Active trachoma (n= 9)				Scarred trachoma (n=9)			
	US	SV	SLG	BM	US	SV	SLG	BM	US	SV	SLG	BM	US	SV	SLG	BM
I	+	+	+		+++	+++	+		+++	+	+		+	+	+	
III	+	+	+		+++	+++	+		+++	+	+		+	+		
IV																
E				+				++				++				+++
VE				+				+++				++				++
LG				+				+				+				+++
V	-	-	-		+++	+++	++		+	+	+		+++	++	+++	

VKC	vernal keratoconjunctivitis
US	upper stroma
SV	around stromal vessels
SLG	stroma around accessory lacrimal gland
BM	basement membrane
E	epithelium
VE	vascular endothelium
LG	accessory lacrimal glands
-	no staining
+	thin and/or patchy discontinuous staining
++	thicker homogenous continuous staining
+++	very dense staining

formation of Type V collagen leads to conjunctival scarring. Type V collagen appears in patches in the upper substantia propria and around blood vessels and accessory lacrimal glands. It can also be seen in the cytoplasm of fibroblasts. Type V collagen is even more predominant in those with marked tarsal scarring (see Table 7.2).

Macrophages seem to play a central role in the pathology of inflammation and scarring. In active trachoma, various inflammatory cytokines released by macrophages IL-1, TNF-α and Platelet Derived Growth Factor (PDGF) are found in the substantia propria (401). Gelatinase B or matrix metaloproteinase 9 (MMP-9) is also released by macrophages and thus digests Types IV and V collagen, elastin and fibronectin (411). In addition, connective tissue growth factor (CTGF) and basic Fibroblast Growth Factor (bFGF) are released by macrophages and can be found in high levels in subepithelial tissues in active trachoma (400). CTGF is profibrotic and stimulates fibroblasts, collagen and extracellular matrix production and the growth of new vessels. Also bFGF stimulates fibroblasts and endothelial cells. Endothelial cells express VEGF and CD105 (endoglin), a marker of proliferation of vascular endothelium. Finally,

tenascin is increased under the epithelium and around blood vessels. It controls cell migration and adhesion during embryogenesis and wound healing (see Table 7.3).

Together these studies show trachoma is associated with intense inflammation and the recruitment and activation of many macrophages. These macrophages release a number of cytokines that have now been identified and can lead to formation of new collagen (especially Type V) leading to scarring and new blood vessel growth. The latter may help explain papillae formation on the one hand and corneal pannus formation on the other (400).

Changes in the cornea include oedema of the epithelium and underlying tissues, infiltration by polymorphonuclear leukocytes and subsequent vascularisation and pannus formation (412). Limbal follicles also form. Later, of course, corneal opacification and scarring can occur as a result of trichiasis or as a consequence of microbial keratitis.

It is important to remember the changes that can occur in the nasolacrimal duct with cicatrization and dacrocystitis (413,414). Inclusions have been found in surgical specimens of the lacrimal sac (415). Punctal occlusion has also been described in

Table 7.3: Summary of staining results (400)

| | Trachoma specimens (n=6) | | | |
	Epithelium	Vascular endothelium	Macrophages	Stroma
CTGF	-	-	+ +	-
bFGF	-	-	+ +	-
VEGF	+ + +	+ +	-	-
CD105	-	+ +	-	-
Tenascin	-	-	-	+ +

CTGF, connective tissue growth factor; bFGF, basic fibroblast growth factor; VEGF, vascular endothelial growth factor.

-, No staining; +, weak staining; + +, intense staining; + + +, very intense staining.

association with trichiasis. Involvement of the lacrimal gland, dacryoadenitis, is also reported from time to time (4,15).

The histopathology of trachoma has been well described over the last 120 years (see summary by Duke-Elder, 1965) (412). The early writers were convinced of the occurrence and importance of central necrosis of the follicles (4,32). "Necrotic" material could be expressed from inflamed lids, and the expression of this was part of basic trachoma treatment dating back to ancient Greece. This central necrosis was not seen histopathologically. It was thought that "The follicles either ruptured spontaneously ... or else gradually absorbed with or without the formation of scar tissue. Usually the necrotic tissue is replaced by scar tissue which invades the follicles from without" (32). This concept underlies the notion of the beneficial induction of scarring as a way of reducing or eliminating harmful inflammation. This interesting thinking is the reverse of our current understanding whereby development of scar tissue is a conse-quence of the ongoing presence (and severity) of inflammation. The modern aim is to minimise (or avoid) inflammation and so reduce the likelihood of scarring and its severity.

The progression of disease

The implicit understanding in all the early descriptions is that trachoma was a chronic disease and once acquired would proceed relentlessly through four stages (25) (see Figure 7.8). In fact, MacCallan postulated three outcomes of a follicle:

"a gradual change into tough connective tissue with absorption of the contents", "rupture of the follicle on its epithelial surface, evacuation of its contents and cicatrization" or "further development of capsule, common cutting off of blood supply and resulting necrosis of the contents of the follicle" (25). The last process led to post trachomatous degeneration. However, some noted the periodic nature of infection and the propensity for relapse and occurrence of reinfection (91,315,316,416). The epidemiologic observations that indicate the importance of reinfection were addressed in some detail in the previous chapter.

The concept of reinfection leads to significant changes in pathogenetic pathways that are likely to be involved. Implicit in the deterministic or persistent infection approach is the inevitable

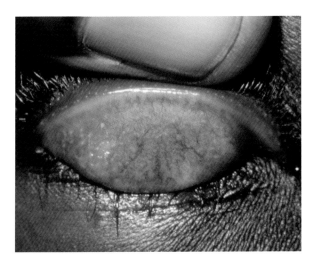

Figure 7.8 The evolution of trachoma follicles to scars. In this child, both follicles and early scarring can be seen.

progression from follicular trachoma to severe scarring and trichiasis. The concept of repeated episodes of reinfection predicts the cumulative development of increasingly severe cicatricial changes that are dependent on the intensity and duration of exposure to infection and induced inflammation. In either case, the response could also be tempered by genetic variation.

The deterministic approach to progression still surfaces periodically and will be discussed in more detail. This arises in discussions of the interaction between the presence of infection (NAAT test +) and clinical disease (233). The model put forward is "latent" trachoma (infection +, clinical disease -), active trachoma or "patent" trachoma (infection + and disease +), and a recovery phase (infection - but disease +). This simplified linear model not only overlooks the occurrence of episodes of reinfection and the periodic presence of infection, but overlooks the possibility of the ongoing presence of a chronic, delayed-type hypersensitivity reaction to occasional exposure to chlamydial antigens. It is well recognised that clinical signs of active trachoma, particularly follicles, may persist for months, even years after "infection" has been eliminated (196,221,227,233,235,236).

Immunopathogenesis

Much of our understanding of the pathogenesis of trachoma has developed from the notion that disease processes in trachoma result from the immune response to chlamydial infection. Art Silverstein drew attention to the likelihood that a long-standing immunopathologic response gave a consistent explanation of the pathogenesis of trachoma: "The subepithelial immune response is unable to clear the organism, so that the disease continues for long periods of time in ever increasing severity" (417). We will come back to the question of what maintains the ongoing presence of the organism in the epithelium. Silverstein's five points support the notion of immunopathogenesis (417):

1 Chlamydia are found only in the conjunctival epithelium.

2 The infection appears to be chronic and chlamydia are present for a long period of time.

3 Chlamydia are not efficiently cleared by the host immune response.

4 The disease process is "not marked by overt signs of epithelial cytopathogenecity by the organism but rather by subepithelial conjunctival infiltrates of lymphocytes and plasma cells with the formation of extensive lymphoid germinal centres".

5 The disease progresses towards corneal and conjunctival scarring. "Given the chronic infection of conjunctival epithelium by an otherwise non-virulent trachoma organism, one can conceive of the persistent release of antigens from this organism into the subepithelial tissue, stimulating a long standing immunopathogenic response" (417).

Chan Dawson has also pondered over the problems of the pathogenesis of trachoma and asked two key questions, "How does the chlamydial agent persist for so long in the conjunctiva to cause prolonged and repeated bouts of inflammatory disease?" and "Why is the inflammation of the subconjunctival connective tissue, while in chlamydial infection, confined to the epithelium?" (121).

Most now accept the notion of immuno-pathogenicity: "Like other intracellular bacterial pathogens, chlamydiae possess little intrinsic toxicity and manifestations of disease appear to result from immune recognition of chlamydial antigens" (418). Even in the 1950s before chlamydia was isolated, the follicular reaction in the subepithelial tissue was seen as an indirect result of infection possibly induced by a toxin released by the "virus" (383).

To better understand how the extraordinarily successful intracellular parasite C. trachomatis causes disease, we will turn to experimental infections in animal models and humans.

Animal and human studies

Animal models

The earliest animal model of trachoma was recorded by Vetch in 1807 (16). He caught a dog after he collected discharge from the eye of a soldier with Egyptian ophthalmia. He then applied the discharge "to the eye of a dog, and so produced a considerable degree of irritation, which continued for some hours, when the loss of the dog prevented farther examination" (16). Chlamydia was first demonstrated during the experimental infection of orang utans (142). Early on Nicolle, Cuénod and others in Tunisia undertook an impressive range of studies in chimpanzees, barbary apes and a range of monkeys (143). Other animals seemed to resist infection, but monkeys became quite widely studied (155). MacCallan also describes some more unusual animal studies in which different authors implanted trachomatous material into the vitreous chamber of rabbits and chickens with mixed results (4).

Much valuable information has come from animal models. MacCallan considered "the experimental disease in monkeys is really trachoma" (4). However, with characteristic bluntness Thygeson stated "At the present time, conclusions based on monkey studies in trachoma must be confirmed by inoculation experiments in human volunteers" (419). Thygeson considered that a single inoculation of infectious material in monkeys "bore little or no resemblance to human trachoma" because the infection was mild, did not involve the tarsal plate or cornea, failed to cause scarring and invariably healed spontaneously. Thygeson conducted a number of human volunteer studies that reflected quite different ethics in research at the time. One study in 1935 involved a one-eyed 50-year-old man who was inoculated in his only seeing eye (150). The volunteer was identified in the acknowledgements and said to be in poor health.

Several reviews have been written on the types and role of more recent animal models used to study chlamydial infection that have included mice, cats, guinea pigs and monkeys (420,421,422, 423,424).

In selecting an animal model it is essential that the features or characteristics of both the animal and the infectious agent are relevant to the particular question being addressed. With each host and agent there will be some properties or characteristics that are similar to the human disease being studied, but other characteristics or responses may be quite different. Picking and interpreting which phenomenon is which is critical. This distinction becomes increasingly important as more is learnt about both the fine variation in the

immune response of different hosts, and subtle differences between species and strains of chlamydia. For example, studies of intravenous injections of chlamydia in mice will involve a range of systemic immune responses that may be very different from the mucosal immune responses invoked by infection confined to the ocular or genital mucosal surface. Studies using invasive lymphogranuloma venereum strains capable of growing in macrophages are likely to be very different from studies of other strains of C. trachomatis confined to epithelial cells. Recent studies have shown significant differences in susceptibility to interferon-γ between the C. trachomatis mouse pneumonitis agent (now classified C. muridarum) and human ocular and genetic strains of C. trachomatis (425). Further work has shown enzymatic differences in tryptophan metabolism between ocular and genital strains of C. trachomatis (426). Some host responses are quite different in different animals. Reflecting a certain degree of frustration, the cryptic comment has been made that "the immune response against C. trachomatis in humans is much more complex than in mice" (427). Given these great variations, one should be cautious when interpreting the results of various animal models and extrapolating for human trachoma. Ideally, studies should use an ocular strain of C. trachomatis, and the only successful ocular hosts for these strains are human and subhuman primates. Although not practical for all experimental work, ultimately key findings probably should be confirmed in a monkey model.

Monkey models of trachoma: single infections

The most consistent subhuman primate model seems to be the cynomolgus monkey (Macaca fasicularis) (see Figure 7.9). It is a better model than the rhesus monkey (M. mulatta) (424). Other species studied in depth include the Taiwan monkey (M. cyclopsis) (428) and the pig-tailed monkey (M. nemestrina) (429). In general, the inoculum used in monkey experiments is comparable to that used in human experiments and is of the order of a human infectious dose of 10^1 or 10^2 organisms (191,430, 431,432,433,434). This serves as a contrast to some other animal models where infectious doses of 10^6 organisms or greater are frequently required.

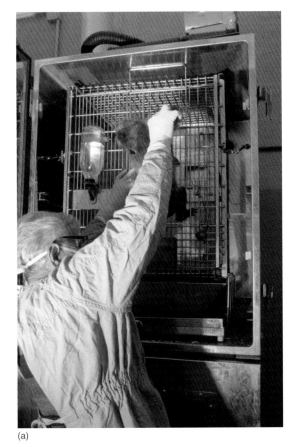

(a)

Figure 7.9 The monkey model of trachoma
(a) monkeys were housed in positive pressure isolation
cages and anaesthetised prior to handling
(b) an infectious inoculum of 20 microlitres was used.
Typically, it contained about 10^3 EB
(c) animals were examined with a handheld slit lamp.

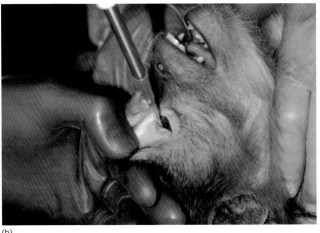

(b)

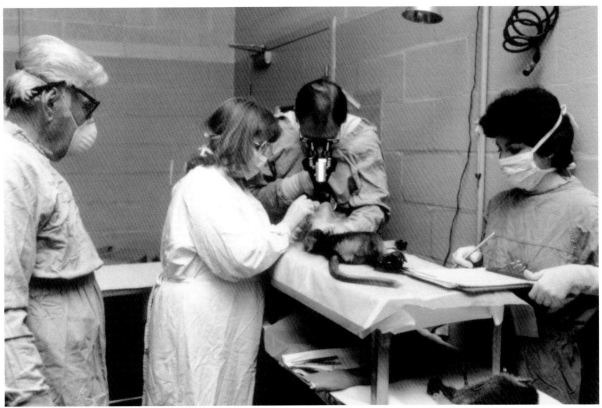

(c)

Response of monkeys to a single chlamydial infection

It is hard to estimate how many hours of argument, pages of journals, or numbers of monkeys were used from mid 1800 until the 1970s to resolve the difference between inclusion conjunctivitis and trachoma. A lot of this distinction became moot after chlamydia was cultured, and as thinking moved from the deterministic model for trachoma to a model driven by repeated reinfection.

Before chlamydia could be cultured, the results of experimental infection were quite variable and difficult to interpret. There were problems in determining the inoculating dose of chlamydia. The ability to track the infection was greatly handicapped, relying solely on Giemsa cytology and the clinical response. The *sine qua non* of clinical response was seen by some to be the development of cicatricial changes, especially corneal pannus. However, the ability to culture chlamydia revolutionised the scope for animal studies.

The response of naïve animals to a single inoculum with *C. trachomatis* is quite consistent and leads to an acute self-limited episode of "inclusion conjunctivitis" (143,315,435,436,437, 438,439,440,441,442). Chlamydia can be cultured within one week of inoculation, and acute follicular conjunctivitis develops rapidly and resolves over a three to four month period (see Figure 7.10). Cultures become negative after about one month.

If animals are rechallenged after recovery from primary infection they show some partial protection. After secondary challenge they have an abbreviated infection which is less productive and resolves more rapidly. This partial immunity gives some protection to higher inoculations (see Figure 7.11).

Ocular infection is accompanied by the development of serovar-specific IgM and IgG antibodies in serum and IgM, IgG and IgA in tears (442) (see Figure 7.12). Subsequent studies showed the tear antibodies to be specifically directed against the species-specific MOMP (443) and serovar-specific T and B cells were demonstrated in the conjunctiva (403,444).

The response was similar in monkeys given a single inoculation with the following ocular and genital serovars A (HA 13), B (TW3 and HA 36), C (TW3) and E (BOUR) (445). Partial protection was seen with rechallenge with the same serovar, but the response to heterologous challenge was similar to a primary infection (315,445).

The length of time after inoculation that chlamydia could be reisolated varied greatly with the sensitivity of the laboratory test (446). Giemsa cytology would be positive for three weeks, culture with iodine stain for four weeks, culture using monoclonal immunofluorescence for six weeks, and DFA cytology for 10 weeks (see Figure 7.13). Later studies showed DNA PCR was positive for 14 weeks while an RNA probe was still positive in several animals at 20 weeks (210).

Quantitative tissue culture and DFA cytology (210) showed a marked reduction in shedding of organism after secondary infection. Reisolation by tissue culture was delayed (first positive cultures at two to three weeks instead of one week after primary infection) and shortened (those animals that were positive by culture were only positive for one to three weeks). The number of inclusion-forming units was reduced by one to two log units. Similar changes were seen with DFA cytology, DNA PCR and RNA blot testing. This is the same phenomenon observed in the field when attributed to a change in immunity to chlamydia because of increasing age (126).

To explore the mechanisms involved in clearance of infection, a group of animals was given cyclosporin A to specifically block IL-2 function.

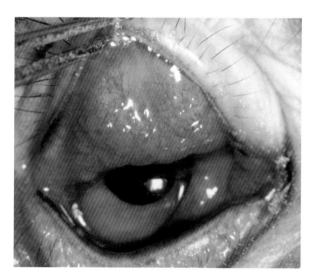

Figure 7.10 The eye of a cynomolgus monkey five weeks after being inoculated with *C. trachomatis* (BOUR strain) showing marked tarsal and follicular follicles.

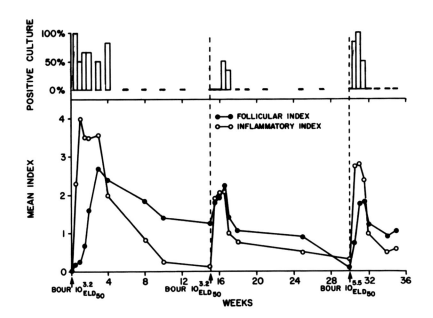

Figure 7.11 Clinical response of naïve cynomolgus monkeys to an initial inoculation of *C. trachomatis* and their mean response to rechallenge at 15 and 30 weeks (Taylor et al 1982 (442). Reprinted with permission from the Association for Research in Vision and Ophthalmology, © 1982).

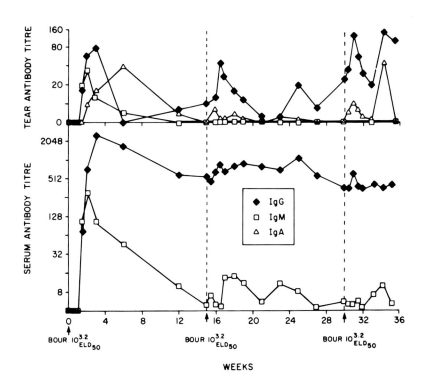

Figure 7.12 Mean serotype-specific antibody levels in tears and serum of six cynomolgus monkeys receiving three single inoculations of C. *trachomatis* BOUR strain 15 weeks apart (Taylor et al 1982 (442). Reprinted with permission from the Association for Research in Vision and Ophthalmology, © 1982).

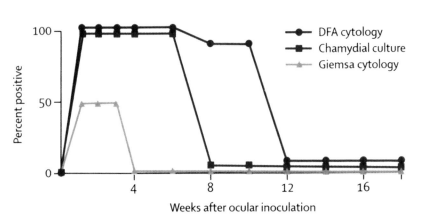

Figure 7.13 Frequency of positive identification of organism in experimentally infected cynomolgus monkeys using three different types of laboratory tests (Taylor et al 1988 (190). With kind permission of Springer Science and Business Media).

This inhibited T helper cells and the primary B cell response. Treated animals had a prolonged primary infection, although it eventually cleared (447). After recovery, they responded normally to a subsequent secondary challenge. Cyclosporin A did not alter the response to secondary challenge in ocular immune animals.

Infant pig-tailed monkeys developed acute self-limited inclusion conjunctivitis when infected with B or C serovars of *C. trachomatis* (448). When rechallenged three or four months later, they showed a more marked response with the development of follicles. It was unclear whether their increased responsiveness was related to further maturation of the animals or a heightened response to reinfection. In general, children are unable to develop follicles before the age of three or four months due to immaturity of their immune systems (449).

Dorothy Patton at the University of Washington in Seattle also developed the conjunctival pocket model which used subcutaneous implants of conjunctiva in pig-tailed monkeys (422,450). These implants formed small cysts that could then be inoculated or infected with chlamydia. These "eye" pockets showed a similar response to infection and showed worse disease with reinfection. Adult monkeys, in fact, show partial protection to cervical reinfection similar to that seen in the ocular model (451).

Human volunteer studies

"Volunteers" had been infected with purulent ocular secretions since the early 1800s. Some studies were quite heroic. For example, in 1956 Tsutsui infected himself, three co-investigators, three nurses and his wife (452). After a period of time they were treated with antibiotics, but Tsutsui reinoculated himself 11 times. These studies are somewhat hard to interpret, although the authors conclude that the immunity induced by a primary infection was not enough to give solid protection to subsequent inoculation, and increasing the time between reinoculations increased the likelihood of a more severe reaction. Tsutsui also noticed that although one eye was infected, the infection frequently spread to the other eye.

A new era of human volunteer studies started once chlamydia could be cultured. After a single inoculation, most investigators reported that eyes

became positive for chlamydia within two to 14 days and cultures remained positive for five to six weeks (148,431,453,454). Once a patient was treated with antibiotic it took two to four months for the clinical disease to resolve. A number of investigators, particularly the San Francisco group, commented on the frequent development of superficial punctate keratitis; pictures of which are strongly reminiscent of adenoviral keratoconjunctivitis, although a response to adenovirus was not demonstrated by serology (431,455). The time taken for symptoms to develop, but not the severity of symptoms, varied with the size of the inoculum (431). After a single infection none of the 41 volunteers developed scarring.

Some serovar-specific resistance was noted to reinfection (432,454). The response to serovar-specific rechallenge was more variable and gave milder and short-lived disease. However, sometimes a hypersensitivity response was seen with rechallenge and corneal changes could be more marked (455). Lymphadenopathy was reported quite commonly in infected volunteers and 14% developed otitis media. In one volunteer, inclusions could be found in fluids withdrawn from the ear (455). This latter finding must have relevance to the frequent occurrence of otitis media in trachoma endemic areas such as outback Australia (456).

Early studies show that some chlamydia produced a free toxin and Mitsui undertook a series of quite heroic studies with two teenage boys who were inoculated 36 times every 24 hours for 18 and 28 days respectively (457). No significant disease developed, and Mitsui concluded that a free toxin was unlikely to be important in trachoma. This toxin is now known to be elaborated by *C. muridarum*, *C. caviae* and *C. pecorum* but not by *C. trachomatis* (266).

Some studies gave unusual findings. Hanna recounts a blind volunteer who had been reinfected 11 times over a five-year period (458). He had been exposed to three different serovars, F, Ba and D, and inoculated with doses of up to 10^6 Egg Infective Doses$_{50}$. After each infection, he was treated for eight weeks with systemic sulpha drugs and topical tetracycline. This volunteer developed long-term positive cytology, although chlamydia could not be cultured, and he was presented as a case of persistent infection. This was similar to a report of two monkeys that had been variously infected and immunised (459). After challenge with an E serovar they developed chronic disease. Chlamydia could be cultured over a 10-year period and the monkeys developed pannus, trichiasis and corneal opacity.

Repeated reinfection and chronic disease

So far we have reviewed the effect of single episodes of infection. In animal studies, the occurrence of reinfection can be controlled in ways that are not possible in the field. How do observations from animal studies align with field observations? Can they help to resolve the relative importance and occurrence of persistent infection versus reinfection in trachoma?

Relying on my field impression of the likely importance of repeated reinfections, I began experiments on cynamolgus monkeys at the Wilmer Institute. Animals were housed in individual containment cages and inoculated once a week with an E serovar (BOUR) (108). As long as reinoculation continued, these animals had a marked, persistent follicular disease with large follicles on their upper tarsus and a papillary response with inflammatory thickening for as long as reinoculation continued (see Figure 7.14). Limbal follicles also developed, although corneal pannus was not evident. By nine months definite tarsal conjunctival scarring was present, both clinically and histologically (see Figure 7.15). Chlamydia could be isolated by culture for the first six weeks and seen on Giemsa cytology for eight weeks. Animals showed a brisk IgM and IgG serum and tear antibody response that was serotype specific. Biopsies confirmed epithelial changes with infiltration of the disrupted epithelium, the development of follicles with germinal centres and an intense cellular infiltrate in the conjunctiva with later scarring (see Figure 7.16).

A number of subsequent studies were undertaken to further characterise and define this monkey model of trachoma—chronic follicular conjunctivitis and tarsal scarring induced by repeated reinoculation. Similar results were obtained with A serovar organism (HAR-1) inoculation (442). The infecting chlamydia had been grown in egg culture, but repeated inoculation of egg yolk did not induce similar disease (442), nor did formalin-killed elementary bodies (434).

Ocular immune animals that had recovered from a primary infection and were partially immune to high dose single challenge still developed chronic disease with weekly reinfection (460). The presence of partial ocular immunity was not sufficient to protect against the development of chronic disease with repeated reinfection. For us, this modelled all the important features of trachoma.

Even though repeated reinoculation with live organism was needed to maintain chronic disease, the presence of the organism could not be demonstrated after the first eight weeks or so. New, more sensitive tests such as DFA cytology and the use of immunofluorescent antibody for culture identified lower levels of productive infection for a longer period, but after 10 weeks even DFA cytology became negative (446). Unfortunately at that time NAAT testing was not available to test chronically reinoculated animals.

In the 1950s topical corticosteroids were considered a "provocative test" for trachoma. The concept was that steroids would "light up" persistent or undetectable chlamydial infection (419,461). Animals with chronic disease were given remarkably large doses of dexamethazone (2mg) subconjunctivally every second day (462). This dramatically reduced the inflammation and by two weeks the animals were essentially normal, both clinically and histologically. Cultures and cytology remained negative throughout. This at least confirmed the immune nature of the clinical disease. Steroid injections were given to a second group of animals in whom repeated reinfection had been stopped five months previously. They also remained culture and cytology negative. It is not clear whether the steroid reactivation test has any clinical validity, but it certainly did not reveal persistent infection in this model.

Bacterial cultures had been taken from animals with chronic disease, bacteria were rarely seen and common bacterial pathogens were not isolated (442). Animals with chronic disease were inoculated with one of three common bacterial pathogens: *Haemophilus aegyptius, H. influenzae* Type B and *Streptococcus pneumoniae* Type 3. This did not produce any exacerbation of disease. These results strongly suggested that bacterial infection was not necessary to produce active disease observed in monkeys which could be explained by the ongoing presence of chlamydia alone. However,

Figure 7.14 The effect of repeated reinfection in the monkey model RIGHT clinical response seen to weekly reinoculation with C. *trachomatis* BOUR strain (E serotype), with mean follicular and inflammatory indices for six cynomolgus monkeys and frequency of positive chlamydial reisolation cultures. Reinfection was continued for more than 40 weeks BELOW RIGHT clinical response to weekly reinfection with C. *trachomatis* HAR-1 strain (A serotype), with mean follicular and inflammatory indices for five cynomolgus monkeys and frequency of positive chlamydial reisolation cultures. Reinfection was discontinued after 17 weeks (Taylor et al 1982 (442). Reprinted with permission from the Association for Research in Vision and Ophthalmology, © 1982).

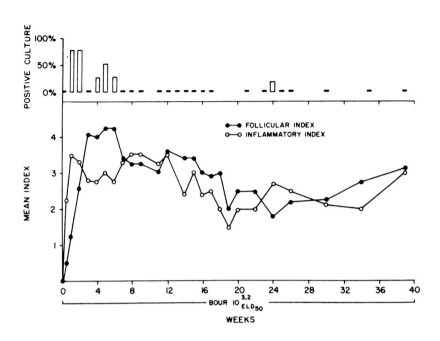

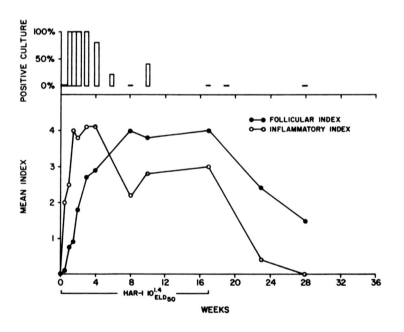

Figure 7.15 The monkey model of trachoma showing persistent follicles and scarring in the tarsal conjunctiva after 30 months of weekly reinoculation.

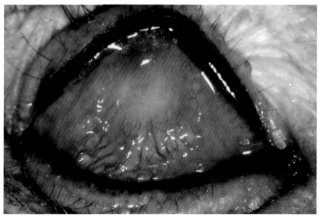

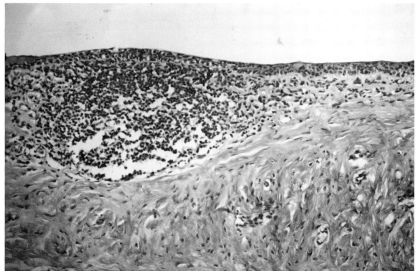

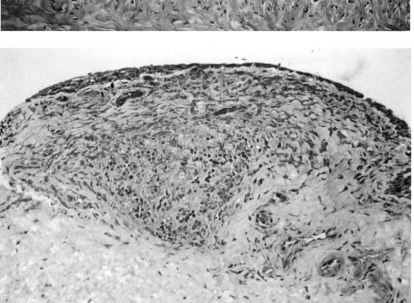

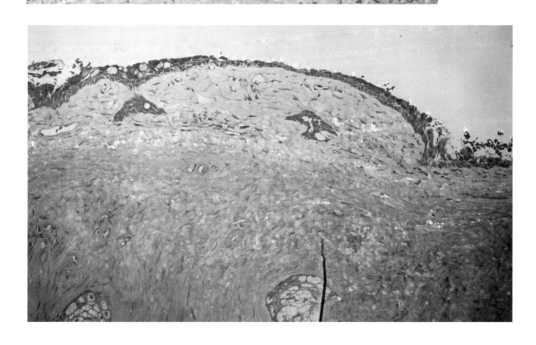

Figure 7.16 Changes in the superior tarsal conjunctiva of cynomolgus monkeys

TOP follicle at 17 weeks after starting weekly inoculation infection, with infiltration of the overlying epithelium (x250)

CENTRE follicle at 35 weeks, demonstrating central necrosis and the presence of elongated spindle cells and dense extracellular material around the follicle (x180)

BOTTOM proliferation of long spindle cells resembling fibroblasts with an increase in thickness of the subepithelial tissue seen at 35 weeks in an area of clinically apparent scarring (x185) (Taylor et al 1981 (108). Reprinted with permission from the Association for Research in Vision and Ophthalmology, © 1981).

in a cat model, more severe disease was produced with the simultaneous inoculation of C. *felis* and a streptococcus species isolated from feline keratoconjunctivitis, rather than inoculating either organism on its own (420).

A series of studies were undertaken to characterise the immune response in the monkey model. Repeated inoculation led to more severe disease with much heavier cellular infiltrate that persisted for as long as reinoculation continued (405). When reinfection was stopped, the inflammation resolved over some months, but reappeared when reinoculation restarted. As with single inoculation, the follicles in the trachoma model contained B cells and serovar-specific IgA and IgG producing B cells that could be isolated from the conjunctiva (403). Large numbers of T-cells were also seen, particularly between follicles and beneath the epithelium. These cells were pre-dominantly CD8+ (405). Conjunctival lymphocytes showed serovar-specific proliferative responses to elementary bodies *in vitro* (403). T-cells did not respond to either purified MOMP or Hsp60. The latter was extracted with a Triton detergent and residual traces may have influenced these proliferation assays.

These studies conclusively show that the monkey model of trachoma can be induced by weekly, repeated inoculation with live chlamydia, even though live chlamydia cannot be recovered from the eye after a period of time. If dead chlamydia are used or if reinoculation stops, the disease will wane and disappear within two to four months. If animals are then rechallenged they will again become culture positive and develop clinical disease. The next challenge was to identify what component of viable chlamydia could cause this immunopathologic response.

Purified antigen preparations

The chlamydial genome codes for 894 proteins (272). However, immuno-blotting studies show that only a small number of these proteins elicit an immune response (443). The major antibody response is directed to the major outer membrane protein (MOMP). This 39 kDa protein is the predominant surface antigen and is used as the

basis for serotyping. MOMP accounts for almost two-thirds of the total protein mass of the chlamydial outer membrane. Antibodies to MOMP are neutralizing *in vitro* (179,463,464). Our studies also showed partial neutralisation *in vivo* in monkeys (465).

Another immuno-dominant molecule is the chlamydial lipopolysaccharide (LPS). Antibodies against LPS are neither neutralising nor protective. Weaker bands are seen for proteins with molecular weights of 60 kDa and 68 kDa. These proteins have been shown to represent the heat shock proteins Hsp60 and Hsp70 (see Figure 7.17). In serum a weak response can also be seen to a 32 kDa protein which has been shown to be an EB specific DNA binding protein (HctB) (418). There is an additional 57 kDa chlamydial antigen, the cysteine-rich outer membrane protein (OMP-2). This protein is not exposed and does not generate an antibody response (418).

Nancy Watkins with Harlan Caldwell used a weak detergent, Triton X-100, to extract an antigen from live chlamydia. When instilled into the eyes of previously infected guinea pigs, this extract stimulated a marked inflammatory reaction (466). Animals that had been infected at distant sites, such as the vagina or the gut, also showed a delayed hypersensitivity response when challenged in the eye with Triton extract. It was exciting to repeat these experiments in monkeys (467).

We tested the ability of a variety of antigen preparations to elicit an ocular inflammatory response in immune animals by inoculating different antigens into the eye once a week and then once a day (468). Purified elementary bodies inactivated with either formalin or UV irradiation produced no response, nor did UV-irradiated infected tissue culture material. Dead elementary bodies did not induce a response. In an attempt to explore the effect of live chlamydia without an established infection, animals were pre-treated with co-trimethoprim and while still receiving this antibiotic they were given a single inoculation of live EB under antibiotic cover. Only a minimal response was induced. The ocular instillation of MOMP or purified chlamydial LPS did not induce inflammation, nor did the subconjunctival injection of LPS (468).

However, a single inoculation of Triton extract

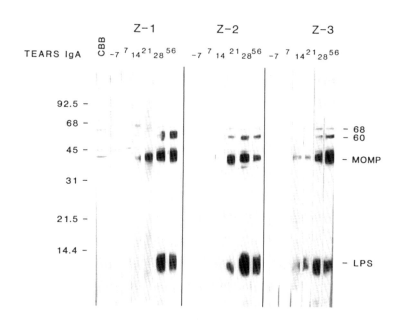

TEARS IgA

Figure 7.17 Immunoblotting analyses of the temporal tear antibody response of cynomolgus monkeys with experimental C. *trachomatis* conjunctivitis. Immunoblots of tears from the three monkeys probed for IgA and IgG antibodies. Tears were collected from animals at seven days before infection (-seven) and at weekly intervals post infection (seven, 14, 21 days, etc). CBB, Coomassie brilliant blue-stained sodium dodecyl sulphate-polyacrylamide gel electrophoresis polypeptide profile of the infecting C. *trachomatis* serovar B. The immunoreactive polypeptides are identified on the right side of the figure (Caldwell et al 1987 (443). Reproduced with permission from the American Society for Microbiology).

gave a marked response with no reaction to the Triton buffer (468). When monkeys were inoculated every day with the extract they developed a marked response (see Figures 7.18, 7.19). However, there was also a significant but much smaller response to the daily inoculation of the Triton buffer. Presumably there was sufficient detergent remaining in this initial preparation so the daily inoculation was like putting dilute soap in the monkeys' eyes, although the single control inoculation had no noticeable effect. Nevertheless, the difference between treated and control eyes was striking. Once the monkeys' eyes had settled, a further single inoculation of the extract again produced a marked response and again there was no response to the buffer. The ocular inoculation of Triton extract had no effect in naïve animals (403). Subsequent experiments showed no ocular response to the Hsp70 antigen in immune animals (469). The characteristics of the immune response induced in the conjunctiva by the Triton extract was the same as that seen with chlamydial infection (403,444). The Triton extract antigen was subsequently identified to be the heat shock protein 60 (Hsp60) and cloned (470). It is the second most abundant protein in chlamydia.

Skin testing of immune monkeys gave a marked positive response to MOMP and chlamydial LPS,

but gave an even stronger response to the Triton extract; two of the three monkeys that were tested with the Triton extract developed areas of necrosis (468). Normal animals did not respond to skin testing with live or killed EB, the control Triton buffer or other antigens.

These monkey experiments used an extracted antigen preparation with the potential for some contamination with residual detergent. The studies in guinea pigs were repeated with the recombinant Hsp60 antigen and produced the same results as those with the Triton extracted antigen (470). More recently, these results have been confirmed in studies using recombinant Hsp60 in the monkey pocket model with fallopian tubes (471). They basically repeated the ocular challenges and only Hsp60 induced delayed-type hypersensitivity reaction. We did not repeat the monkey experiments with the recombinant antigen and no studies of this nature have been carried out in humans.

Chlamydial Hsp60 shows strong homology to the GroEL protein in *E. coli* and also with human heat shock proteins. Several authors have commented on the homology and possibility of developing an autoimmune disease process in humans (418,470), although later human studies of the immune response in trachoma showed no evidence to suggest the presence of an autoimmune

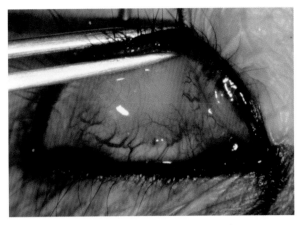
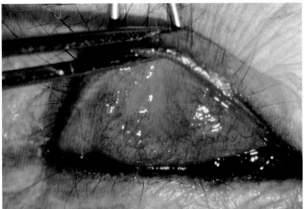
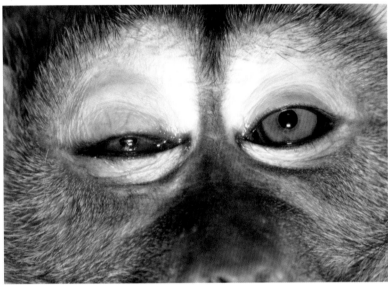

Figure 7.18 The marked clinical response of an ocular immune monkey to Triton X-100 extract inoculation to the right eye. Inoculations were given at day one and then daily from day seven
ABOVE LEFT pre-inoculation, right eye
ABOVE RIGHT day 14, right eye
RIGHT day 14, full face.

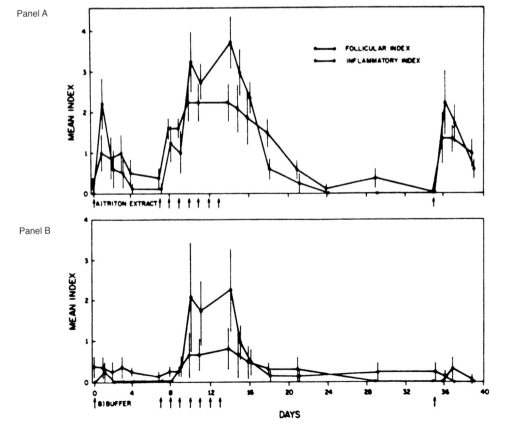

Panel A

Panel B

Figure 7.19 Ocular response of groups of four monkeys given 20μl ocular inoculations of Triton X-100 extracted chlamydial serovar B antigen (1mg per ml) (Panel A) and triton buffer (Panel B). The mean follicular and inflammatory indices are shown. Error bars represent SEM (Taylor et al 1987 (468) © 1987 The American Association of Immunologists Inc).

component (472). Hsp60 can also induce an immediate or innate inflammatory response (473).

From these experiments we concluded the presence of antibodies to Hsp60 in either tears or serum were not protective, but the exposure of immune animals to Hsp60 stimulated a tissue response indistinguishable from trachoma. This intense delayed-type hypersensitivity reaction to a chlamydial antigen was entirely consistent with the notion that trachoma was a disease of immunopathology. This was further supported by the resolution of inflammation with intense local steroid treatment. Copious quantities of Hsp60 are produced during chlamydial replication, but residual Hsp60 is easily removed from the surface of elementary bodies in purified preparations. Hypersensitivity is the undesirable or damaging response of the presensitised immune system on re-exposure to a given antigen. These hypersensitivity responses are grouped in four types (see Table 7.4).

The concept of trachoma as a disease of delayed-type hypersensitivity totally changes one's thinking about the interaction between infection and disease. The classic example of delayed-type hypersensitivity taught in medical schools in the US and elsewhere is poison ivy. Almost everybody in America seems to have had experience with poison ivy, poison sumac or poison oak and can relate to this analogy very well. The same is true for other contact allergies induced by plants or other allergens. The mere touch of a leaf by somebody previously sensitised will lead to the development of a painful skin reaction within a day or so that will take one to three weeks to resolve. There are marked skin changes in the absence of any antigen. The antigenic contact is fleeting and occurs days or weeks before the inflammatory reaction finally resolves.

If one tries to translate this concept to trachoma, one would only need to postulate the occasional, transient infection of a few epithelial cells with chlamydia to allow sufficient time for chlamydia to elaborate and release some Hsp60. It is quite clear that partially immune animals (whether monkeys or humans) are still susceptible to reinfection, and only short bursts of infection would generate sufficient Hsp60 to maintain active inflammation. To my mind, the analogy with poison ivy is compelling. Another analogy would be the way in which the occasional, appropriately aimed and well-timed tap with a stick will keep a hoop rolling along more or less indefinitely, or until one gets bored. An important corollary is that the disease process is related to a cell-mediated immune response. As far as pathogenesis is concerned, the presence or absence of a humoral response seems to be of little importance.

Guinea pig inclusion conjunctivitis (C. *caviae*) has been a useful model to study genital tract infection. Guinea pigs received recurrent subcutaneous immunisation with recombinant Hsp60 with or without ocular boosting (474). This induced significant serum and ocular IgG titres when the animals were challenged. After ocular challenge, immunised animals had somewhat less severe disease, as measured by conjunctival erythema, oedema and exudate, rather than an exacerbation of disease. The number of inclusions

Table 7.4: Classification of hypersensitivity response

Hypersensitivity response	Classification
Type I	Immediate or anaphylactic – mediated by IgE with mast cell degranulation (e.g. asthma, allergic conjunctivitis, anaphylaxis
Type II	Antibody-dependent – IgG or IgM bind to surface antigens and activate the classical complement pathway to lyse the cell (e.g. pemphigus transfusion reactions)
Type III	Immune complex – soluble immune complexes containing IgG or IgM form are deposited in tissues (e.g. serum sickness, glomerulonephritis)
Type IV	Delayed-type hypersensitivity or cell-mediated immunity where T-cells react to antigen presented by cells, usually macrophages, leading to the release of cytokines and recruitment of more cells (e.g. contact dermatitis, temporal arteritis, tuberculosis)

in conjunctival scrapings and their response to further rechallenge was not altered. This study showed that immunisation with Hsp60 neither gives consistent or significant protection, nor in the presence of infection did immunisation induce greater disease. However, it did not assess whether exposure of an immune animal to Hsp60 would induce disease.

Studies of Hsp60 in humans

A number of serologic studies were undertaken to examine the role of Hsp60 in human female genital tract infection (see review by Brunham 418 and 473). Both the prevalence of antibodies to Hsp60 and their titre increased progressively in women with increasingly severe chlamydia pathology; that is, comparing fertile women with positive chlamydial serology to women with chlamydial cervicitis, women with chlamydial pelvic inflammatory disease and women with chlamydial tubal obstruction who had the highest titres (418). Brunham also noted that although many women may have developed chlamydial infection, only a subset developed severe disease, and he wondered whether the antibody response to the Hsp60 was genetically determined. Brunham suggested the possibility of autoimmune inflammation as a result of molecular mimicry.

There were very few studies of human cell-mediated immunity to Hsp60. Women with salpingitis had higher lymphoproliferative responses to Hsp60 (475). The longer women were exposed to chlamydia, the more severe their disease, and the greater their cellular response to Hsp60. In women with STD, the presence of serum antibodies was not linked with a CMI response to either EB or Hsp60, but women who had cell-mediated immunity to Hsp60 were strongly protected against incident infection (476). Another study reported increased responsiveness to Hsp60 in women with tubal factor infertility and suggested that this response was regulated by HLA-D2 and IL-10 genes (477). Hsp60 will stimulate CD4+ T helper cells *in vitro* (478,479), and cytokines released by Th-1 cells such as interferon-γ play an important role in protection. Hsp60 from C.

pneumoniae is also thought to play an important role in the pathogenesis of arteriosclerosis (480).

What do we know about the role of Hsp60 in causing damage in human trachoma? A study using affinity purified Hsp60 showed no increase in proliferative responses in Gambian children with active trachoma, but significantly increased responses in those who had recovered from active disease (481). The responses to MOMP showed a similar pattern. Further studies also showed peripheral blood cells in people with scarring (TS) when exposed to Hsp60 responded with the production of the Th-1 cytokine IFN-γ and Th-2 cytokines Interleukin IL-4 and IL-10 (482). Th-2 cells and their cytokines are associated with fibrosis, a finding that further supports the role of Hsp60-driven fibrosis.

A correlation has been found between the presence of trachomatous scarring (TS) and increased levels of Hsp60 antibodies (483). Those with antibodies doubled their risk of TS but only 32% with TS had Hsp60 antibodies. However, there was a poor correlation between serologic response and cell-mediated immunity to Hsp60 (476). The importance of a delayed-type hypersensitivity reaction to Hsp60 in humans with trachoma awaits further testing, but current data are either supportive or they do not refute it.

At the molecular level, the story of chlamydial Hsp60 became more complex as three homologues of Hsp60 have been identified (484). Chlamydial Hsp show strong similarities to bacterial and mammalian heat shock proteins such as GroEL from *E. coli*. They belong to a group of chaperonins that form heptameric rings with other chaperonins. These proteins are responsible for the folding and refolding of proteins and their correct delivery into assembling cell membranes. It appears that the second homologue of Hsp60 has a relative inhibitory effect to the function of the first, and is therefore produced in increased quantitites during persistent or non-productive growth including that induced by IFN-γ (485,486,487).

Cells and cytokines

So far we have looked at the pathogenesis of trachoma from a relatively broad perspective, but we will now look inside the "black box" and examine some of the cellular and molecular events described to date. This is a rapidly evolving field and the development of new technology can lead to rapid advances in knowledge. There is a current and broad review of this in a recent textbook (488).

As mentioned, the interpretation of animal data is fraught with difficulty in relating changes in one infection/host model system to another due to differences between different chlamydia (their sensitivity to interferon (IFN-γ), for example), the site of inoculation (superficial mucosal or systemic) and the animal host (human, subhuman primate, mouse or guinea pig). In animal studies, the timing and frequency of ocular challenge is controlled, but human studies in the field cannot control for reinfection. The latter also suffers from difficulties in disease definition; people with mild but definite and unequivocal active trachoma may be classified as not having "active trachoma" (TF/TI or F_2/P_3) and regarded as "normal". The detection of infection will vary with the type of test (PCR, LCR or EIA) and the handling of specimens. Despite all these difficulties some very interesting and important advances in our understanding have been made over the last 10 years or so.

Human trachoma is almost invariably caused by serovars A, B, Ba or C (296). Although there is regional variation as to which serovars predominate, only these four "ocular strains" are associated with trachoma. Harlan Caldwell and his group have shown that there is a specific biochemical difference between ocular and genital strains of *C. trachomatis* (426). As we will see, one of the key responses to chlamydial infection is the production of IFN-γ (489). IFN-γ induces the expression of indoleamine-2, 3-dioxygenase (IDO). IDO in turn depletes intracellular levels of tryptophan, essential for the metabolism of chlamydia. The genomes of ocular and genital strains share 99.6% identity and the area that is not identical is known as the plasticity zone (268), which codes for tryptophan biosynthesis, toxin production and purine metabolism. As it turns out,

the genital strains are able to encode for tryptophan synthetase, but this gene is mutant in the ocular strains. Having this functional enzyme enables the genital strains to use exogenous indole to escape from the inhibitory effects of IFN-γ. It has been postulated that the bacterial flora in the genital tract produce sufficient levels of indole to provide this exogenous supply (273,426).

Although bacteria are present in even the normal conjunctiva, they are present in vastly smaller numbers than in the heavily colonised genital tract. There would seem to be insufficient ocular bacterial flora to generate sufficient indole. Without this mechanism it is unclear as to how the ocular strains cope with the relative depletion of tryptophan, or how this process may interact with productivity or persistence of ocular infection. Tears do not provide a source of tryptophan either as tryptophan is not found in human tears (490,491).

The inflammatory response in active trachoma has multiple components: one stimulates inflammation, another damps down inflammation and a third stimulates fibrosis and scar formation (see Figures 7.20, 7.21).

An extensive series of studies including those using specific genetically modified "knockout mice" have shown the importance of Type 1 T helper cells (Th-1) or a pro-inflammatory response in the resolution of infection (492). Th-1 cells characteristically release IFN-γ, TNFβ and other cytokines. They are involved in delayed-type hypersensitivity. Conversely, Type 2 T helper cells (Th-2) are thought to have contributed to the disease resolution and were considered to be anti-inflammatory, although scarring and "repair" are part of the process of the resolution of inflammation (493). Th-2 cells release IL-4, IL-5 and IL-I3 and other cytokines. They also stimulate B cells and antibody production. Studies in Tanzania and The Gambia have shown the presence of mediators released by Th-1 and Th-2 cells as part of a pro-inflammatory delayed-type hypersensitivity response in the conjunctiva of children with active trachoma (494,495). Burton concluded that the presence of active disease is associated with the expression of pro-inflammatory cytokines (IL1/TNFβ), noted an anti-inflammatory

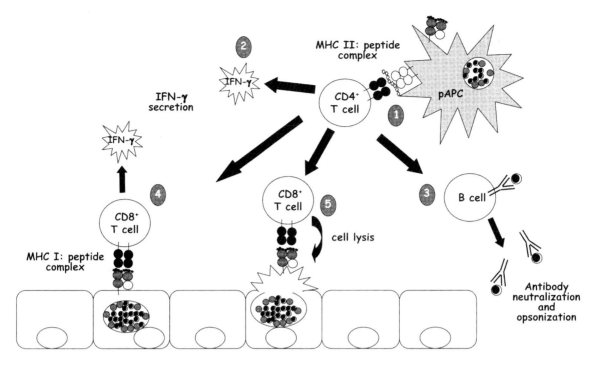

Epithelial cells

Figure 7.20 All arms of the adaptive immune system help to control *Chlamydia* infection. (1) Professional antigen presenting cells (pAPC) process and present *Chlamydia* antigen on their cell surface in complex with MHC class I and II molecules. When antigen-specific CD4⁺ T cells recognise MHC class II: foreign peptide complexes at the surface of pAPC, these T cells become activated. (2) Effector CD4⁺ T cells produce cytokines, especially IFN-γ, which help to control *Chlamydia* infection. Not only does IFN-γ stimulate the bactericidal activity of macrophages, but it also helps to reduce replication of *Chlamydia*, presumably by depriving the organism of tryptophan and iron. (3) Activated CD4⁺ T cells can also direct the activities of B cells and CD8⁺ T cells. A subset of circulating B cells express antigen receptor molecules that recognise surface components of the *Chlamydia* elementary body (EB). This subset of B cells becomes activated by effector CD4⁺ T cells to proliferate and differentiate into antibody-secreting plasma cells. These secreted antibodies bind EBs and prevent them from infecting host epithelial cells in a process termed "neutralisation". Additionally, through a mechanism known as "oposonisation", antibody binding of EBs facilitates the uptake and destruction of organisms by pAPC. (4) Via their T cell receptors, CD8⁺ T cells recognise *Chlamydia* peptides complexed with MHC class I molecules. However, in order to become fully activated, antigen-specific CD8⁺ T cells often require "help" from CD4⁺ T cells. Once activated, effector CD8⁺ T cells that recognise *Chlamydia*-infected cells will respond by secreting the inflammatory cytokine IFN-γ, which helps to control *Chlamydia* infection. (5) Upon recognition of a *Chlamydia*-infected cell, it is also possible that effector CD8⁺ T cells directly lyse the host cell and deprive *Chlamydia* of its intracellular niche (Balsara ZR, Starnbach MN. CD8⁺ T cell recognition of cells infected with *Chlamydia*. In: Bavoil PM, Wyrick PB, eds. Chlamydia Genomics and Pathogenesis. Norfolk: Horizon Bioscience; 2006:381–411. Reprinted with permission from Horizon Scientific Press and Michael Starnbach).

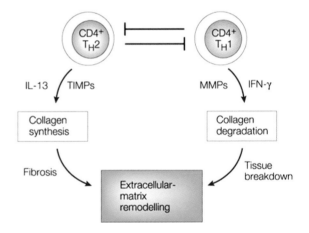

Figure 7.21 Opposing roles for T_H1 and T_H2 cytokines in fibrosis. The T helper 1 (T_H1)-cell cytokine interferon-γ (IFN-γ) directly suppresses collagen synthesis by fibroblasts. It achieves this through regulating the balance of matrix metalloproteinase (MMP) and tissue inhibitor of matrix metalloproteinase (TIMP) expression, thereby controlling the rates of collagen degradation and synthesis, respectively, in the extracellular matrix. IFN-γ and/or interleukin-12 (IL-12) might also indirectly inhibit fibrosis by reducing pro-fibrotic expression by T_H2 cells. The main T_H2 cytokines (IL-4, IL-5 and IL-13) enhance collagen deposition by various mechanisms; however, IL-13 seems to be the crucial mediator (Wynn 2004 (493). Reprinted with permission from Macmillan Publishers Ltd: Nature Reviews Immunology, © 2004).

"back-lash" (IL10) and evidence of changes in the regulation of the extra cellular matrix with increased MMP9. In cases with active chlamydial infection, an activated cell mediated immune response produces IL12, IFNβ and perforin. This suggests the occurrence of down regulation of the cell mediated response with the clearance of infection. Cytokines were at their highest levels in children with intense trachoma (TI) and in those with the highest loads of infection. They were also elevated in adults with TS. Bobo postulated that levels of mediators may be high in those who were unable to control high levels of infection and would therefore develop more severe disease (494). Gambian children who recovered from infection, for example, had higher levels of cell-mediated immunity to chlamydial antigens (481).

These pro-inflammatory cytokines can lead to activation of the epithelium as mentioned above and the expression of matrix metallo proteins (MMP)—enzymes released to digest collagen and other proteins and ground substance that forms connective tissue. Specifically activated was MMP-9 (411,495) which degrades the extracellular matrix, especially basement membrane (Type IV collagen), and facilitates the migration of cells including polymorphs and fibroblasts (473). MMP-9 can also activate TGFβ and so promote the formation of scar tissue and increases 10 fold in children with intense inflammatory trachoma (P$_3$) (496).

Th-2 cytokines that have an immune regulatory and/or anti-inflammatory role are also released, specifically IL-10 (495). In mice IL-10 is thought to be predominantly released by T regulator (or suppressor) cells (493). IL-10 limits IFN-γ production and tissue damage caused by pro-inflammatory Th-1 mediators, but may also impede the effective clearance of infection. IL-10 normally suppresses collagen synthesis and scar formation (493). A specific genetic change in the IL-10 haplotype in some people was associated with an increased risk of scarring and trichiasis (320,497). Similar findings come from genital tract infection (477). People with this apparently less active IL-10 haplotype expressed higher levels of IL-10 during infection, and this may alter their subsequent risk for developing scarring (498). Why their risk was increased, however, is unclear. In knockout mice,

the absence of IL-10 enhanced the clearance of chlamydia, but also increased the severity of inflammation (499). More needs to be written about this complex interaction.

The expression of different cytokines changes with the evolution of active trachoma. IL-1β, IL-10, TNFα and MMP-9 correlate with the presence of clinical active trachoma; whereas IFN-γ, IL-4, IL-12p40 and perforin were increased in children with demonstrable infection (495,500). IL-4 is expressed by Th-2 cells, other T helper cells, natural killer (NK) cells and mast cells. IL-4 may be indicative of damaging inflammation. In mouse models IL-13, also released by Th-2 cells, may be responsible for more fibrosis than IL-4 (493). IL-12 is released by dendritic cells and macrophages. It drives Th-1 cells and the production of IFN-γ. Perforin is indicative of the presence of CD8$^+$ cytotoxic T-cells.

IFN-γ is a key molecule in the inflammatory response to chlamydia and has the direct effect of impeding chlamydial development by limiting tryptophan availability. In *in vitro* studies this leads to laboratory defined "persistent infection" or non-productive infection (489). Cultured chlamydia can be kept in the equivalent of suspended animation until tryptophan levels are restored. In the laboratory this state can be maintained for about 30 days with care. This is as long as the infected cell cultures remain viable. During this time, ribosomal assembly is blocked and the production of chlamydial antigens such as MOMP stops, although the production of Hsp60 is augmented (478,485,501). Hsp60 can be detected in persistent *C. pneumoniae* found in atheromatous plaques (480,502). In trachoma areas, high levels of IFN-γ and IDO were evident in the conjunctival scrapings of those who were infected, whether they had clinical disease or not (503). IL-10 was also high in those who had both clinical disease and infection. These data suggest that the increasing antigen load stimulates high levels of IFN-γ that eventually leads to the control of infection with a balancing IL-10 response to reduce inflammation (503). Alternatively, chlamydia could evade the IFN-γ /IDO pathway and continue to grow despite high levels of the cytokines. It is still unclear what mechanisms ocular serovars use to cope with tryptophan deficiency induced by IFN-γ and IDO (273). Once infection cleared but clinical disease persisted (resolving disease), the levels of a T regulatory cell (T$_R$) marker FOXP3 were elevated (503). T$_R$ cells are thought to limit and encourage repair.

Holland used some clever new technology to detect antigen specific CD8$^+$ T lymphocytes in the peripheral blood (319). HLA peptide tetramers to epitopes of chlamydial MOMP were used to identify HLA I restricted CD8$^+$ cells present in low numbers in peripheral blood. They were related to the presence of infection but not related to the load or resolution of infection, development of new infection or the presence of clinically active trachoma. The significance of these findings is still to be determined. Human T-cell clones can recognise surface exposed chlamydial antigens (504).

As mentioned previously, Th-2 cells have been linked to the production of scarring. Both MOMP and recombinant Hsp60 stimulate cells to produce IFN-γ from normal control subjects and those with trachoma (482). However, Hsp60 also stimulated cells from patients with trachoma scarring (TS) to produce IL-4 and increased amounts of both IL-10 and IFN-γ (482). An association with TS and HLA DR (Class II) histocompatibility antigens was not seen by Holland (482) or Conway (505), although Conway did find an association with increased scarring and Class I HLA *6802. A subsequent study of adults from The Gambia showed an increased response to Hsp60 by those with HLA DRB1*0701 and a decreased response with both DQB1*0301 and DQB1*0501 (506). A study in Omanis with blinding trachoma showed susceptibility and was linked to the presence of HLA-DR16 (a DR2 subtype) (507). Other HLA II antigens (HLA-DQA1x0102 and DQB1x0602) and the IL-10-1082AA genotype have been associated with scarring in the genital tract causing tubal infertility (477). With studies such as these chance findings are possible and associations require confirmation. However, they open the door to further studies of differences in genetic susceptibility as do studies of IL-10 haplotypes.

Holland demonstrated that low levels of circulating CD8$^+$ cells also recognise both MOMP and Hsp60 (472). He could find no evidence for autoimmunity. The antigen specific CD8$^+$ cells seemed to have little role in the inhibition of local infection. His group postulated that changes in the balance between T regulatory and T effector cells, both cytotoxic CD8$^+$ cells and Th-1 and Th-2 cells, may lead to chronic infection (505).

Ultimately, this complex inflammatory soup of T-cell cytokines from the cell mediated immune response controls the recruitment and activation of macrophages and fibroblasts (493). As previously mentioned, there is strong evidence for the ongoing activity of macrophages and deposition of new collagen by fibroblasts which forms the scars we recognise clinically and distort the tarsus to cause trichiasis and blindness.

Progression of cicatricial changes from scarring to trichiasis

As previously mentioned, the presence of severe inflammation is a clear risk factor for the development of scarring (138,322). Dawson observed that "children with severe or moderate disease develop sufficient scarring by the age of 15 to make blindness an inevitable consequence for at least some of them" (138). Negrel has been even more succinct: "scars today, trichiasis tomorrow" (53) (see Figure 7.22).

There is variation in the rate of progression from scarring (TS) to trichiasis (TT) with estimates ranging between 2% and 7% per year (323,508, 509). The level of endemicity may also influence these rates. The two Gambian studies showed approximately one-third of those with minor trichiasis developed major trichiasis within four or 10 years. In Tanzania, the five year incidence for trichiasis varied with age and gender and ranged between 3.2% in women with TS (aged 15 to 19 years), to 15.1% in women with TS (aged 55 to 59 years) (510). The presence of chlamydia detected by PCR doubled the risk of developing trichiasis (511). Once trichiasis was present, up to 40% of older women developed corneal opacity (CO) within 10 years (510). The four year incidence of CO in The Gambia was 5% for those with minor trichiasis and 10% with major trichiasis (509). Significantly, the risk of CO was increased eight times if TT was present (512). An important study in Ethiopia showed that having trichiasis for two or more years increased the risk of CO more than twofold, and the risk of total CO more than sixfold (513).

Many have stressed the importance of ongoing inflammation as a risk factor for the development of trichiasis, often associated with bacterial infection (407,509,510). Pathogenic bacteria are much more commonly isolated from those with trichiasis (106,514). Anyone examining people with trichiasis is familiar with the discharge so commonly seen. In addition, about half of those with trichiasis have significant tarsal inflammation. More recently Burton has demonstrated increased expression of inflammatory cytokines (TNFα, IL-1β, MMP-9 and TIMP-2 in those people with trichiasis who also have bacterial infection) (515).

The relevance of persistence: infection versus reinfection

How does this information further our understanding of the pathogenesis of trachoma and the relative importance or contribution of reinfection compared to persistent infection?

It is quite clear that animals (human and experimental animals) that have recovered from a chlamydial infection remain susceptible to secondary challenge infections, even though they may show partial resistance or immunity compared to naïve subjects. With secondary challenge, the duration of clinical disease and chlamydial shedding (infectious load) is reduced. This pattern was characterised almost 100 years ago by Nicolle (143) and 30 years ago by Grayston (288) and observed in detailed longitudinal studies (126). Grayston first drew attention to the importance of reinfection (315). Bailey attributed the decreased duration of infection in older people to a changed immunity relative to ageing, rather than an age-related change in exposure to reinfection. The highest load of infection is seen in the youngest children (122,168,298) and they also have the poorest facial hygiene and ocular promiscuity. They are at maximum risk of reinfection, and it would seem that the apparent longer duration of infection seen in children, may well represent the effect of multiple episodes of re-exposure/reinfection rather than a true immunologic difference.

Observations of the kinetics of infection are

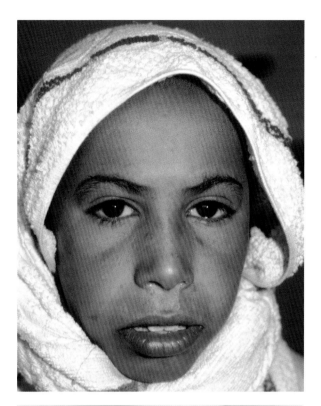
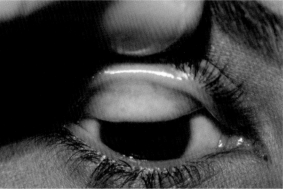
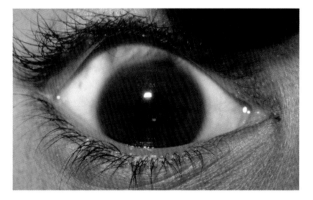

Figure 7.22 Early onset of cicatricial trachoma
TOP a teenage Tunisian boy who already has
CENTRE severe scarring and
BOTTOM trichiasis.

thwarted by the infrequent examination interval of most field studies typically at two, six or 12 months. We conducted a study with three monthly examinations (195); Bailey examined people every two weeks (126) and in her impressive work in Tanzania, Bobo collected weekly specimens (124). However, even this may be too infrequent. Immediately replicated PCR swabs may have a 5% variation and a 1% false positive rate (217) and DFA smears taken every two days may show a 25% discordance (195). Is this artefact or is it real variation in shedding?

The ability to finally resolve the importance of reinfection in trachoma areas will require much more careful field studies with more frequent examination, stringent attention to the possibility of sample contamination, and the use of the most sensitive tests for both the detection of infection and importantly measurement of clinical disease. For programmatic control activities, the outcome may not be critical—trachoma may disappear before this conundrum is finally resolved. However, for those attempting to develop computer models of trachoma, it is a central and critical issue (516).

It seems apparent that instances of persistent infection of chlamydia may occur at least occasionally. It is important to differentiate the laboratory term "persistent infection" from the clinical concept "continuing infection". In the laboratory we know that chlamydia can be held in suspended animation for several weeks instead of completing their life cycle within two to four days. Persistent or continuing infection in humans relates to either the ongoing presence of infection (months or years) after notionally effective antibiotic treatment, or the prolonged presence of demonstrable organism in the absence of exposure to reinfection.

Prolonged infection has been observed in infants infected at birth, who have persistent chlamydial infection of the eye and nasopharynx over two years (517). Cervical infection in women has been reported to last for two to five years despite various treatments, although the possibility of multiple episodes of reinfection cannot be excluded (518). Without treatment 54% of women with cervicitis are clear of infection within one year and 94% within four years (519). Another study found

persistent infection in 8% of women with chlamydial cervicitis who had been treated and denied having sexual contact (520). This suggests primary treatment failure with ongoing infection. Women whose partners had not been treated had a 25% rate of infection, suggesting the occurrence of reinfection. It has also been suggested that persistent *C. trachomatis* infection may be important in arthritis (521), and persistent *C. pneumoniae* infection may occur in atheroma (502) and possibly even in age-related macular degeneration (522,523,524,525).

An examination of naturally occurring infections in animals does not resolve this issue. Certainly the vast majority of infections in animals with *C. psittaci*, *C. abortus* and *C. suis* are asymptomatic (260). It is unknown whether these common, unapparent endemic infections result from slow host elimination of infection (or persistence) or from reinfection.

Information about trachoma is less clear, and certainly no study has been able to control for the possibility of reinfection. Ongoing or "persistent" infection is commonly seen after antibiotic treatment especially with community-based studies of azithromycin. These studies have not treated the youngest children in the first few months of life and many have not treated any children under 12 months. These little children are known to have the highest levels of infections and will remain as sources of reinfection. The rate of return of infection after azithromycin treatment in Ethiopia is an astounding 12.3% per month (526).

Persistent infection was suggested in Tanzania when half the women with infection at two PCR tests taken three years apart had either no infected children or no children (323). These women may have had persistent infection, but without controls for specimen collection and more detailed behavioural information, the possibility of artefact or reinfection cannot be excluded.

As discussed, Tom Lietman and his group have reintroduced discussion about the concept of the latent period of infection where infection is present and the eye is normal; the period of clinically active trachoma with the presence of infection (the "patent" period); and a recovery phase when infection can no longer be demonstrated, but clinical disease is maintained or slowly resolves (233). Implicit in this linear model is the concept of a single defining episode of infection. If one is to entertain the possibility of reinfection, one needs to break the patent and recovery periods into a series of alternating episodes of ongoing clinical disease with the intermittent presence of infection. Further, one could suggest episodes of infection sufficient to release Hsp60 to stimulate cell-mediated immune response.

Therefore we can deduce that in trachoma it is not the infection that causes blindness, but the inflammation. It is important to remember that as the prevalence of trachoma decreases, the first thing to be reduced is the intensity of infection and inflammation; the second is the incidence; and the last is the prevalence of follicles or active disease. If one considers trachoma as a chronic, delayed-type hypersensitivity with subsequent fibrosis, one also needs to remember that only the occasional exposure to antigen may be enough to sustain the ongoing clinical disease.

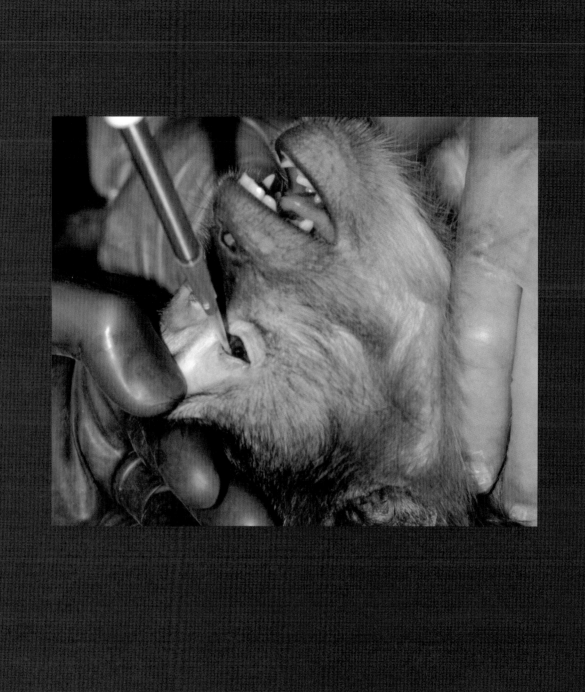

CHAPTER EIGHT

Trachoma vaccine development

The possibility of making with the trachoma agent a preventive and therapeutic
vaccine was contemplated in 1960 when the problems connected with the isolation
and the cultivation of the agent were solved

GIAMBATTISTA BIETTI, 1967

THE IDENTIFICATION OF chlamydia by Giemsa cytology and confirmation that trachoma resulted from infection opened the way for the first trachoma vaccine studies. This was a path previously followed for other infectious diseases.

Chlamydia were identified in 1907 by Halberstaedter and von Prowazek (142). In the same year Nicolle and his group in Tunis began their experimental studies (143) inoculating human volunteers and a range of subhuman primates including chimpanzees, various apes and monkeys. They confirmed the infectious nature of trachoma and noted that once animals had recovered from a single infection they were relatively resistant to infection but could be reinfected. As previously mentioned (see chapter four) Nicolle's group confirmed that trachoma should be classified as a virus because it was small enough to pass through the pores of a Berkefeld V filter and the "virus" was destroyed by heating it to 50 °C for 30 minutes or by drying on cloth for one hour at 32 °C. The virus could be stored for one week in glycerine.

They then initiated a series of quite extraordinary vaccine studies using subconjunctival or intravenous injections of filtered material collected from conjunctival scrapings of patients with trachoma (143). These studies were undertaken in humans and monkeys and vaccines gave variable and inconclusive results. They must have experienced great difficulties in standardising immunising doses and the infectious challenges. They noted some resistance to rechallenge suggesting immunity in some cases but in others, the response to rechallenge led to worse disease, a finding frequently reconfirmed over the next 100 years.

There seemed to be little further work on vaccine development between the two world wars, although a lot of experimental work was undertaken in both humans and subhuman primates to identify and culture chlamydia (46).

MacCallan opined that in humans:
"There is absolutely no immunity against reinfection by the virus of trachoma for an individual who has apparently recovered from the disease. [However] when … the normal epithelium has been replaced by scar tissue epithelium and a delicate layer of cicatricial tissue has been laid down beneath the epithelium of the major part of the conjunctival extant, reinfection is rare" (4).

Early vaccine studies

The isolation of chlamydia in 1957 spurred another burst of interest in a trachoma vaccine. The ability to culture chlamydia improved the quality of research by several orders of magnitude. It was now possible to determine and quantify the size of immunising doses, infectious challenges and the infectious load recovered after ocular challenge. The availability of organism made it possible to develop antibody assays and it became possible to track serum and tear antibody responses and after the introduction of microIF in 1967, to serotype different strains and determine the serovar-specificity of antibody responses.

In the 1960s four major groups worked on trachoma vaccine development; Leslie Collier's London-based group working in The Gambia, Tom Grayston's Seattle-based group in Taiwan, Roger Nichols' Boston-based group in Saudi Arabia and Giambattista Bietti's Rome-based group in Ethiopia. Each conducted initial studies in subhuman primates and undertook clinical trials of varying size. Small trials were also performed in South Africa (527). The Italian studies led to the full-scale commercial production of a vaccine.

The London group in the Medical Research Council Trachoma Unit studied baboons immunised with a so-called "fast strain" of chlamydia, and subsequently this strain was shown to be LGV. They used live vaccine and showed partial resistance of baboons to rechallenge for two to six months (528). Some studies used intravenous

immunisation but this led to the widespread dissemination of live LGV agent, particularly in the lymph nodes and spleen (529). Three human trials were undertaken in The Gambia, but results were not clear-cut, showing neither a protective nor therapeutic effect (170,530). A further trial testing both live and formalin-killed bivalent vaccines (with a total of 3.7×10^6 or 4.3×10^8 organisms) was undertaken by this group in Iran. These vaccines were given intramuscularly with a booster two weeks later. They showed a mild transient reduction of infection at one year, but had no effect at two years. "This short-lived, moderately beneficial effect of trachoma vaccines is, however, not sufficient to be of practical value" (91).

The Seattle group worked at the Naval Medical Research Unit No 2 (NAMRU 2) in Taiwan. Extensive studies in the Taiwan monkey (*M. cyclopsis*) showed the development of partial protection after primary infection and immunisation (315). Formalin-killed EB were used and vaccines of high titre (10^9 organisms) gave some initial protection, although this protection decreased by nine months and had disappeared by two years (531). However, lower-dose vaccines (5×10^7) did not protect consistently and the monkeys that became infected developed more severe disease. Partial protection was serotype-specific, although there was some cross reactivity related to the evolutionary cascade of chlamydial antigenic changes in MOMP, the so-called senior and junior antigens (531). Animals that had a hypersensitivity reaction to challenge infection developed pannus and scarring was observed. Grayston also noted that the hypersensitivity and increased disease with rechallenge lasted longer than the partial protection (316). This was a particularly significant finding that clouded the future use of trachoma vaccines.

Several vaccine trials were carried out in Taiwan that had a clever design. The youngest siblings of first grade schoolchildren with active trachoma were immunised with a purified vaccine (532). An alum adjuvant was used. Although the results at one year showed a reduced incidence, any protection had disappeared by two to three years and no protection was seen at six years. In those who received the monovalent vaccine infections were more severe and occurred more frequently (316). Another trial with 100 children using an oil adjuvant (incomplete

Freund's adjuvant) caused considerable reactions to the booster injection (533). More immunised children developed trachoma at two and a half years than placebo children.

The Seattle group also conducted a trial in the Punjab assessing a very high dose bivalent formalin-killed vaccine (>10⁹ EB) (534) administered to 450 children aged three months to five years who did not have trachoma. Booster injections were given approximately three months later. At one year, vaccinated children had approximately half the incidence of trachoma. When followed up at 12 years, there was no difference between vaccinated and placebo groups (535). Significantly, vaccinated children had not developed more severe disease. At that time Grayston predicted the future "hope for the control of trachoma would seem to lie in the explosive advances being made in immunology" (536).

The third major group working on a trachoma vaccine was the Boston group who worked with Aramco in Saudi Arabia. In the laboratory they mainly studied owl monkeys (Aotus trivirgatus), a new world monkey that had a more florid response to chlamydial eye infection (439). Animals again showed a short-lived, partial resistance to reinfection that correlated with the presence of tear and serum antibodies (537). A major vaccine trial assessed a bivalent vaccine in children under the age of three years. Although there was less clinical disease at six months, the effect was reduced at 12 months and disappeared by 18 months (538). However, children who had received the higher dose aqueous vaccine were three times more likely to develop clinical disease than those in the control group.

The Italian group working in Ethiopia initially studied Grivet monkeys (Cercopithaecus griseoviridis) and undertook a series of vaccine studies evaluating aqueous vaccines, and alum or incomplete Freund's adjuvants. They used a monovalent formalin-killed vaccine with 5 x 10⁸ EB; half this dose was given as a booster at six weeks (539). Between 1960 and 1962 three separate studies in several thousand children showed this vaccine could prevent the acquisition of new infection. The vaccine also showed a therapeutic effect as it "hastened healing" and subsequently more vaccinated children moved from active trachoma (Stages II or III) to inactive (Stage

IV) disease with scarring. In these double-masked studies, the rate of development of new disease was halved with vaccination and about twice as many vaccinated children showed a therapeutic benefit.

In 1964 Bietti conducted a large field trial vaccinating 5000 children with the same number of children as controls. This was the first of Bietti's trials to use computer analysis. At 12 months, less vaccinated children had acquired trachoma and more had resolved. Summarising his experience, Bietti noted that the preventive benefit of the vaccine lasts for approximately one year, whereas the therapeutic effect could be observed at three years. The effects were more marked in children over the age of six and in areas with mild trachoma or where a large number of children were immunised. Each of these could be an indicator of areas where trachoma might decrease because of secular changes. Bietti noticed no gender difference and the vaccine was more effective in Grade II disease and had no effect in Grade III disease.

Based on these findings, a commercial vaccine was developed with approval from the Italian Ministry of Health. Bietti considered the vaccine would be useful for several purposes: it would prevent infection in those entering the endemic areas such as expatriates; it could be used with antibiotic treatment to shorten the duration of disease; it could be used to prevent reinfection in those already cured; and to protect the very young from developing infection. Bietti found no sustained benefit by combining vaccination with treatment with oral sulphonamides (539). Similar findings also came from Taiwan (540). Bietti died sometime after this and although commercial quantities of his vaccine were made, it was never really taken up because the vaccine was only partially effective.

After about 15 years, the intense interest and activity in a trachoma vaccine ran out of steam. A vaccine could produce partial, short-term protection both in experimental infections and in the field. The protection in either subhuman primates or human volunteers was comparable to that seen after the recovery from a primary ocular infection. In some instances, immunised individuals developed more severe disease. As mentioned, a commercial vaccine had been developed, but was not used.

Monkey experiments with purified vaccines

The vaccines studied in the 1950s, 1960s and early 1970s used whole elementary bodies. With the development of the monkey model of trachoma at Johns Hopkins, we had the opportunity through the 1980s to examine the role of a number of purified antigen preparations that became available. Also we were able to examine the immune response of immunised and challenged animals with much greater precision, and follow the antibody response and the development of cell-mediated immunity both systemically and locally. The various vaccine approaches for immunising antigens are summarised in Table 8.1. These extensive studies showed:

- none of the immunising regimes or vaccines that were tested gave better protection than that seen after recovery from a single, primary ocular infection

- intramuscular immunisation induced cell-mediated immunity and a serum antibody response

- oral immunisation gave good serum antibody titres, but usually did not give tear antibody titres. The "maximal" immunisation gave very high serum antibody titres and there was some spillover with low levels of tear antibodies

- ocular immunisation or ocular boosting gave high titres of antigen-specific tear IgA, IgG and

Table 8.1: Summary of vaccine studies in monkeys, 1986–94

Vaccine trials include:

	Reference
• Oral	
★ Live L2 serovar (challenge with B serovar)	(555)
★ Maximal immunisation Live B serovar (challenge with E serovar)	(555)
★★ UV inactivated L2 serovar (challenge with B serovar)	(555)
Formalin-killed L2 serovar (challenge with B serovar)	(555)
Live B serovar (challenged with B serovar)	(555)
Chlamydial LPS (challenge with B serovar)	(556)
MOMP-B +IP + Cholera toxin (challenge with B serovar)	(557)
OGP-MOMP-C +IM (challenge with C serovar)	(558)
• Ocular	
★ MOMP-B (challenge with B serovar)	(557)
★ MOMP-B Ocular and Oral (challenge with B serovar)	(557)
★ MOMP Ocular and IP + Cholera toxin (challenge with B serovar)	(557)
VS-1 + Cholera toxin (challenge with C serovar)	(559)
VS-2 + Cholera toxin (challenge with C serovar)	(559)
VS-1 + 2 + Cholera toxin (challenge with C serovar)	(559)
★ OGP-MOMP-C + Cholera toxin (challenge with C serovar)	(558)

★	Gave partial protection
★★	Induced worse disease
VS	Variable segment, an epitope of MOMP
MOMP	Major outer membrane protein
Chlamydial LPS	Chlamydial lipopolysaccharide expressed by recombinant *E. coli*
	Maximal immunisation, rectal and oral live EB, intramuscular EB with Freund's adjuvant
OGP	A mild detergent used to extract MOMP

IgM, with antigen-specific conjunctival IgA and IgG B cells and antigen-specific conjunctival T-cells. After challenge ocular boosting gave an amnestic antibody response with increased CD4$^+$ cells in follicles and intrafollicular CD8$^+$ cells

- the presence of tear or serum antibodies did not prevent infection

- the presence of either chlamydial EB or MOMP antigen-specific T-cells or B cells in the conjunctiva did not prevent ocular infection

- vaccination could induce an antibody response to Hsp60, but this was neither protective nor harmful.

The results of these studies were disappointing and failed to induce immunity better than that seen following recovery from a primary ocular infection (see Figure 8.1). They emphasise the imperative of comparing the response of immunised animals with the response of "naturally immune" animals receiving secondary challenge. Naturally immune animals have recovered from a primary infection. These vaccine trials did not lead to examples of worsening of disease.

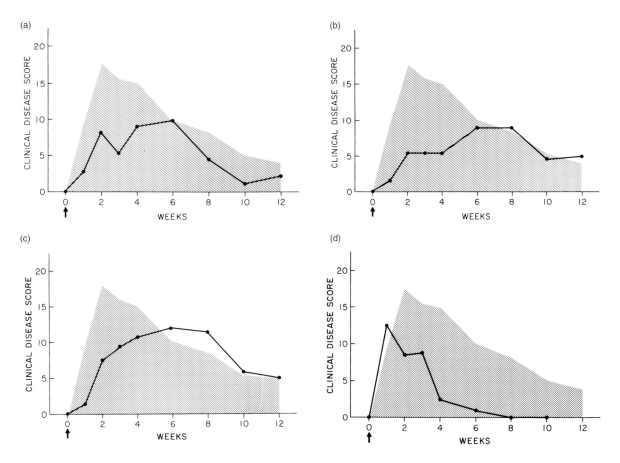

Figure 8.1 Mean clinical disease score of: (a) four monkeys that received ocular vaccination with MOMP; (b) four monkeys that received enteric vaccination with MOMP; (c) four monkeys that received combined vaccination with MOMP; and (d) five ocular-immune monkeys challenged 18 weeks after primary infection (Taylor et al, 1988 (557). Reprinted with permission from the Association for Research in Vision and Ophthalmology, © 1988).

Current status and future developments

It is important to remember that vaccines against chlamydia are widely and effectively used in veterinary practice (260). These vaccines against *C. psittaci*, *C. abortus* and *C. cati* contain either live or killed whole EB. The fact that whole EB vaccines in animals are successful when they were clearly not effective against trachoma, show major differences must exist in immune mechanisms that operate in different situations.

With the explosion in tools and reagents available for cellular and molecular studies and genetic manipulation, the mouse has become the prime experimental animal for chlamydial research (423). Mice are easy to handle, cheap, and inbred strains can be studied in large numbers and provide a good model to study genital tract infections (541). Although some work in mouse models has used human pathogens (542,543), most studies have used the mouse pneumonitis agent MoPn, a mouse biovar that was initially classified as *C. trachomatis*, but has subsequently been reclassified as *C. muridarum*. MoPn can cause respiratory infection when inoculated intranasally, or genital tract infection can occur in female animals after treatment with high doses of progesterone. These two model infections have been used extensively and have advanced our understanding of the response to chlamydial infection in many ways.

However, when extrapolating these findings for human trachoma, one has to recognise that MoPn differs significantly from human ocular strains of *C. trachomatis*. For example, MoPn is quite different in its response to IFN-γ and the reduction in available tryptophan (273,544). There are also significant differences between human and mouse immune responses. Newer techniques allow us to dissect the immune response in even greater detail and characterise finer components. This makes even subtle differences between infective organisms and host responses potentially more significant. An example would be a study in women with tubal infertility where the Th-2 response was found to be as important as the Th-1 response (427). The authors observe "the results also suggest that the immune response against *C. trachomatis* in humans is much more complex than in mice, where a strong Th-1 response correlates with the elimination of bacteria and resolution of disease".

Most recent studies in the mouse model have looked at the mechanisms of systemic immunity rather than mucosal immunity. Systemic mechanisms are strongly involved in the lung infection model. The salpingitis model also induces strong systemic immune response. This focus is understandable as much of the drive for a chlamydial vaccine comes from STD and respiratory fields. Trachoma on the other hand is an infection confined to the mucosal surface and significant differences exist between the systemic and mucosal immune responses.

Given the necessary caution when extrapolating findings from the mouse model to human trachoma, studies both in mouse and humans indicate the importance of a strong Th-1 response in the resolution of infection (492,494,495). Darville recently reviewed this field summarising a large number of experiments including those in knock out mice and other mouse models that demonstrate the importance of the Th-1 response (544). These findings are also consistent with the studies of cytokine expression in humans (494,495). Genetic factors that regulate the induction and activation of Th-1 cells and perhaps IL-10 producing T regulatory cells may be important in directing human immunity towards protection or pathology (498,544).

A CD8⁺ T-cell response seems to be less important in protecting against infection both in the mouse model and in humans, although the role of these cells in clearing human infection is less clear-cut. Cloned human CD8⁺ cells found in the blood of people with trachoma (319) are capable of recognising chlamydial outer membrane complexes on the surface of infected cells (504). The relevance of antibodies in protecting against secondary infection is quite unclear (476,482,503) although in the mouse model antibodies play an important role (545).

It would take a braver man than I to look into the crystal ball and predict the successful development of a vaccine to control blinding trachoma before 2020. Although MOMP may be the immunodominant antigen and antibodies against it are neutralising, it seems most unlikely that an effective MOMP-directed vaccine could be developed. After all the negative results with

MOMP vaccines despite evidence of good priming, it is unlikely that conformational or adjuvant adjustments (546,547) will make the quantum change in protection required for an effective and useful vaccine. Anti-MOMP-specific antibody can be neutralising *in vitro*. In tissue culture systems when one needs centrifugation and the use of high molecular compounds to make EB attach to cells, an antibody that attaches to the surface of the chlamydia may provide sufficient non-specific interference to block this artificial cell attachment. *In vivo* studies in animals suffer a similar problem when relatively huge titres of antibodies can be used to neutralise purified elementary bodies prior to inoculation. Clearly in both humans and animals the presence of tear antibodies against a range of chlamydial antigens including MOMP does not prevent infection or even the culture and re-isolation of viable organism. However, the presence of tear antibodies may control the shedding of infection and reduce the titres of organism that are recoverable in culture.

Another antigen currently being studied is the polymorphic membrane protein D (PmpD) (548,549). This cleaved protein is highly conserved and surface exposed. It seems to be more specifically involved with the attachment of chlamydia than MOMP and antibodies to PmpD can be neutralising (267). This makes it an attractive vaccine. Attention is also being directed to the immunity-related guanosine triphosphatases (IRG or p47 GTPases). These IFN-γ induced enzymes are involved in the intracellular control of intracellular pathogens such as tuberculosis (550) and chlamydia (551). Another vaccine candidate

could be attachment targets for chlamydia and Type III Secretion System (552,553).

A wide range of adjuvants is now available and it may be possible to deliver chlamydial vaccines that are much better targeted and so induce a more specific immune response (543,546,547). Based on the cytokine studies, a vaccine should aim to induce a strong Th-1 response and reduce or minimise the Th-2 response. Toll-like receptors (TLR) are pathogen-recognition receptors that enhance the presentation of antigens to T-cells. Vaccines that stimulate TLR signalling may be more effective although this is not yet well established (554).

So far we have examined the role of a protective vaccine. I do not see how a therapeutic vaccine as such is likely to help. These vaccines were trialled by Bietti and based on the concept of an ongoing chronic disease following a single episode of infection. However, another approach would be to look at a tolerising vaccine that reduced the host immune response to deleterious chlamydial antigens. Immune tolerance is a concept that has been studied for 40 years, especially in tissue transplantation, but is still not fully understood. However, if the hypothesis that trachoma is a hypersensitivity response to the Hsp60 antigen were correct, in theory a vaccine that specifically down-regulated this response should reduce the severity and intensity of disease. However, a more pragmatic approach in the foreseeable future is the public health approach embodied in the SAFE Strategy outlined in the following chapter. This offers a more likely way to eliminate blindness due to trachoma than the development of a vaccine.

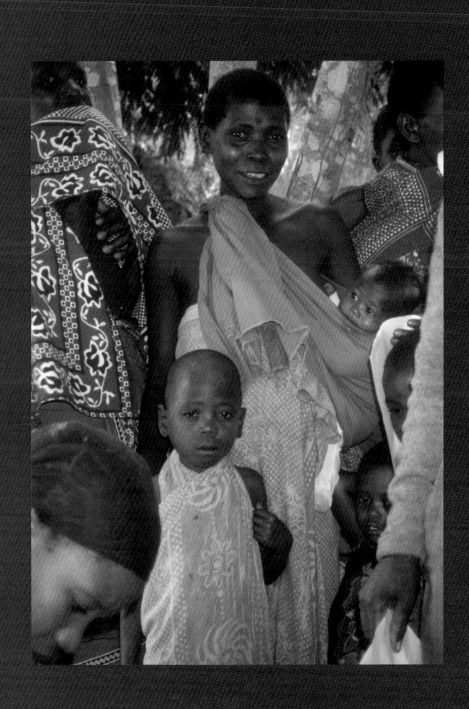

CHAPTER NINE

Trachoma control and the SAFE Strategy

Drugs? I'd prescribe water. If governments were to
put water on nobody would have trachoma!

IDA MANN, 1966

Past treatments

THE EBERS' PAPYRUS (1553–1550 BC) was basically a collection of ancient Egyptian prescriptions of which about 70 were for the treatment of eye disease. Much Egyptian medicine was based on topical treatment; a variety of animal, vegetable and mineral products were applied to the eye, often with the feather of a vulture.

The Greeks had a different notion of disease. They related most disease to humoral causes and so treatments were used to divert inflammation from the affected eye to other organs. By and large topical medications were not favoured. Hippocrates and the Greek physicians in the fourth century BC advocated curing ocular disease by drinking wine, bathing, purging, bloodletting, and with cleansing medications. Three types of operations were used to treat trachoma: the scarification of the granular conjunctiva or ophthalmoxysis by a variety of means followed by the application of copper compounds such as copper oxide and copper sulphate (Discordes 60 AD, Celsus 43 AD); the surgical excision of the fleshy granular tissue in thickened lids, followed by cautery with a heated iron and copper treatment; and various surgical methods to correct entropion and trichiasis.

These principles were subsequently followed by Greek and Roman practitioners (10), taken up by Byzantine and Arabic physicians and passed back again into western European medicine in the Middle Ages. These principles formed the basis of the treatment of trachoma until the introduction of the first effective antimicrobials—the sulphonamides—in 1937.

Certainly for millennia copper sulphate and silver nitrate were the standard worldwide treatment including China (8), Egypt (12), Europe (4,29,46) and the USA (130). Cautery or bloodletting was also advocated to reduce inflammation (see Figure 9.1). An analysis of traditional medicines used in Egypt in the 1980s showed many of the compounds listed in Ebers' papyrus were still in regular use (12). Itinerant healers in the Middle East also continued to perform traditional lid surgery (see Figure 9.2). However, surgical interventions were less emphasised and almost forgotten by European writers until the early 1800s when army surgeons were confronted by troops with the Egyptian ophthalmia. Tarsal excision became quite popular and was widely practised for a time. For example, it was the recommended treatment in the US into the 1920s with disastrous results (74). Irradiation with X-rays and radium was tried with limited success in the London Trachoma Schools at the end of the 19th century (30).

The Greco-Roman medical management we have inherited has three pillars: surgery, medicines, and lifestyle and diet. These components bear a striking similarity to the elements of the current SAFE Strategy. Now our approach to trachoma control is based on the notion of repeated episodes of reinfection and the need to use multiple interventions to break the vicious cycle (see Figure 9.3).

Sulphonamides and tetracyclines

Sulphonamide drugs were the first effective antimicrobial agents and they became available in 1937 and were rapidly used to treat trachoma. Their use in England is said to have led to the closure of the British Trachoma Schools in 1944 (65). In Egypt their use in the treatment of select children was found to be disappointing having little impact on trachoma, although corneal ulceration rapidly responded to treatment (300). In 1949 Lindner wrote "A few years ago trachoma was one of the most serious diseases of the eye. That this is no longer the case is due to the sulfonamides" (560).

In Indian reservations in the south-west of the United States they replaced the use of topical copper sulphate, and when used to treat the whole community, they led to a marked reduction in trachoma (79). Their distribution was stopped when the USA entered the Second World War in 1942 as drugs were requisitioned for military use (see chapter two and Figure 2.15). A rebound in trachoma in Indian communities was noticed in the 1950s (359) and a new program began in 1967 (79). All school-age children were examined and any found to have trachoma and their family members were treated with triple sulphas for 21 days (561). Those who were sensitive to sulphas (or sulfas in America) were treated with topical tetracycline. Rates in schoolchildren were reported to be as high as 74%. A nurse also made home visits and gave further hygiene education. Improved distribution of drugs, examination of all community members and significant improvements in housing led to an accelerated reduction (80). The prevalence of trachoma in people of all ages fell from 16% to 7% in just three years, and further dropped to 3% by 1976, and the program was stopped in 1985 when prevalence was less than 1% (398).

In 1944 Father Frank Flynn, an Australian ophthalmologist and army chaplain in Central Australia during the Second World War, treated people living in at least five Aboriginal communities in Central Australia with oral sulphanilamide he had requisitioned from army stores (562). Having done this once without proper authority it seems he was unable to convince the authorities to provide more of this precious drug. After the war, he conducted large scale treatment with oral sulphas administered for two weeks with variable results (383).

Following the surveys of Ida Mann in Western Australia and the identification of trachoma in Aboriginal people, all Aboriginal children were treated with sulphadimidine in 1959 (563). The next year there were only a few cases of trachoma. Following a high rate of side effects with longer acting sulpha drugs used in 1961 and 1962, targeted treatment continued in 1963 and 1964 but enthusiasm had waned:

The reason for the lack of success in controlling trachoma is, in my opinion, that we have expected too much from drugs alone. We have relied on tediously

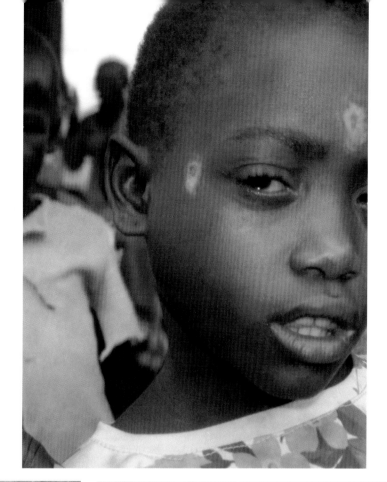

Figure 9.1 Burns applied to the
forehead and temples of a Tanzanian
child to treat trachoma follows the
traditional treatment first set out by
Hippocrates (1990).

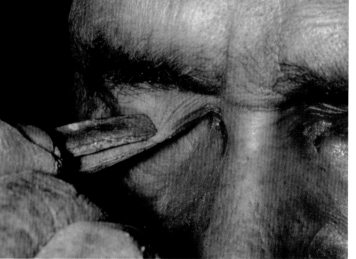

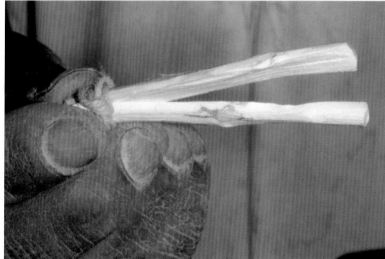

Figure 9.2 Traditional surgery to correct
trichiasis as performed in Oman
the lax eyelid skin was tented upwards with a
large pair of forceps
a split stick was then tied over the "redundant"
skin causing pressure necrosis and so shortening of the anterior
lamellar of the lid (courtesy, Mark Reacher).

Epidemiology of Trachoma

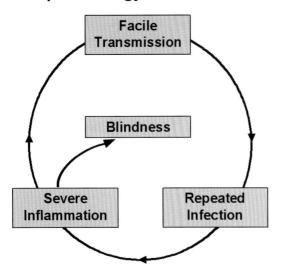

Figure 9.3 Now our approach to trachoma control is based on the notion of repeated episodes of reinfection and the need to use multiple interventions to break the vicious cycle of trachoma (redrawn from West S, Taylor HR. Community-based intervention programs for trachoma control. Int Ophthalmol 1988; 12:19–23. With kind permission of Springer Science and Business Media).

long courses of not very efficient drugs while next to nothing has been done to improve the native environment which, with its overcrowding, dirt and flies and absence of personal hygiene remains ideal for spreading the disease (563).

However, sulphas continued to be widely used in Australia. In 1972 Hollows treated all the members of an Aboriginal community over the age of six weeks for one month with oral co-trimethoxazol (103). Two months later there was a marked reduction in the amount of inflammation and at three years active trachoma had dropped from 75% to 5% and residual cases had minor follicles only.

Based on this experience, Hollows and the NTEHP used co-trimethoxazol for their massive treatment campaigns (103). A total of 25,000 people over the age of three months were treated in four large programs. The average dose distributed was 26 out of 40 possible doses, with the target being twice daily doses for 20 days. The poorest

compliance was amongst 20 to 40 year old men. Side effects occurred in about 5%; three-quarters of which were mild, the most common being nausea and vomiting or a rash. Over 2000 children were re-examined between six to 12 months post treatment. There was a 48% reduction in the overall prevalence of active trachoma in children from 52% to 27% and an 80% reduction in severe disease. Commenting on these interventions, Hollows considered antibiotic treatment to be an interim measure until adequate home health hardware became available (318) (see Figures 9.4, 9.5).

The mass distribution of oral sulphas was also one of the key components to the elimination of trachoma in Malta (343). Extensive studies with oral sulphas were also undertaken in Ethiopia including the use of lower doses of long-acting drugs administered every second week (539). This treatment was still troubled by recurrent episodes of infection.

The use of topical sulphas was associated with frequent allergic reactions. The new antibiotic tetracycline, first discovered in 1945, was effective against chlamydia and well tolerated when applied to the eye. In Pakistan topical treatment with silver nitrate, copper sulphate, sulphacetamide, chloramphenicol, three tetracyclines and three combination treatments of antibiotic and curettage were compared (564). The best results were achieved with tetracycline ointment combined with curettage and copper sulphate which gave a 55% cure at six months. A large study in South Africa involved some 10,000 children in 36 schools who were treated with a range of topical medication that included sulphacetamide, tetracyclines, neosporin and steroids (565). Only children attending school were treated. No difference was observed between the various antibiotics and at six or 12 months trachoma rates were reduced by about 25%. The addition of steroids did not seem to enhance or impede antibiotic treatment. A study in China found topical tetracycline to be superior to copper sulphate and although oral sulphas were helpful with acute treatment, they were not needed for long-term control (158).

Dawson undertook two studies in Tunisia comparing topical tetracycline, topical erythromycin and boric acid as a control. The first

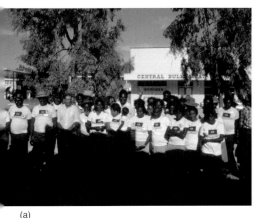

(a)

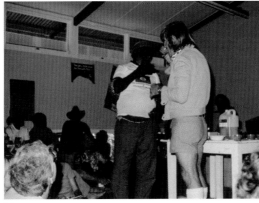

(b)

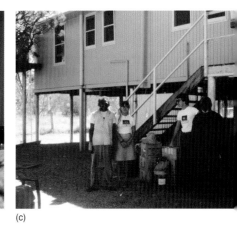

(c)

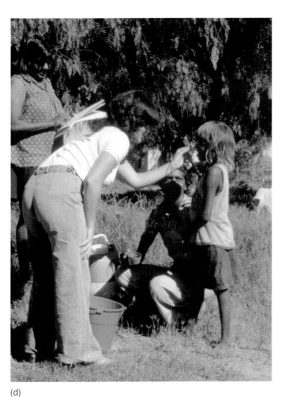

(d)

Figure 9.4 Community-wide treatment was given on a large scale during the NTEHP (1977)
(a) aboriginal health workers assembling for a training course in Alice Springs
(b) Fred Hollows and a Pintupi elder (whose first encounter with Europeans was less than 10 years before) during the training session
(c) teams of medical students and Aboriginal health workers arriving at a community with three weeks supply of drugs
(d) Septrin suspension given to a young girl.

Areas of mass systemic trachoma treatment programs 1976–1977–1978

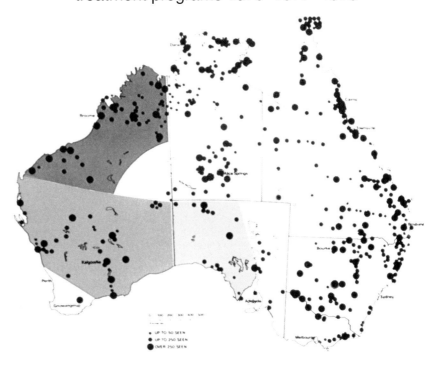

Figure 9.5 Area covered by mass antibiotic treatment during the NTEHP (NTEHP 1980 (103); courtesy, Royal Australian and New Zealand College of Ophthalmologists).

study used daily treatment for 60 days in six to nine year olds. Although the antibiotic reduced bacterial colonisation and suppressed chlamydial infection, no difference was observed at four months between the three groups which all showed a reduction in trachoma (566). The second study used intermittent treatment applied twice daily for five consecutive days each month for six months (567). Again, no difference was observed and trachoma decreased and then rebounded in both groups. A further study in American Indian high school children compared oral tetracycline for three weeks and a placebo (568). A dramatic fall in infection was noted with immunofluorescent cytology in both groups. The intensity of inflammation rapidly reduced, but follicles changed more slowly. These temporal changes mirror those seen today with azithromycin.

In 1952, the WHO recommended topical tetracycline four times a day for two months and oral sulphas were administered for two months (20). If the disease had not resolved, tetracycline was to be continued, and the three-week course of sulpha treatment was to be repeated on two or three occasions as necessary. Silver nitrate and copper sulphate were still advocated for selected cases. The recommended frequency of topical tetracycline was reduced to twice a day in 1956 (33) (see Figure 9.6). In 1962 erythromycin was also suggested as an alternative and the intermittent use of topical tetracycline for three to six days a week each month for six months was advocated (49). The assessment of the impact of treatment should be delayed for at least three or possibly six months after the cessation of treatment.

The WHO had supported major trachoma control activities in countries such as India, Pakistan, Burma, Morocco and Egypt. The intermittent topical tetracycline schedule was also tested in India (302). Overall, each treatment was more effective when given under supervision. Better results were noted at six months in older people

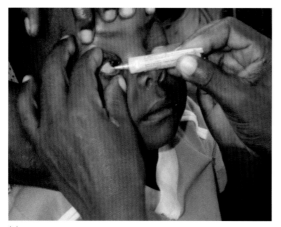
(a)

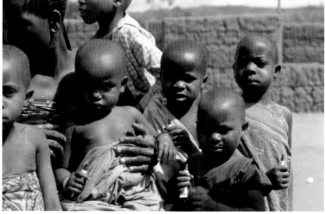
(b)

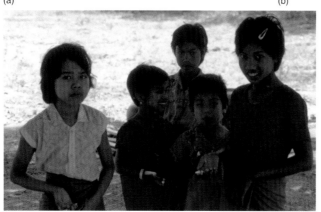
(c)

Figure 9.6 Topical tetracycline has been one of the mainstays of trachoma control for 50 years (Tanzania and Burma 1986)
(a) being applied by healthworkers
(b) & (c) more commonly, tubes are normally given to children with the expectation they will be used properly.

and those with less severe disease. There was a tendency for relapse at 12 months. The results are difficult to interpret as the MacCallan grading was used, but an overall cure rate of about 35% was recorded. The intermittent schedule was recommended as it was as effective and considered more practical. Primary schoolteachers assisted with the treatment of schoolchildren. Antibiotic treatment campaigns were also linked with health education activities that included village meetings, leaflets, posters and the screening of a special film "Trachoma".

Impressive work was reported from southern Morocco where Reinhards compared intermittent treatment using tetracycline ointment twice a day for three days each month for six months using oral treatment with triple sulphas administered over four days (139). The impact of fly suppression and the combination of different modalities as well as untreated control villages were assessed. Extensive studies were conducted in three areas over a 10 year period. The copious amounts of data are again difficult to interpret, in part because of the use of the MacCallan grading, and in part because of the lack of computing power to produce the multivariant analyses that have now become standard. Overall, Reinhards found no benefit for trachoma from fly control alone although fly control did reduce the amount of bacterial conjunctivitis (381). Only a small benefit was observed with the addition of oral sulphas to topical tetracycline therapy (139). Reinhards observed that intermittent treatment delayed the onset of infection and reduced both the intensity and gravity of infection. One outcome measure was the age at which cicatrization was first observed; this was used as an indicator that active trachoma was resolving. In one study this had decreased from eight to three years—a significant improvement. The onset of active trachoma was also markedly delayed from three months to three years. Attention was drawn to the difficulty of treating infants, although treatment "has not immediately been sufficiently directed towards the infants and young children" (139). This 10 year study also showed that treatment needed to be repeated each year "for many years". Although initially topical tetracycline had been distributed to families each month, in the second year of the program, families

were given a supply at the start of each summer and subsidised ointment was also made available in local tobacco shops.

The report from Morocco was the largest and most detailed of the WHO studies, but in 1976 Yuri Maitchouk summarised the experience with topical tetracycline treatment in 15 countries in the Eastern Mediterranean Region (569). Different intermittent treatment regimes had been used including once daily for six consecutive days each month for six months, once daily for two weeks each month for three months, one or twice daily for five days for six months, or once daily for 10 days for six months. All had an equal therapeutic result and the particular regime seems to have been determined by local considerations. However, after 10 years of treatment in the Sudan, for example, the rate of active trachoma in children under the age of 10 had fallen from approximately 60% to less than 10%. Severe trachoma had almost disappeared from Syria with three years of treatment and bacterial conjunctivitis was greatly reduced in several study areas. Similar results with topical tetracycline were reported in Ethiopia (570). One community health worker was assigned to treat 25 to 30 people and in one year there was a 45% reduction in severe active disease.

As an alternative to topical tetracycline, studies were conducted with oral doxycycline, a long-acting tetracycline. In Iran, Jones conducted a community-based study distributing doxycycline twice a week for three weeks and the rate of moderate and severe active trachoma was halved at two years (571,572). Again using family-based treatment, a study in Palestine found that oral doxycycline was as effective as tetracycline or oral sulphas and all gave an 80% cure at one year (573).

Hollows and the NTEHP used community-based distribution of oral doxycycline to treat trachoma in one Aboriginal community. A dose of 100mg was administered three times a day for two weeks to capitalise on the ability of higher doses of doxycycline to also treat holoendemic syphilis. This unpublished study was inconclusive due to poor compliance. Many suffered gastrointestinal complaints as the morning dose almost universally was taken on an empty stomach.

A single oral dose of doxycycline administered

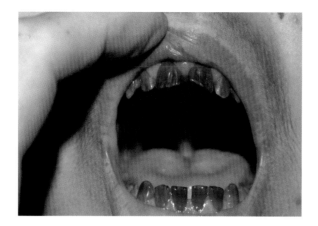

Figure 9.7 The dental changes associated with use of oral tetracyclines in childhood.

once a day for two or three weeks was a viable alternative to the prolonged and difficult treatment program required with intermittent topical tetracycline (574). When Schachter and Dawson balanced the cost benefit advantages of the reduction of the likeliness of blindness against the side effects of oral doxycycline (dental changes, long bone deposition and photosensitisation), they concluded that doxycycline treatment "is warranted for treatment of active infectious trachoma in children" (574). When the prevalence of active trachoma had dropped below 20%, for example, they suggested it would be cost-effective to give doxycycline to all children with moderate or severe disease (575) (see Figure 9.7).

Some clinical trials were also conducted with rifampicin (105,576). However, they were only moderately successful and this important drug for the treatment of tuberculosis was not widely used to treat trachoma.

Trachoma control programs

I have thus far concentrated on the assessment of antimicrobial agents. Usually, although not always, antimicrobial treatment was combined with other health intervention measures (20,52). In 1952 the WHO recommended that control activities should focus on both the disease itself and the associated epidemic bacterial conjunctivitis. This involved (i) case finding and treatment, (ii) health education,

and (iii) the destruction of possible vectors together with environmental sanitation measures (see Figure 9.8). There was a need to emphasise prevention. Health education programs, for example, might use teachers and other measures. A vertical program to initiate trachoma control would be needed for at least two years and thereafter yearly follow-up to maintain control. The successful model developed in Egypt by MacCallan was taken as the prototype (52) with a central national institute to co-ordinate activities of static and mobile eye hospitals. It used teams of nurses and doctors and had active programs in schools and in the media. Interestingly, the group reiterated that in Tunisia (with a population of 3.8 million people) 20 million working days were lost a year through trachoma and they used this as an argument for action (52).

In 1956, the WHO Expert Committee emphasised the need for preliminary epidemiologic information; the conduct of pilot studies, the desirability of mass campaigns as a way of reducing costs; further cost reduction through co-ordination with other programs and the use of "lay people"; and the ultimate integration of the program of normal activities of public health services (33).

These messages were very much taken to heart in China during the Great Leap Forward where Professor Chang listed the five ways in which trachoma programs had been incorporated into the patriotic health movement (158). First, the health system in the people's commune provided the foundation for anti-trachoma work. Second, the "Four Combinations" provided the principles for anti-trachoma work: (i) closely combined with the health movement, (ii) education to improve personal hygiene, (iii) health linked to increased production and (iv) the combination of traditional and modern therapies. Third, the training of cadres to increase numbers of anti-trachoma personnel was needed. Fourth, education propaganda together with the patriotic health movement provided the knowledge of prevention and treatment of trachoma to the people (via films, radio broadcasts, television, newspapers, etc.). Each person was to have their own washing towel and wash their face and hands with running water. Fifth, continuing scientific research considered essential for anti-trachoma work. Chang spoke with authority as one of the group that had first isolated chlamydia. In 1964 he estimated that the prevalence of trachoma in China was 50%.

Eye health promotion campaigns "anticonjunctivitis fortnight" (Quinzaine ANTI-RMAD) were held in Tunisia prior to the annual epidemic (52). They focused on simple hygiene methods and used a variety of media and school programs. Intermittent tetracycline was later combined with health education and the provision of trichiasis surgery (577). Subsidised ointment was also made locally available. Over a 20 year period, in 13 of 18 governances, the prevalence of trachoma in five to seven year olds had dropped from an average of 24% to 1.4%.

In Australia, three small studies combined bathing at school with antibiotic treatment using oral sulphas and topical tetracycline (578), topical tetracycline (579) and co-trimethoxozol (365). The latter two showed a reduction in trachoma at one year of more than 50%, but none were sustained.

In 1973, the WHO published *Field Methods for the Control of Trachoma* (102) that dwelt on the role of antibiotics, but also outlined the importance of trichiasis surgery, training the health cadre and the need to promote health education. It mentioned the role of education of school-age children, and the delivery of messages in maternal and child health clinics. Only a few examples of the areas to be covered under health education were given, but personal hygiene and the provision of water were included.

The WHO also published an updated *Guide to Trachoma Control* in 1981 (107) setting out seven elements that should be included in programs to control trachoma:

1 Assessment of the problem and establishment of priorities.

2 Allocation of resources.

3 Chemotherapeutic intervention.

4 Surgical intervention to correct lid deformities.

5 Training and utilisation of local health aids and other non-specialised health workers.

6 Health education and community participation.

7 Evaluation of intervention programs.

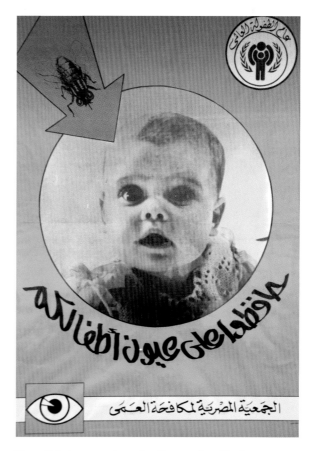

Figure 9.8 A poster advocating fly control and hygiene in Egypt from the 1960s (© WHO, reproduced with permission).

Elements 1, 2, 6 and 7 really dealt with process issues. The chemotherapy recommended was either six weeks of topical tetracycline ointment or one of two variations of the intermittent schedule (either twice daily for five days or once daily for 10 days each month for six months and repeated as required). Alternatives included oral tetracyclines or doxycycline for three to four weeks or the use of oral sulphonamides for two to three weeks. Erythromycin was given as a further alternative. For the correction of trichiasis, epilation, electrolysis and cryotherapy were suggested and eight different operations were recommended for entropion and trichiasis.

The recommendations on health education were of a high level and quite general. Mothers of young children were identified as the prime target for health education which emphasised the provision of water, the reduction of crowding and the

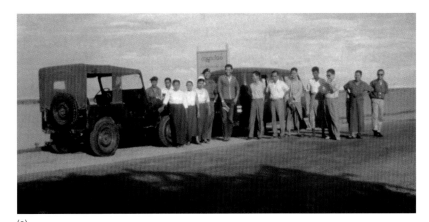

(a)

Figure 9.9 Trachoma control activities.

In Burma in the 1960s (courtesy, Dr Thein Dan)

(a) the assembled trachoma team on the road

(b) conducting examinations in the village. Note the military presence

(c) trichiasis surgery being performed in a community setting

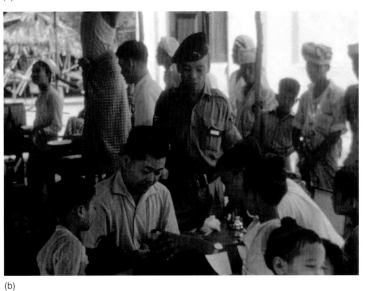

(b)

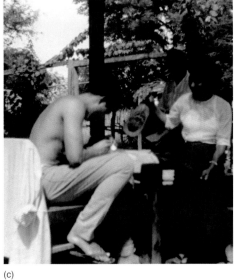

(c)

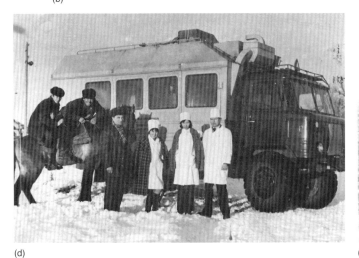

(d)

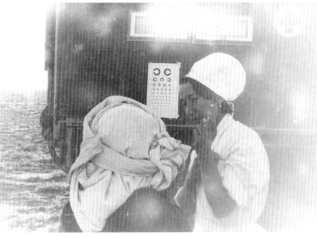

(e)

Figure 9.9 *continued*

In Kazakhstan, USSR in the 1980s (courtesy Bagdad Suleyeva and Galina Makeyeva)

(d) the mobile team from the Kazakhstan Institute of Eye Diseases in winter near the Chinese border

(e) testing visual acuity in summer.

identification and control of breeding sites of eye-seeking flies. The improvement of personal hygiene should be actively encouraged and assisted. Movies, schoolchildren and teachers were all suggested as a means of delivering the message. These were somewhat diffuse and ephemeral recommendations for a trachoma control program and with the exception of a few countries such as Burma, Thailand, Tunisia, USSR and Vietnam (54), little programmatic trachoma activity continued on an organised national basis (see Figure 9.9).

The observations of the importance of facial cleanliness in the 1980s led to calls for more targeted trachoma intervention programs that focused on a more specific "motivational message" (388). The need for such programs to be sustained and long term required appropriate sociomedical research within the community (368,580). Others also recognised that the widespread use of antimicrobial agents on their own would not reduce endemic disease in the absence of socioeconomic improvement or behavioural changes (581).

The SAFE Strategy

In the early 1990s, a number of factors were coming together. Since 1985 the Edna McConnell Clark Foundation, a New York-based philanthropic organisation, had provided support for new trachoma research (582). Epidemiologic studies had identified specific risk factors; new diagnostic tests were being used; clinical trials had assessed trichiasis surgery and facial cleanliness; and studies of new antibiotics, especially azithromycin, were in progress. This collective activity and progress led to a resurgence of interest in trachoma similar to that seen in the 1810s, 1910s, 1930s and 1960s.

In 1993 a new field guide was developed by the WHO called *Achieving Community Support for Trachoma Control, a Guide for District Health Work* (583) which became known as the "green book". This guide brought together the results of recently completed controlled clinical trials on trichiasis surgery and facial cleanliness. It built on the WHO Simplified Grading for Trachoma (128), the recently released publication *Final Assessment*

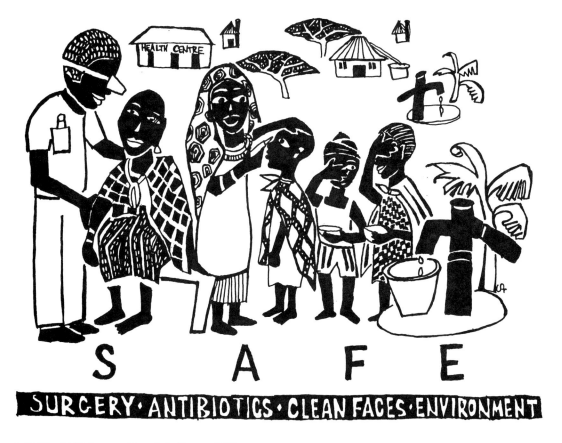

Figure 9.10 The SAFE Strategy (Francis & Turner, 1993 (583) © 1993 WHO, reproduced with permission).

Table 9.1: Treatment of trachoma, WHO, 1993 (583)

Proportion of children aged 1–10 years with trachoma	Basic treatment	Additional treatment
TF: 20% or more, or TI: 5% or more	Mass topical antibiotic treatment	Selective systemic antibiotic treatment of severe cases
TF: 5% to 20%	Mass or individual/ family topical antibiotic treatment	As above
TF: Less than 5%	Individual topical antibiotic treatment	Not indicated

Mass treatment: (all members of all families in the community) tetracycline one per cent eye ointment applied twice daily for six weeks, or as intermittent treatment, with ointment applied twice daily for five consecutive days per month, or daily for 10 consecutive days per month for at least six consecutive months per year.

Family treatment: identify and treat families where there are one or more members with TF or TI; treat the whole family in accordance with one of the topical antibiotic regimens for mass treatment, as above.

Selective systemic antibiotic treatment: identify individuals with TI. Give one of the following:

either	oral tetracyclines: 250mg x four/day for three weeks
or	doxycycline: 100mg daily for three weeks
or	erythromycin: 250mg x four/day for three weeks
or	cotrimethazole: two tablets x two/day for three weeks

Encourage general improvement in family and personal hygiene, especially keeping children's faces clean. General useful measures include mproved water supply, fly control and distribution of antibiotic ointment for cases of acute conjunctivitis with discharge from the eyes.

of Trichiasis Surgeons (584) and environmental risk factors identified by epidemiologic studies. The authors came up with the **SAFE** Strategy including **S**urgery for trichiasis, **A**ntibiotic treatment for active trachoma (tetracycline), **F**ace washing to keep children's faces clean, soon changed to **F**acial cleanliness, and **E**nvironmental improvements that focused on water provision, toilets and general cleanliness leading to fly reduction. The Strategy incorporated the clever acronym, SAFE, although it gave the elements in the reverse order to their public health importance. The acronym EFAS was far less catchy. Fortunately SAFE also translated well into French as CHANCE. The treatment recommendations did not yet include azithromycin (583) (see Table 9.1, Figure 9.10).

In 1996, the WHO convened the first Global Scientific Meeting to review trachoma since 1966 (257). Using available data (in many cases quite out of date), the group identified 47 countries where blinding trachoma was known to exist, 13 countries in which blinding trachoma was suspected, and a further 16 countries plus "some

Pacific Islands" where non-blinding trachoma was suspected. These were distributed in Sub-Saharan Africa, the Middle East and Crescent, Latin America and Asia. In total, 10% of the world's population (or 590 million people) were at risk, with 146 million active cases of trachoma, and 10.6 million people with trichiasis and 5.9 million people who were blind from trachoma.

This group strongly supported the adoption of the SAFE Strategy. It also reviewed newly available results of recent studies with azithromycin and recommended its use in trachoma prevention. This working group declared that the Global Elimination of Trachoma as a Blinding Disease by 2020 was an achievable goal, and called on the WHO to take a lead in developing and co-ordinating international efforts and on member countries to address trachoma.

Following this meeting and after a lot of work, a resolution was adopted by the World Health Assembly in 1998 calling for the Global Elimination of Blinding Trachoma (585). Subsequently blinding trachoma was defined as:

active inflammatory trachoma of a duration and intensity sufficient to cause tarsal conjunctival scarring, which leads to trichiasis and visual loss. Elimination of blinding trachoma in a specific geographical area is achieved and sustained when the prevalence of active inflammatory trachoma is maintained at less than 5% in children aged one to nine years, and no operable cases of trichiasis are left uncorrected in that area (586).

In addition, the WHO Alliance for the Global Elimination of Blinding Trachoma was established to oversee this ambitious program that became known by its own acronym, GET 2020. Since 1997, the Alliance has met annually. It includes country representatives, NGOs, WHO staff and other experts in the field. With representatives from Pfizer it has formed a successful public private partnership. The Alliance has reviewed and guided the progress of trachoma control activities, integrating the results of ongoing operational research and other field studies. To support this work, the WHO and various NGOs developed a suite of manuals and reports (3,127,240,248,584, 586,587,588,589,590,591,592,593,594,595, 596,597,598).

In 1999 the WHO and the International Agency for the Prevention of Blindness (IAPB) jointly launched a new global initiative, "Vision 2020: The Right to Sight" that aims for the global elimination of avoidable blindness by 2020 (57). Vision 2020 has three major strategies: disease control, human resource development and infrastructure and technology development. Five areas have been identified under disease control, one of which is

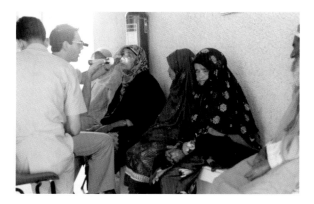

Figure 9.11 Mark Reacher examining patients during his study on trichiasis surgery in Oman (1989).

trachoma, and Vision 2020 has fully adopted the GET 2020 program and the SAFE Strategy. The SAFE Strategy has also been endorsed by the International Council of Ophthalmology and is included in their international clinical guidelines series (599).

The S component: surgery for trichiasis

The surgical technique

The surgical component of the SAFE Strategy was built around the bilamellar tarsal rotation procedure described in the 1993 WHO publication (587).

Mark Reacher, a young British ophthalmologist working in Oman, was confronted by many cases of trichiasis (see Figure 9.11). His review of the literature showed more than 47 different techniques were currently advocated (600). Some were modifications of ancient techniques dating back 100 years, but many had been advocated in the preceding 20 or 30 years. He undertook an initial study examining the five most common procedures with about 30 people in each group (601). Based on the outcomes of this study, he undertook a more definitive study that included people with minor trichiasis (less than five lashes touching the eye), major trichiasis (more than five lashes touching the globe) and those with defective lid closure who had had previous unsuccessful surgery (116). The bilamellar tarsal rotation was clearly the superior procedure for both minor and major trichiasis; at two years 82% of patients with major trichiasis had no recurrence (see Figures 9.12, 9.13, 9.14). In three-quarters of the recurrences, less than five lashes were touching the globe. He also showed that two years after surgery there was a small but significant improvement in visual acuity that averaged half a Snellen line of visual acuity, approximately the same as the overall decreased acuity observed with 10 years of ageing of that cohort. Following bilamellar tarsal rotation, no patients had lid closure defects and only two of 150 had a poor cosmetic result.

Based on these results, bilamellar tarsal rotation became the recommended procedure in the SAFE Strategy (587). In francophone West Africa a

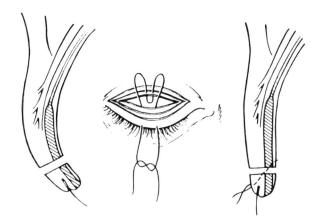

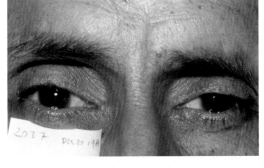

Figure 9.12 Schematic of the bilamellar tarsal rotation (Reacher 1990 (601), reprinted with permission of the BMJ Publishing Group Ltd © 1990).

Figure 9.13 Good result one year after right bilamellar tarsal rotation (courtesy, Mark Reacher).

Figure 9.14 Outcomes of randomised controlled trial of trichiasis surgery (Reacher et al 1992 (116). Reproduced with permission © 1992, American Medical Association. All rights reserved).
RIGHT Kaplan-Meier survival analysis of operative success following surgery for minor trichiasis in lids completing randomly allocated surgery. The relative hazard for electrolysis was 6.1 (95% confidence interval [CI], 2.9 to 12.8); and the relative hazard for cryoablation was 7.5 (95% CI, 3.6 to 15.4)
BELOW RIGHT Kaplan-Meier survival analysis of operative success following surgery for major trichiasis in lids completing randomly allocated surgery. The relative hazard was 3.1 (95% CI, 1.9 to 5.2).

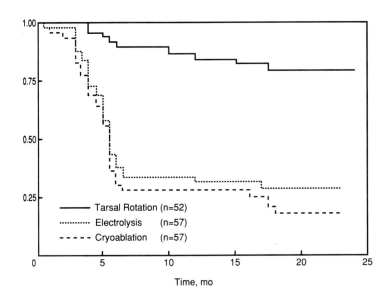

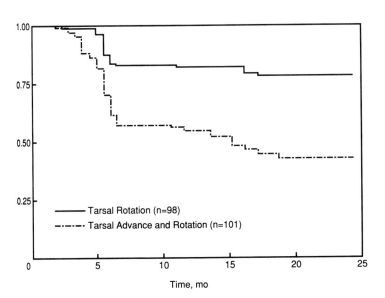

variation, the Trabut procedure, was commonly used, whereas in Vietnam another variation, the Cuenod Nataf procedure was used. Both these procedures had been long established in their ongoing national programs. There was discussion as to whether they should be compared with the bilamellar tarsal rotation in clinical trials. Such comparative trials have not been published, but good one year results have been reported with the Cuenod Nataf procedure (602).

Good results with bilamellar tarsal rotation were reported for Morocco, where 84% were trichiasis free (603). Of the others, 13.4% had minor recurrences and 2.4% had lashes touching the cornea. Most recurrences occurred in the first year after surgery. Overcorrection was seen in 2.3%, 18% reported their vision had improved significantly and 52% reported decreased lacrimation.

The GET 2020 Alliance initially concentrated on the provision of surgical kits and ensuring that surgery was provided at a community level (248). Attention was directed to the importance of training and certification of surgeons and ongoing monitoring and evaluation of the surgical program (592,593). Subsequently, recurrence rates ranging from 15% to 50% were reported and this caused considerable concern (594). Some reported that between 10% to 30% of people who were offered surgery refused (586). With a 50% failure rate this refusal might not be considered unreasonable.

Factors influencing a recurrence of trichiasis

Following reports of quite unacceptably high recurrence rates, a number of specific studies were undertaken to identify why this might occur and what could be done to prevent this. Women usually have higher rates of scarring trichiasis or ongoing exposure to reinfection, so one obvious factor to examine was gender. Although one study found women had a 30% increased risk of recurrence (604), another found a 60% increased risk in men (605). People over the age of 40 had a somewhat high risk of recurrence, although this was not significant (53,604), and those with more severe trichiasis had an approximately three-fold increased risk of recurrence (106,605).

The presence of inflammation at the time of surgery was the major risk and led to a two- to six-fold increased risk of recurrence (106,605). At times this was associated with bacterial conjunctivitis (106,514). The presence of chlamydia on PCR testing did not increase the risk of recurrence (106,604,605), although a small study in Nepal found a significant association (606). Similarly, there was no association with the presence of trachoma in the household (604), although if two or more people had active trachoma there was some increased risk.

Due to the potential importance of ongoing bacterial or chlamydial infection, three studies were undertaken to assess the impact of azithromycin administered at the time of surgery. One study in The Gambia found no effect (106) with a high recurrence rate, 41% at one year. It may be that the surgical technique of the nurses involved was less than optimal, masking the possible impact of the antibiotic treatment. In the study in Ethiopia, the one year recurrence rate was reduced from 10.3% in those who received tetracycline ointment to 6.9% with azithromycin—a statistically significant reduction (605). The final study in Nepal also found a reduction in recurrence with azithromycin treatment of those with major trichiasis, even with an overall rate of recurrence at one year of 29% (607).

These results suggest that the presence of inflammation is an important risk factor for recurrent surgery. Inflammation is more common in those with severe trichiasis and is often associated with chronic bacterial conjunctivitis (515). Chlamydia do not seem to play a significant role in maintaining this inflammation in surgical patients, as there is no change in surgical outcome with PCR detection of chlamydia, or family presence of trachoma (either someone with active trachoma in the family or family-based treatment) (605). Previous histologic studies also failed to demonstrate the presence of chlamydia in the eyes of those having trichiasis surgery, even if they were inflamed (407). It seems likely that the perioperative use of azithromycin exerts an effect on conjunctival bacterial pathogens rather than a specific anti-chlamydial effect.

Another important risk factor for recurrent trichiasis seems to be the surgeon, their level of training and attention to technique. Some studies have shown no significant surgical variation (605) and others have confirmed that excellent surgical results can be obtained by nurses (608,609). However, some studies have shown huge variations in recurrence rates between different surgeons (509,604) and variations in surgical technique (610).

Surgical factors found to be important in influencing the risk of recurrence include the length of the incision, meticulous surgical sterility and attention to suturing (598). Higher recurrence has been observed in the left eye and recurrences are more common temporally in the left eye and nasally in the right eye, consistent with increased difficulty in the accurate placement of sutures by right-handed surgeons (611).

A useful review of trichiasis surgery has recently been completed for the Cochrane database (612). This review has the strengths and weaknesses of the Cochrane evaluation approach but concludes that the bilamellar rotation is probably the best technique.

Despite the outcome of the randomised trial in Oman (116), a number of programs continued to advocate the use of epilation for people with minor trichiasis. Certainly this is a time-honoured procedure widely used by the people themselves, for example, 78% of those presenting for trichiasis surgery used epilation in Ethiopa (513). A study in The Gambia showed that in 12 months one-third of patients with less than five lashes had increased the severity of their trichiasis, and one-third also had progression in corneal scarring (508). Bowman also noted that after surgery patients were twice as likely to show an improvement in vision compared to those who had not been operated upon. Epilation was usually performed by a friend or family member, although one-quarter of the time the individual epilated themselves. Most of the time locally-made forceps were used, but fingers were also used, 20% of patients used hot ash as an adjunct and 20% used traditional eye medicine (see Figures 9.15, 9.16).

A large case control in Ethiopia showed that in eyes with mild entropion (trichiasis) epilation did not reduce the likelihood of corneal opacity (613). However, in eyes with more severe trichiasis, epilation may have reduced the frequency and progression of corneal opacity.

Both studies suggest that people with minor trichiasis should proceed to trichiasis surgery as expeditiously as possible. However, it would seem to make good sense to epilate lashes while patients wait for surgery and epilate any recurrent lashes post surgery. Care must be taken with epilation not to damage the cornea or break the lashes. Broken lashes can be even more damaging than intact lashes rubbing the eye because they often form stiff bristles that rapidly abraid the cornea.

Surgical uptake

Studies have shown that many patients will decline trichiasis surgery. The numbers can vary greatly but may range between 8% to 35% (240). Having surgery performed in the village can increase uptake (614,615) and several studies have shown that women were less likely to have surgery than men. In central Tanzania only 18% of women with trichiasis had had surgery in a two-year period (616). Barriers that prevented these women from having surgery included cost, the provision of care for children left at home and having someone accompany them to a health centre. Of those who had had surgery, two-thirds reported a decrease in pain, a subjective improvement in vision and an improved ability to carry out their activities of daily living. A further study in Vietnam showed that even though the rate of trichiasis was two to six-fold higher in women, the rate of surgery was approximately equal between men and women (333). This was a further indication of gender disequity.

In a study in Malawi, Courtright found that accessibility to surgery and knowledge of other people who have had successful surgery were important indicators of the likelihood of women accepting surgery (617). In Nigeria cost was the main barrier (251). Similar findings come from India where the average duration of symptoms before people came for surgery was 30 months (SD ± 46 months) (618). Unoperated trichiasis has a major impact on quality of life independent of the reduction of visual acuity (619) (see Figure 9.17). It affects physical, psychological and environment domains but not the social relationships domain. After surgery these three affected domains each showed a significant improvement.

An economic analysis in The Gambia found the average cost of untreated trichiasis to the community was US$89 in 1998 (620). Surgery, including

Figure 9.15 Epilation forceps
(1979 and 1990)
RIGHT available from a local
market in Kenya
FAR RIGHT worn around the neck
in Tanzania.

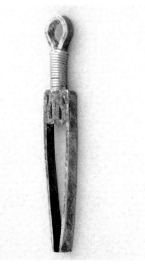

BELOW **Figure 9.16** Epilation
can frequently lead to broken
lashes. These short stubby lashes
can be even more damaging than
the normal inturned lashes.

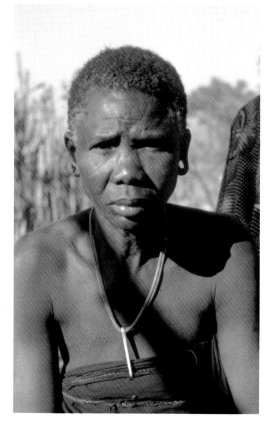

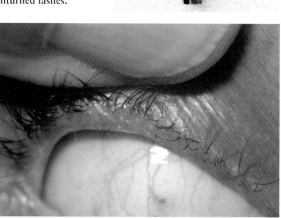

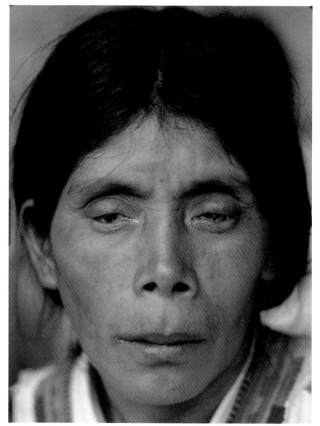

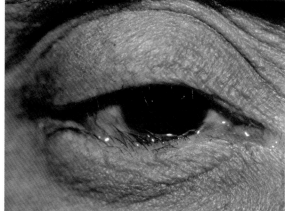

Figure 9.17 A relatively young Mexican woman with
LEFT severe ocular discomfort, reduced vision and
photophobia from quadrilateral trichiasis, and with
ABOVE her right eye also showing broken lashes from
failed epilation.

transport, cost US$6.13 per case and patients' expressed willingness to pay was assessed to be US$1.43. This showed a lack of individual perceived value in trichiasis surgery at a community level.

The way forward

In 2003, the WHO (3) estimated there were 7.6 million people with trichiasis who required surgery. Even the largest current national programs are only making a small impact on the number of trichiasis operations needed. Clearly there is a growing need for trichiasis surgery. Accordingly programs need to boost their capacity and expand their services. The number of people who require trichiasis surgery will continue to increase as the numbers of older people in endemic areas increase (304). A three-fold increase in 30 years has been projected (309). Surgery will be needed long after active trachoma disappears as the last cohorts who had severe active trachoma as children progressively age.

It makes good sense to treat patients who have active conjunctival inflammation at the time of surgery. As much of this inflammation seems to be due to bacterial infection, the use of azithromycin or another convenient antibiotic at the time of surgery is good practice. Surgeons who are trained need to actually undertake the surgery they have been trained to do. The surgical output was examined in 95 surgeons trained in the preceding 10 years and a further 28 trainees could not be located, had died or retired (621). The median trichiasis operations were only seven per year, ranging from 0 for 22 to over 100 for five surgeons. Those surgeons who were linked with outreach activities undertook more surgery. Good supervision and complete surgical kits were important factors for increased output.

There is a tremendous range in surgical outcome with recurrence rates varying from 5% or 6% to 40% in one year. There is an urgent need to ensure that every surgeon is properly trained in both surgical procedure and the use of sterile techniques. The WHO has developed a new publication *Final Assessment of Trichiasis Surgeons* (584) that should improve standardisation and quality of surgery. Clearly the challenge for the foreseeable future is for programs to ensure that quality trichiasis surgery is consistently carried out and strive for recurrence rates below 10%.

Finally, each surgeon should actively monitor patients they have already operated on for the following two reasons. A surgeon should monitor or audit their own surgery to provide important feedback to themselves as a means of quality control. This is basic surgical best practice. Of even more importance, it must be remembered that scarring and trichiasis can be a progressive disease and trichiasis is likely to recur.

Data from Oman would suggest that with a 17 year follow-up, some 47% of patients with mild trichiasis may eventually have recurrence, even when short-term (two year) results are excellent (622). Over half of the unoperated eyes that initially did not have trichiasis also developed trichiasis. This underscores the progressive nature of this disease.

Unfortunately many of those involved in trachoma field programs have been influenced by their experience with the delivery of cataract surgery. On the one hand, modern intra-ocular cataract surgery is a miracle; significant sight can be restored within hours of surgery and the patient, their family and the whole village celebrate this restoration of vision. However this is not the case with trichiasis surgery. Post-operatively the eyelids look funny. Although there may be a statistical improvement in vision and a reduction in the risk of further loss of vision, these indirect future benefits are often not perceived by the patient, their family or community. In contradistinction, the restoration of vision after cataract surgery can be

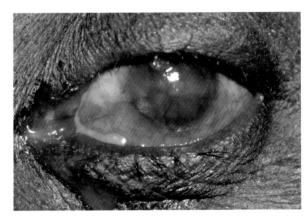

Figure 9.18 Advanced trichiasis and corneal scarring (TT and CO). Lid surgery may make this Tanzanian woman more comfortable but it will not significantly change her vision.

breathtaking and people are lost for words. In addition, by definition, trichiasis surgery is performed in badly scarred and damaged tissue and cannot restore the normal anatomy or function. Negrel has called trichiasis surgery an attempt at "squaring the circle" (53). He sets out the criteria for the ideal procedure as simple and quick; low cost; permanent; effective in terms of function, anatomy and aesthetics; safe; and feasible for paramedical staff to perform in the community setting (see Figure 9.18).

Trichiasis surgery is really a last resort in badly damaged and distorted tissue. Some have suggested that new trichiasis operations should be developed. Many of the cleverest surgeons have tried for over 2000 years to develop new and better surgical techniques. Cataract surgery benefited from the development of anaesthesia, aseptic and microsurgical techniques as has trichiasis surgery. The quantum leap taken by cataract surgery was the development of the intra-ocular lens. I see no such major breakthrough on the near horizon for trichiasis surgery. The way forward seems to be to use the tools and techniques we currently have and extend the coverage and quality of surgery. With trachoma control activities trichiasis should cease to be a public health problem long before a new breakthrough in trichiasis surgery appears.

The A component: antibiotic treatment

In trachoma, antibiotics are used to reduce the level of chlamydial infection and break the cycle of repeated episodes of repeated reinfection. Of course, they will also reduce any concomitant bacterial infection. For whatever reason, a single course of antibiotics may not totally eliminate chlamydia. This is true in trachoma and also in genital tract infection (623,624). It is unclear whether this is due to poor compliance, reinfection, levels of antibiotic lasting less than the slowest replication time, the presence of organisms in a true "persistent" and insensitive state, or the use of antibiotics that are really only bacteriostatic for chlamydia rather than being bacteriocidal. Whatever the reason, 70 years of experience shows that antibiotic treatment needs to be repeated a number of times. If the only change in an endemic area is treatment with antibiotics then once antibiotic distribution has stopped there is nothing to stop the recrudescence of trachoma to its previous levels. There are many examples from Sub-Saharan Africa through the Middle East to Central Australia.

For these reasons, the WHO supported antibiotic treatment with the other three components of the SAFE Strategy to achieve

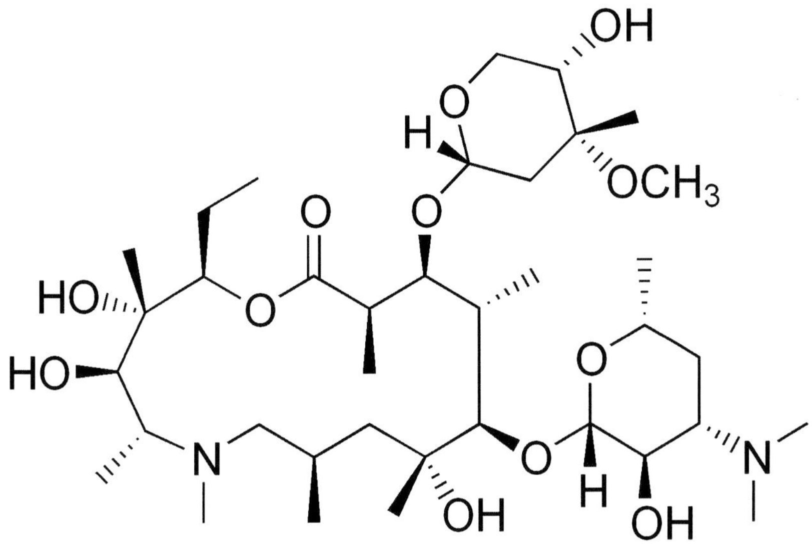

Figure 9.19
Molecular structure of azithromycin.

sustainable trachoma control. When the SAFE Strategy was first promulgated tropical tetracycline was the only realistic option available. However, by the time the Global Alliance first met in 1997, azithromycin had already undergone successful clinical trials against trachoma and its use was recommended (248). In 2004, azithromycin was added to the WHO model list of essential drugs and to the WHO model formulary (597).

Azithromycin and its mechanism of action

Azithromycin was the first member of a new azalide subclass of macrolide antimicrobials derived from erythromycin with a methyl-substituted nitrogen in the lactone ring (625). Azithromycin possesses a broad spectrum of activity against Gram-positive and Gram-negative bacteria and is more effective than other erythromycins against *Haemophilus influenzae* and *Moraxella catarrhalis* (see Figure 9.19).

Azithromycin is effective against chlamydia and binds to the 50S RNA ribosome and so blocks translation of RNA and protein synthesis (625,626). *In vitro*, it prevents the growth of chlamydia at all stages of development (627). Unlike conventional antibiotics that are only effective if introduced to the culture system in the first six hours, azithromycin can block chlamydial replication in cultures up to seven days after infection. Unlike penicillin which blocks the development of chlamydia and leads to persistent infection, azithromycin causes the development of ghost-like particles (627).

Azithromycin has high acid stability and approximately 30% is absorbed. It can easily be taken with food. The assumed half life is greater than 60 hours and it is primarily excreted unaltered through the biliary and faecal routes (625). The mean inhibitory concentration (MIC) for chlamydia is given at 0.125µg per litre.

Early studies in genital tract infection showed that a single dose of azithromycin (1g or 20mg per kg) was effective as a full seven-day course of doxycycline (628). Azithromycin has high tissue selectivity and becomes concentrated in macrophages, polymorphs and epithelial cells (625,629). Intracellular levels are 100 times higher than serum levels. This is especially important given the intracellular growth of chlamydia. Pharmaco-

kinetic studies have shown that serum levels are above the MIC for 24 hours in serum. However, in tears levels they are more than 10 times the MIC and remain above the MIC for at least six days (630). In conjunctival biopsies of uninflamed eyes azithromycin levels far exceed the MIC for at least 15 days (631).

Azithromycin is the treatment recommended by Centers for Disease Control in the USA for chlamydial genital tract infection including in pregnant women (624). Although erythromycin is the recommended treatment for chlamydial infection in infants, the Morbidity & Mortality Weekly Report (MMWR) notes:

> Data on the use of other macrolides (eg. azithromycin and clarithromycin) for the treatment of neonatal chlamydial infection are limited. The results of one study involving a limited number of patients suggest that a short course of azithromycin, 20 mg/kg/day orally, 1 dose daily for 3 days, may be effective (624).

They also point to treatment failure rates of 4% for genital infections and up to 20% in neonates. CDC also recommends azithromycin for the treatment of infants with pertussis in preference to erythromycin (632).

Azithromycin meets the criteria for the ideal drug for trachoma: "A drug that is chlamydicidal, non-toxic and readily administered as a single dose would be ideal for mass treatment" (580). In addition, it also has high intracellular penetration (53). Because azithromycin provides a safe single oral dose treatment, individual diagnosis is not required and its distribution can be integrated into primary health care. However, one must remember that repeated treatment will be required and for a sustainable impact, antibiotic distribution needs to be accompanied by other components of the SAFE Strategy.

Azithromycin is registered for use in the treatment of infections caused by *Staphylococcus aureus*, *Streptococcus pneumoniae*, *H. influenzae*, *Moraxella* and chlamydia that cause community-acquired pneumonia (mild or moderate severity), pharyngitis, tonsillitis, otitis media, skin infection, urethritis, cervicitis and genital ulcers (629). It is contraindicated in those with severe pneumonia and in people with demonstrated hypersensitivity.

There is little interaction with other drugs and there is no need to change its dosage with the concomitant use of other drugs. Importantly, there is no evidence of mutagenicity. It is not teratogenic at maternal toxic doses and teratogenicity has not been reported in over 15 years of human clinical use. A recent study shows no adverse effects of azithromycin treatment during pregnancy on malformations, spontaneous abortion, foetal distress, gestational age or birth weight (633). Although azithromycin has not been tested specifically for safety in children under six months, it has been found to be safe and effective in children over six months. It is listed as a Class B1 drug, which means it can be used in pregnancy when the benefits outweigh the risks associated with being untreated (629).

Adverse reactions are rarely reported with azithromycin and include diarrhoea or nausea in 5% or less, and less frequent reports of vomiting or abdominal pain. Azithromycin has fewer side effects than many oral antibiotics previously used to treat trachoma such as the sulphonamides and tetracyclines (625). This has also been the experience in the field and most studies report few if any side effects (634).

Due to its broad spectrum, especially for Gram-positive organisms, azithromycin also offers the additional advantage of concurrently treating many respiratory, skin and genital infections (635,636). This is often perceived in the community as the

major benefit of mass treatment. The use of systemic medication also leads to the treatment of chlamydial infection in other mucosal surfaces, and this may prevent chlamydial reinfection from autoinoculation (637). Despite the advantages of a single oral dose, azithromycin eye drops have also been developed and are effective in treating bacterial conjunctivitis (638). When used twice a day for three days they are as effective against trachoma as a single oral dose (639).

Field trials with azithromycin

The first three trials of azithromycin treatment in trachoma compared the drug against topical tetracycline ointment (203,640,641,642). Although Gambian and Saudi studies examined the effect of a single dose, the study in Egypt also examined three repeat doses at weekly intervals and six doses at monthly intervals. These studies showed that azithromycin treatment was as effective as topical tetracycline (see Figure 9.20). No advantage was seen with multiple doses of azithromycin. Both of these studies treated individual selected children. No treatment was given to other family members and so there was no control for the possibility of reinfection. Both studies assessed clinical disease and the presence of infection in conjunctival smears, and both showed a more dramatic decrease in the presence of chlamydia and a slower decrease in the reduction of clinical trachoma.

A subsequent multi-centred trial was conducted

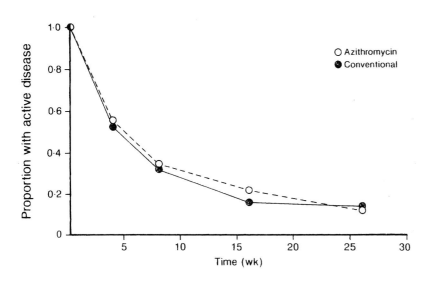

Figure 9.20 The decrease in clinical signs of trachoma seen in The Gambia following a single oral dose of azithromycin compared to a six-week course of "conventional therapy" (topical tetracycline and erythromycin for severe cases) (Bailey et al 1993 (203). Reprinted from The Lancet, Vol 342, Bailey RL, Arrullendran P, Mabey DCW, Whittle HC. Randomised controlled trial of single-dose azithromycin in treatment of trachoma, 453–6, © (1993), with permission from Elsevier).

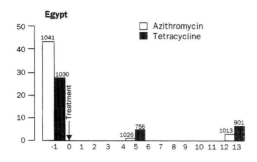

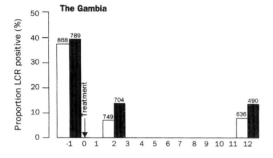

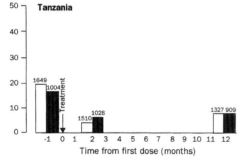

Rates of *C trachomatis* infection in the conjunctiva, by country and by treatment group, before, at first follow-up, and at 1 year after treatment

Figure 9.21 The results of the ACT Study. Rates of C. *trachomatis* infection in the conjunctiva, by country and by treatment group, before, at first follow-up and one year after treatment (Schachter et al 1999 (221). Reprinted from The Lancet, Vol 354, Schachter J, West SK, Mabey D, Dawson CR, Bobo L, Bailey R, Vitale S, Quinn TC, Sheta A, Sallam S, Mkocha H, Mabey D, Faal H. Azithromycin in control of trachoma, 630–5, © (1999), with permission from Elsevier).

in Egypt, Tanzania and The Gambia, the Azithromycin Control of Trachoma (ACT) study (221). This trial randomised villages to receive either community-wide distribution of oral azithromycin with three doses given one week apart, or topical tetracycline daily for six weeks. In the azithromycin villages women of childbearing age were treated with either erythromycin or amoxicillin for two weeks. Compliance was reported to be over 90% except for tetracycline treatment in Egypt. Clinically active trachoma was reduced more effectively by azithromycin than topical tetracycline at three and 12 months. Infection as determined by LCR was also reduced more effectively by azithromycin in each of the three countries at three months. A detailed analysis of clinical trachoma was not presented, although the overall amount of trachoma in each area was reduced by about half at one year, and the prevalence of severe inflammation was reduced to one-third or one-sixth of pre-treatment levels. This study analysis was based on LCR positivity, but interpretation of these results is hampered because in two study sites 30% of children without disease were LCR positive. In the third site the rate was 1.8%. This strongly suggests the possibility of false positivities or specimen contamination at two sites and this would significantly reduce the ability to determine the effect of a treatment (see Figure 9.21).

A 10 year follow-up of Egyptian villages in the ACT study showed a marked reduction in trachoma in all three villages irrespective of treatment allocation (643). This was attributed to socioeconomic development. The household clustering of disease was noted to be even more obvious as rates declined, emphasising the need for family-based treatment.

A Cochrane Review has been undertaken looking at the impact of antibiotic treatment on trachoma (642). It included some 15 studies dating back to 1966, half of which had been completed before 1973. This study concluded that "there is some evidence that antibiotics reduce active trachoma but results are not consistent and cannot be pooled" (642). Selected studies were "consistent with there being no effect of antibiotics but are suggestive of a lowering of the point prevalence of relative risk of both active disease and laboratory evidence of infection at three and 12 months after treatment". Further, this analysis suggested that oral treatment was neither more nor less effective than topical treatment.

The Cochrane Collaboration brings great strength by the rigorous assessment of prospective randomised controlled trials and uses openly disclosed criteria. This provides a firm evidence base of efficacy. However, the rigorous criteria and procedures of a Cochrane Review have strengths and weaknesses (644,645,646). Since the Review, four large cohort studies have been reported, each showing a decrease in the prevalence of active trachoma and infection following community-wide treatment. Several other cohort studies were excluded from consideration in the Cochrane Review. The Review neither assesses the method of identifying and treating individuals, nor the possibility of study subjects being exposed to continuing episodes of reinfection. Students who are starting the school year in a boarding school, for example, are removed from the family pool of infection. The interpretation of placebo-controlled studies using these students is therefore difficult. Similarly, treating individual school-age children who continue to live at home is difficult because these children are likely to have falling rates of trachoma, although they still may be exposed to reinfection at home. Studies of "mass treatment"

that do not treat children less than one year or six months leave untreated significant sources for reinfection within the family.

The design of antibiotic trials needs to reflect that trachoma is "a disease of the crèche". This means it is the family unit that should be treated, not the individual. Another corollary of this is that community-based studies may not be necessary to evaluate the impact of antibiotic treatment, as the unit of transmission is the family, not the community. The study of families instead of villages or communities would greatly simplify the design of future studies. Currently studies usually randomise a relatively small number of villages. They end up with a very large study but still with only limited statistical power. If families were used, one could randomise a much larger number of families which would both decrease the size and complexity of the study and greatly increase its statistical power.

A cohort study in the mesoendemic Rombo district of northern Tanzania showed a striking reduction in infection (226). At baseline the prevalence of active trachoma was 20% and rates of active disease at each of the follow-up examinations were approximately half the baseline prevalence. Each age group of children showed a marked initial drop and then some variation. Trachoma was graded using the simplified grading

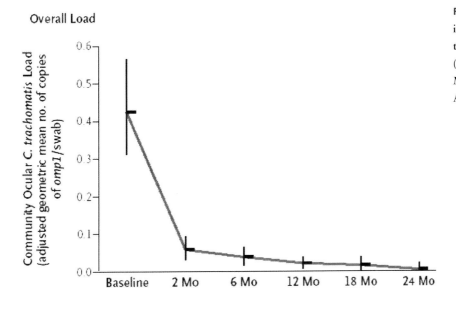

Figure 9.22 Community load of infection determined by PCR over time in the Rombo Study (Solomon 2004 (226) © (2004) Massachusetts Medical Society. All rights reserved).

scheme, but information is not given as to how this was carried out in the field, nor the steps taken to control observer variation or bias. Most of the data analysis was based on PCR including quantitative PCR. There was dramatic and progressive reduction in infectious load after treatment so at two years only one child was still positive by PCR, whereas 91 people had been PCR positive prior to treatment (see Figure 9.22).

In this study all those over the age of 12 months were offered azithromycin. Children under the age of 12 months and pregnant women were given tetracycline ointment for six weeks. Treatment coverage was quite extraordinary at 97.6%. Importantly, in addition at each re-examination round, any person found to have active clinical disease at any exam was given a further course of tetracycline ointment. This study did not actually examine the impact of a single dose of azithromycin, but rather azithromycin supplemented by six monthly retreatment of any active trachoma with topical tetracycline. This study has been misinterpreted by some to show that a single oral dose of azithromycin can eliminate infection. Even though there was extraordinarily good compliance with the initial round of treatment, infection was not eliminated and a significant number of children were retreated every six months. The results could be used to support the efficacy of retreatment every six months with either tetracycline or azithromycin. Significantly, this study did not implement any of the other components of the SAFE Strategy.

A report at five years showed no residual infection in one to nine-year-old children in Rombo and rates of TF had finally fallen (647). The community had been retreated with azithromycin at 24 months, although no further tetracycline had been distributed. It was suggested that transmission of chlamydia had dropped below the critical threshold required to sustain episodes of reinfection, the so-called "Allee effect".

Another cohort study in a hyperendemic area in central Tanzania is interpreted quite differently to show that a single dose of azithromycin does not eliminate infection (122). Unlike Rombo, follow-up treatment was not given. This study aimed to treat everybody over the age of six months with azithromycin. Children under six months were not

treated and pregnant women who did not have clinical disease were given topical tetracycline or otherwise they received azithromycin. Overall, the coverage rate was 86%. Baseline prevalence of trachoma in children under the age of 10 years can be calculated as 72%, although data are not presented on the impact of treatment on clinical disease in the initial report. However, at baseline, 57% of participants had chlamydia demonstrated by PCR and this was reduced to 12% at two months. Most of the residual load was in individuals under the age of 10 (122). Further study of this village showed that the prevalence of clinical trachoma in children aged one to seven years had dropped from 77% at baseline to 47% at 12 months, but returned to 57% at 18 months. The percentage of those who were laboratory positive in this age group went from 68% at baseline and stayed around 21% at 2, 6, 12 and 18 months (299). Another report on this study uses slightly different age ranges (298).

Other cohort studies are reported from Ethiopia. One study of 24 villages treated all residents one year and older with azithromycin, pregnant women were offered tetracycline ointment, but children under the age of one apparently were not treated (526). The coverage was 92% of those who were eligible. Follow-up data on clinical grading were not given. The PCR positivity was 56% at baseline, it dropped to 7% at two months and had risen to 11% at six months. Another study published after the Cochrane Review examined eight villages that had been treated and a further 15 untreated villages that served as a non-concurrent control (648). Again clinical data were not given and there was a change in the technique used to collect samples for PCR testing between the baseline examination and the 12 month examination of treated villages, which coincided with the baseline examination of control villages. The treated villages showed a decrease from a mean level of infection of 44% before treatment to 5% at two months, with a modest recrudescence to 7% at 12 months, and 11% at 24 months. In one of the eight villages infection seemed to have disappeared. The control villages showed what was attributed to a strong "secular trend" as their baseline infection rate was only 17%. The change in collection techniques between the two "baseline" collections may have accounted for some of this difference. These studies concluded that a single dose of azithromycin was not enough to eliminate trachoma. In the absence of the other components of the SAFE Strategy or the more frequent use of antibiotic, trachoma would return over a 24 month period. They also showed that infection with trachoma can increase from very low levels. Mathematical modelling suggested that in this area treatment should be repeated every six months (526).

An earlier study of Ethiopian children under 12 months of age who had not been treated and children born after azithromycin distribution showed a significant reduced risk of infection six months after the treatment round (648). In Tanzania no evidence could be found for a protected cohort effect, although after two rounds of treatment given 18 months apart, levels of infection and clinical trachoma were lower in pre-schoolchildren than in the initial cohort (649).

A cohort study was also undertaken in a hypoendemic area in The Gambia where 14 villages were studied (238). The baseline prevalence of active disease was 8% and 7% showed infection with PCR. Everybody over the age of six months was treated, children under six months were given tetracycline ointment and women of child-bearing age were given oral erythromycin for two weeks. Thus antibiotic coverage was 83%. The results were variable with a poor response in two villages attributed to a large number of village residents travelling on a pilgrimage. However, in 12 of the 14 villages the initial mean prevalence of infection fell from 3% to 0.3%. The other two villages had a baseline infection rate of 24% and at 17 months had dropped to 11%. These data suggest that in hypoendemic areas a single dose of azithromycin can have a long lasting effect in the absence of other intervention, although persisting infection was seen especially in younger children who had high loads of infection. In houses with low levels of infection or relatively good hygiene a single dose of azithromycin may eliminate infection, but repeated treatment will be needed where there is a high pressure of reinfection amongst young children.

Another cohort study in Nepal compared the treatment of all children aged one to 10 years with the targeted treatment of the whole family of those children with active trachoma (650). For family treatment, children over the age of six months were treated with azithromycin and pregnant women were offered either erythromycin or tetracycline. The prevalence of trachoma at baseline was 29% and coverage was 95%. No difference was seen between the two treatment strategies and the rates of trachoma approximately halved in each group. LCR testing was also performed but these data were not presented. Other studies have reported the use of azithromycin in selected subgroups, usually schoolchildren and sometimes their families (310, 651). However, the outcomes of these studies are difficult to interpret because of study design issues.

Antibiotic resistance

To date, *C. trachomatis* has not developed acquired resistance to any antibiotic that has been used on a large scale to treat chlamydial infection. These drugs include sulphas that have been in use for 70 years, tetracycline and erythromycin for about 50 years and azithromycin for 15 years. There is a single report in the literature of three isolates of multiple drug resistant *C. trachomatis* for genital swabs (652). Although chlamydia have a plasmid, because of its unique replication cycle, the horizontal exchange of antimicrobial resistance factors is not seen as an issue (653). Some strains of *C. suis* are naturally resistant to tetracycline. Gene insertion techniques indicated that this resistance is conferred by novel resistance genes contained in apparent plasmids that are integrated into the chlamydial chromosome (654).

Concern has been expressed rightly about the possibility of other bacteria becoming resistant to azithromycin. Erythromycin-resistant Gram-positive organisms show cross resistance to azithromycin (625) but despite the extensive use of erythromycin over many years, only limited and sporadic outbreaks of bacterial resistance to erythromycin amongst previously sensitive organisms are evident. The prolonged tissue levels of azithromycin reduce the likelihood of the induction of bacterial resistance following incomplete treatment courses, although it will always favour the selection of pre-existing resistant strains (655). The development of resistance of ocular bacteria to tetracycline was not seen to be an issue after its topical use, although the disappearance of *Moraxella* was noted (656).

Table 9.2: Nasopharyngeal carriage of S. pneumoniae: frequency and proportion of azithromycin (AZM)-resistant strains before and after treatment with AZM for trachoma (658)

	No. of children examined	Total no. (%) S. pneumoniae positive children	Azithromycin-resistant S. pneumoniae		
			No. of children colonised*	Frequency (% of children examined)†	Proportion (% of carriers)'
Before treatment	79	54 (68)	1	1.3	1.9
After treatment 2–3 weeks	38	11 (29)	6	15.8	54.5
2 months	37	29 (78)	10	27.0	34.5
6 months	39	34 (87)	2	5.1	5.9

* Tendency for pneumococcal carriage rate to fall and then rise after treatment: $\chi^2_2 = 13.3$, P < .001.

† Tendency for frequency of resistant pneumococci to rise and then fall after treatment: $\chi^2_2 = 18.9$, P < .001.

' Tendency for the proportion of resistant pneumococci to rise and then fall after treatment: $\chi^2_2 = 22.4$, P < .001.

In The Gambia a significant reduction in *S. pneumoniae* carriage in the oropharynx was noted after oral treatment with azithromycin (657). There was no change in *H. influenzae* frequency and a lesser effect was seen with tetracycline.

An important study was reported from a community in Central Australia where there was a significant reduction in the nasopharyngeal carriage of *S. pneumoniae* two months after azithromycin treatment, although at six months carriage had rebounded (658). Before treatment only one of 54 isolates of *S. pneumoniae* was azithromycin-resistant. Two weeks after treatment, six of 11 isolates were resistant, at two months 10 of 29 and at six months two of 34 (see Table 9.2). The selective effect of azithromycin appeared to allow the growth and transmission of pre-existing azithromycin resistant strains and further surveillance of this effect was strongly recommended. However, there was a significant reduction in invasive *S. pneumoniae* serotypes present at baseline and recolonisation occurred with different serotypes. A subsequent report from the same community found colonisation rates of Group A streptococci had dropped markedly two weeks after treatment but had returned to pre-treatment levels by two months (636). Azithromycin resistance was not seen. At two and six months, the rate of skin sores was halved with treatment (see Figure 9.23). Similar reductions in skin infections and in diarrhoea have also been reported from Nepal (635).

No resistance to *S. pneumoniae* was found before azithromycin treatment in Nepal, but three of seven strains isolated two weeks after treatment were resistant (659). Two of these strains came from children who had had azithromycin-sensitive *S. pneumoniae* at baseline. A subsequent study examined nasopharyngeal isolates one year after azithromycin treatment and showed no residual resistance (660).

A recent report from the Kimberley region in Western Australia shows the continuing sensitivity of *S. pneumoniae* to penicillin, the recommended first line therapy (661). In this area azithromycin is routinely used as the initial treatment for people with suspected sexually transmitted infection and their partners. Azithromycin resistance of *S. pneumoniae* does not seem to be a real issue as azithromycin is not recommended or used to treat *S. pneumoniae* infections (662).

Although there is a global system of monitoring bacterial resistance to azithromycin (593), data from trachoma areas are more restricted. Data are also collected in Australia, but they are not specifically analysed for areas in which azithromycin distribution has taken place (663). In these studies, as elsewhere, resistance to erythromycin is taken to represent resistance to azithromycin (664). Overall, resistance rates of *S. pneumoniae* have increased from 8% in 1994 to 23% in 2005 (see Figure 9.24).

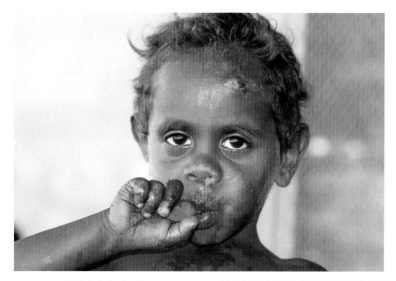

Figure 9.23 A skin infection in Aboriginal child
ABOVE impetigo on the forehead and a dirty face
RIGHT infected scabies (courtesy, Heathcote Wright).

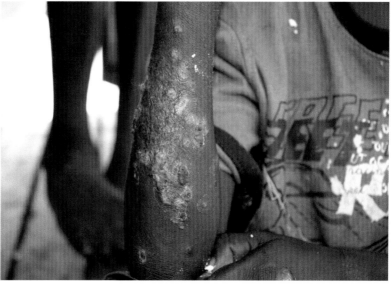

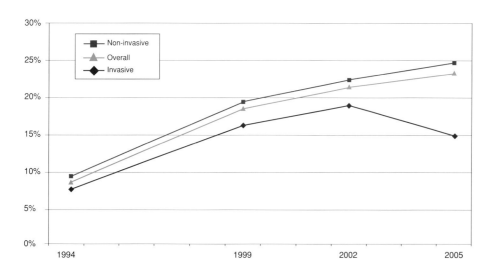

Figure 9.24 Erythromyin resistance in Australia 1994–2005 (663) (reproduced with permission from the Australian Group on Antimicrobial Resistance (AGAR)).

Tom Lietman and colleagues examined overall antibiotic usage in a village in Nepal (665). One-third of children under three years of age and half the children under 10 had taken antibiotics in the preceding year. Two-thirds of these antibiotics were effective against chlamydia. Children received on average 3.0 defined daily doses of antibiotic effective against chlamydia each year. The annual mass distribution of azithromycin would increase this by 2.6.

Recrudescence of infection

The WHO recommendation for the use of antibiotic as part of the SAFE Strategy is to "initially conduct mass treatment with antibiotic preferably azithromycin for a minimum of three years and not stopping until TF in one to nine-year-old children is less than 5%" (3). If the prevalence of TF is more than 5%, mass treatment should continue with subsequent surveys repeated every one to three years as indicated. If the prevalence is less than 5%, individual or family-based treatment should be considered. The intent of these recommendations is to give guidance to develop more effective and efficient programs.
It is explicit that A (antibiotic treatment) is an integral part of the full SAFE strategy.

Despite these recommendations and almost without exception, the studies quoted so far have assessed antibiotic treatment in isolation and have not included the other components of the SAFE Strategy. Facial cleanliness and environmental components are designed to reduce the likelihood of ongoing reinfection and give a sustainable reduction in trachoma. Without these components to reduce the possibility of transmission, trachoma would be expected to soon reappear after antibiotic treatment.

In a hyperendemic area in Ethiopia the astounding, exponential rate of return of infection of 12.3% per month has been observed (526). In this study children under the age of one were not treated and pregnant women were only treated with topical tetracycline. In another hyperendemic area in central Tanzania, infection levels were initially reduced to quite low levels, but started to increase gradually from two months and accelerated after 12 months (298). Incident infection at six months was 3.5 times more likely if another member of the household was also

infected. The risk was not increased by travel, visitors, gender, or whether the individual had been treated. Re-emergent or recrudescent infection occurred within the family. Further analysis using spatial distribution confirmed the household clustering of infection, and only after 12 months spread from one household to another was noticed (299).

The persistence of chlamydial ocular infection after antibiotic treatment in the absence of obvious reinfection has been reported. For example, 32% of neonates who had been treated with both topical tetracycline and oral erythromycin for two weeks had chlamydia recultured in pharyngeal swabs (623). The nasopharyngeal carriage of chlamydia in children with trachoma did not seem to cause infection after treatment in one study in Tanzania (326), although a more recent study in three sites has suggested infected nasal secretions may play a more important role (328).

An unexpected potential complication of antibiotic treatment comes from observing the number of notifications of chlamydial sexually transmitted diseases in British Columbia (666). Brunham has noted an apparent increase in infection and reinfection after an infection control program based on early case identification and treatment had been introduced. He has postulated that early treatment may prevent the development of full protective immunity which would leave the person more susceptible to subsequent reinfection. Some support for this notion comes from animal experiments that show that mice treated within the first three days of inoculation will clear the infection without time to develop the normal partial immunity to rechallenge (667). Therefore on rechallenge they behaved essentially as naïve mice. However, it is unclear whether any human disease management program could identify and treat patients with genital tract infection within three days of inoculation. Others have reported a significant change in the frequency of positive reports following a change in chlamydial testing and have cautioned about the over-interpretation of these trends (668).

When the transmission of trachoma has been reduced, a fall in the intensity of the infection is noticed first, followed by a decrease in the incidence of new infection, and finally a reduction in the prevalence of inactive disease. There has been no suggestion from these trachoma endemic communities of the type of rebound phenomenon inferred by Brunham with one recent exception (666).

In late 2006, a report from Vietnam presented the three-year findings of trachoma control in three intervention villages; one village had S, another S, A and F and the third had S, A, F and E (669). The authors reported a four-fold increased rate of infection detected by PCR in the two villages where azithromycin had been distributed for two years compared to the third village where topical tetracycline had been used. They conclude that "the increasing reinfection rates suggest that treatment may interrupt the duration of infection required for developing immunity, increasing the number of individuals susceptible to reinfection and adversely affecting disease prevalence over time"(669). In other words azithromycin treatment (combined with S and F in both villages and E in one) made trachoma worse. This unusual finding stimulated considerable press and email traffic. Editorials (670) and letters to the editor (671,672) pointed out some of the methodologic weaknesses of this study and analysis. They included questions about the diagnostic accuracy of both PCR testing and clinical grading, the highest prevalence of infection (21%) was in the older age group where there was little active disease (4%) and the prevalence of infection was similar in those with and without disease. The question of contamination of PCR specimens comes up again. The poor overall coverage of antibiotic treatment resulting from the targeting of schoolchildren resulted in the treatment of only 11% with infection (PCR positive) and less than half with active disease. The study villages all have low prevalences of trachoma (<5%), there was only one village in each group and baseline inter-village variances were not analysed. Furthermore, no measures of the immune response were made which makes their inference speculative. It will be most interesting if such exceptional findings can be repeated by other, well-designed and carefully conducted studies.

The next steps

Despite 15 years of trials with azithromycin and tens of millions of doses distributed, there are some major questions about the distribution of azithromycin that need to be addressed, even if one takes a somewhat less acerbic view than the

Cochrane Review (642). There are at least six major issues to be resolved:

1 Who to treat? (what about infants and pregnant women?).

2 How to treat? (family- or community-based).

3 Why treat? (a prevalence >10%, >5% or <5%).

4 When to treat? (six or 12 monthly).

5 What to treat? (infection, clinical disease, blinding trachoma).

6 When to stop? (what test to use and what prevalence?).

Clearly these answers need to be ascertained in areas where F and E components also have been implemented.

1. Who to treat?

Several studies with quantitative PCR (168,122, 227) have confirmed earlier observations (92) that the highest levels of infectious organisms are found in the youngest children, particularly those with intense active disease. In fact, much of this infection is in children under the age of one year. As already noted, many studies have not treated children under the age of one, and almost none have treated children less than six months, even though CDC recommends the use of azithromycin for the treatment of chlamydial infection and pertussis in infants in the first six months of life (624,632). This would seem to be a major gap in our current protocols for the distribution of azithromycin. To leave untreated the family-based infantile fountains of infection seems to me to be totally counter-intuitive.

Equally, a strong case can be made for treating all women with azithromycin rather than relying on their possible use of tetracycline or the complexity of a two-week course of erythromycin or amoxicillin. The WHO noted that azithromycin is a Class B1 drug for which there is no evidence of adverse effects on the foetus, although there is insufficient data to specifically recommend its use in pregnancy except in the absence of adequate

Table 9.3: Estimating Zithromax requirements (588)

	Tablets	Paediatric oral suspension /ml	mg/treatment
Adults	4		1000
Children >35 kg	4		1000
Children 25–35kg	3		750
Children 17–25kg	2		500
Children 15–20kg		10ml	400
Children 10–15kg		7.5ml	300
Children 7–10kg		5ml	200

One bottle POS = four children (under five years of age)
One case POS/48 bottles = 192 children
One bottle tablets = seven adults or 11 children aged five years or over
One case tablets/48 bottles = 360 adults or 528 children

Table 9.4: Standardised height-based treatment schedule for children aged six months to 15 years receiving azithromycin for the treatment of trachoma (674)

Height (cm)	Dose
Children aged six to 59 months receiving oral suspension	
50.6–53.7	80mg (2ml)
53.8–65.4	160mg (4ml)
65.5–76.4	240mg (6ml)
76.5–87.4	320mg (8ml)
87.5–98.3	400mg (10ml)
98.4–110.2	480mg (12ml)
110.3–122.2	560mg (14ml)
122.3–130.0	640mg (16ml)
Children aged six months to 15 years receiving tablets	
74.0–87.8	250mg (one tablet)
87.9–120.3	500mg (two tablets)
120.4–137.6	750mg (three tablets)
≥137.7	1000mg (four tablets)

alternatives (596,633). However, CDC does recommend azithromycin for the treatment of genital chlamydial infection in pregnancy (624). Pregnant women, especially those with other young children with active trachoma, must also be a potent source of potential reinfection within the family. They are also likely to have extraocular infection that may place their unborn baby at considerable risk. A single oral dose of azithromycin makes good sense.

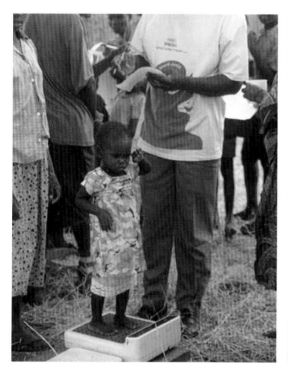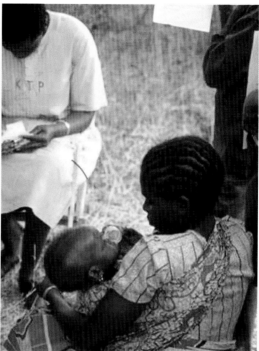

Figure 9.25 Distributing azithromycin (courtesy, Sheila West)
LEFT a child being weighed during azithromycin distribution in Tanzania
RIGHT the suspension being delivered.

2. How to treat?

The importance of family-based transmission of trachoma has been made repeatedly. This also leads to the corollary of the importance of family-based treatment. The recommendation to treat the whole community when prevalence levels are high (>5% or 10%) is really made on logistic grounds; it is cheaper and easier to go ahead and organise a mass treatment of the whole community rather than try to examine and treat every family individually. However, this does not mean that future treatment studies cannot take the family as the treatment unit. It has been clearly shown to be the transmission unit and the source of re-emergence of infection (298,526).

The use of weight-adjusted dose of suspension for young children (20mg/kg) initially required each child to be weighed. Borrowing from an idea used successfully with the distribution of ivermectin to treat onchocerciasis (673), a height-adjusted schedule was also introduced for azithromycin (674) (see Tables 9.3, 9.4, Figure 9.25).

Again borrowing from the experience of ivermectin distribution was the use of community directed treatment (675). Earlier experience in trachoma control activities in South Africa (676) and Tanzania have used community volunteers to distribute antibiotics successfully (677,678). Successful community-based treatment of ivermectin requires community ownership and support of community leaders (679). Coverage was related to the ratio of distributors to people to be treated; two per 250 seemed optimal. Better performance (coverage) was seen when direct incentives (cash or in-kind compensation) were not given. Volunteer distributors seemed to be motivated by political goodwill, personal satisfaction and altruistic fulfilment.

The WHO has set a target coverage of 80% for azithromycin distribution (3). Some studies have reported much higher coverage (221,226) and others have reported lower rates (310,650). Clearly coverage is important and likely to be lower in programmatic activities (680). A meta analysis of treatment impact by coverage suggested a greater impact at six months with coverage over 90%, but this difference was not observed at 12 months (681).

3. Why treat?

The threshold suggested by the WHO for the mass treatment of trachoma has been set at 10% for logistic reasons as it is thought to be cheaper and more efficient to treat the whole community rather than individual families at prevalences of greater than 10%. The initial suggestion of using 20% as the threshold came from programs that used topical tetracycline. However, field experience with azithromycin from large programs in Morocco and Mali suggested 10% was a more appropriate threshold for azithromycin distribution for logistic and cost reasons.

It is important to remember that the thresholds suggested or recommended by the WHO are broad indicators to provide guidance. Often they are misinterpreted to say one must not treat (anybody) if the prevalence of active trachoma is less than 10%, or that after three years one can just walk away, or that three years is the longest any area would ever need to be treated. Both of these positions are clearly wrong.

One of the issues that arises with prevalence thresholds is the definition of the denominator, or base population for whom prevalence is determined. This has been set at the "community" which may typically be 1000 to 5000 individuals in Africa (3,598). This community or village should be the smallest population grouping for whom mass treatment would be given. When prevalence is less than 5% it may not be appropriate to continue community-based mass distribution for a range of reasons. However, it would seem to be both highly appropriate and ethical to continue family-based treatment. Certainly any families that have children with intense disease, or two children or more with active disease, should be given family-based treatment. Remember that trachoma control programs in the UK and the USA were continued until every last case of active trachoma had disappeared. They were not prepared to accept rates of active trachoma of 5%, or even 1%, in *their* children.

4. When to treat?

The rate of recrudescence of infection seems to be linked to the starting prevalence of active trachoma. An argument can well be made for the use of six-monthly retreatment in areas of high endemicity (greater than 50%) (513,682,683). In meso- and hypoendemic areas single antibiotic treatment may be adequate, although success in Rombo was based on ongoing selective repeat treatment every six months (226). Interestingly, the risk of having active trachoma six months after

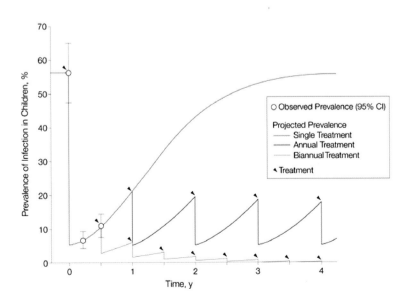

Figure 9.26 Mathematical projections of trachoma prevalence derived from empirical pre-treatment, two- and six-month post treatment results (Melese et al 2004 (526). Reproduced with permission © 2004, American Medical Association. All rights reserved).

azithromycin distribution was significantly reduced (odds ratio 0.3) if the child had actually been treated (649). This effect had disappeared at one year (odds ratio 1.18). This also suggests that repeat treatment every six months may be more appropriate than annual treatment. An interesting modelling analysis using Ethiopian data suggests that to be maximally effective annual antibiotic treatment should be given three months before the "low" season (684). Based on modelling their trachoma data, Lietman has clearly stated "single mass treatment will not eliminate trachoma" (682) (see Figure 9.26).

5. What to treat? and 6. When to stop?

The ultimate objective of trachoma control is clearly the elimination of blinding trachoma. Also the prevalence of active trachoma, particularly TF in children, is a relatively slow indicator to change, particularly if there is any ongoing reinfection. All treatment studies that have measured TI rates have found they will fall much more rapidly than TF. The difficulty with the grading of TI is the problem of over diagnosis (see chapter three). However, it may be that TI should be the clinical indicator used to assess the shorter term efficacy of interventions because it is more sensitive to change than TF and will change more quickly. Also TI is a better indicator of disease severity and the likelihood of scarring and blindness. Proper standardisation of graders and probably the use of photo documentation will be required to increase the precision of this critical sign.

The alternative promoted by many is to use laboratory tests as the indication of the presence of chlamydial infection and thereby trachoma (202,258). Although laboratory tests have been widely used in clinical trials, added expense (685) and technical complexity have been barriers to their widespread use in programmatic activities (206). If they were to be used one might select an indicator group, such as children under the age of one, as a way of monitoring the load of infection in a community. An alternative to NAAT testing might be the newly developed "dip stick" EIA test (205). This may prove a cheap and easy field-friendly laboratory test and the results of the further evaluation of this new test are anticipated with interest. However, the programmatic costs of even the cheapest tests can become significant when

repeated thousands or millions of times.

To help guide the distribution of azithromycin the WHO prepared a manual *Trachoma Control, A Guide for Program Managers* (127) that goes to some lengths to present the method of assessing the requirements for azithromycin and the process of its distribution. This complements an earlier publication by the International Trachoma Initiative (588).

The F component: facial cleanliness

Although facial cleanliness is seen as the critical, final common pathway by which a variety of environmental factors affect the risk of trachoma, facial cleanliness is the component of the SAFE Strategy that has received the least attention. In part this may be because it does require a behavioural change and these are not necessarily easy to induce. It is much easier to drive in, bore a well, or tell people to take a pill, or even build a pit latrine and drive out again. Behavioural change can be hard to achieve and may need prolonged local involvement, but in the end, this is what is needed. As Fred Hollows would have said "It is a hearts and minds job".

An interesting and fundamentally significant change in personal hygiene in western culture has been the adoption of toilet paper (686). Before the 1800s the use of paper was virtually unknown. Specially manufactured toilet paper first appeared in 1857 and by 1900 it was in general use. This dramatic change occurred in the absence of any overt or co-ordinated public health education campaign. What was required was health "hardware". The increased provision of indoor plumbing, for example, was associated with the increased use of toilet paper. In this case, the "software" came naturally.

Many programs that have included facial cleanliness, or the F component, have also included the other components of the SAFE Strategy, and they will be reviewed in the last section of this chapter. In this section, I want to review the evidence that specifically supports the notion of the importance of increasing facial cleanliness.

Several early studies in Australian Aboriginal children that encouraged face washing at school have been mentioned previously (365,578), and a

Table 9.5: Odds of trachoma at one year for children in intervention villages compared with control villages (393)

	Odds ratio (95% CI) for severe trachoma (TI)	Odds ratio (95% CI) for any trachoma (TF/I)
Intervention village	0.62 (0.40–0.97)	0.81 (0.42–1.59)
Age	0.76 (0.68–0.85)	0.85 (0.80–0.90)
Trachoma at baseline*	5.21 (3.51–7.74)	5.07 (3.26–7.84)
Cattle	–	1.62 (1.22–2.15)

*Trachoma of the relevant category

Table 9.6: Effect of sustained facial cleanliness on trachoma in children at one year (393)

	Odds ratio (95% CI) for severe trachoma (TI)	Odds ratio (95% CI) for any trachoma (TF/I)
Sustained facial cleanliness	0.35 (0.21–0.59)	0.58 (0.47–0.72)
Age	0.81 (0.72–0.91)	0.89 (0.82–0.96)
Trachoma at baseline	4.74 (3.28–6.83)	4.69 (2.91–7.57)
Intervention	0.59 (0.38–0.91)	–
Cattle	–	1.45 (1.04–2.03)

similar study was reported from Ethiopia (687). Enforced face washing at school, with or without antibiotic treatment, decreased the amount of trachoma in schoolchildren over one year. A larger study of schoolchildren in 36 Aboriginal communities used a factorial design to assess tetracycline drops and face washing. This incomplete study did not find a change in the rate of trachoma in schoolchildren at three months (688) and was limited by its very short follow-up.

The landmark, randomised control trial on facial cleanliness was undertaken in central Tanzania (393). All members of each village were to receive topical tetracycline daily for 30 days. Three intervention villages were randomly selected to have an additional program focusing on facial cleanliness in children. At the end of 12 months, the proportion of sustained clean faces (on two or more visits) had increased by more than 60% in the intervention villages. The prevalence of intense active trachoma (TI) was reduced by 38% (odds ratio 0.62, 95% CI 0.40–0.97) in all children in intervention villages irrespective of whether or not their face was clean (see Table 9.5). The effect on TF was similar but less marked (0.81, 0.42–1.59). More importantly, in children with sustained clean

faces the rate of active trachoma was reduced by 42% (0.52, 0.47–0.73) and the rate of intense trachoma was reduced by 65% (0.35, 0.21–0.59) (see Table 9.6). It must be remembered that this effect of facial cleanliness was additional to the already significant impact of the community-wide antibiotic treatment in all villages. Again, the more marked reduction in severe disease (TI) before the reduction in milder (TF) disease is noted (see Figure 9.27).

Two studies have been recently published evaluating the additional effect of health education to the distribution of azithromycin. In Ethiopia, 40 villages were randomised into four groups (689). All villages received radio health education messages. Three groups of villages also received azithromycin distribution and "NGO activities". In one of these groups, printed information, education and communication (IEC) materials were distributed and in another group of villages, the IEC package was supplemented with a video prepared by the BBC World Service Trust. The NGO activities included specific attention to face washing and environmental improvements and these were further emphasised in radio and video messages. The starting prevalence of active

Figure 9.27 Health promotion activities in the Kongwa clean face study included
(a) meetings with women and men
(b) play acting to demonstrate face washing
(c) and (d) examples of face washing
(courtesy, Sheila West).

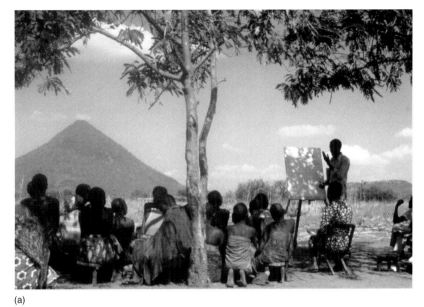

(a)

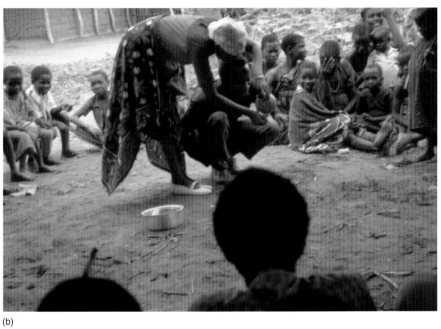

(b)

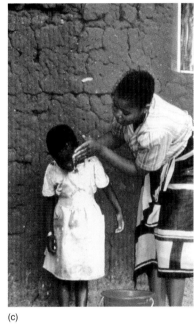

(c)

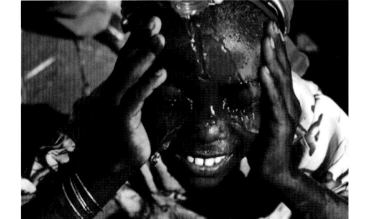

(d)

trachoma in these villages ranged between 64% and 72% and at one year prevalence was between 22% and 24%. There was no significant difference in trachoma rates between the different intervention villages, but there was a marked increase in knowledge about trachoma and eye health, although the change in behaviour was less marked. This study suggests that even more intense, grassroots intervention may be required to influence health behaviour.

The other behavioural study that took place in Vietnam (334) compared two villages that both received S and A components, but the intervention village also had a major program of health education and the provision of health hardware. Over 250 houses were provided with latrines, bathrooms, wells and water tanks. Data on facial cleanliness were not reported. The prevalence of active trachoma in children in the "control village" dropped from 10.2% to 5.5% at one year and 13.8% to 2.3% in the intervention village. These findings support the notion that improved hygiene and facial education are beneficial, although with only two sites, other interpretations are also possible.

Ethnographic studies in Tanzania have shown that mothers tend to overestimate the amount of water necessary to wash a child's face, and that they were not able to change their water use priorities without the consent of their husbands and the support of the community (368). This implied a health education program would need to address misperceptions about the quantity of water required, and also address the community as a whole, rather than focus solely on the women. McCauley recounts how, when given a gourd with a litre of water, the men estimated they could wash one or two faces, but found they could actually wash 12. The women thought they could wash five or six faces, but actually washed between 30 and 35 faces with one litre of water. McCauley goes on to say "When women learn that the men had been able to wash fewer faces they commented that men were always less careful with water than the women who had to carry it" (368). The components required for a health education program were subsequently developed (690) and used in the clinical trial of facial cleanliness (393).

The WHO and members of the Global Alliance have prepared several useful background booklets dealing with F and E components of the SAFE Strategy (127,589,590).

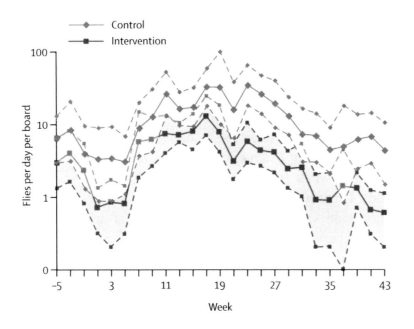

Figure 9.28 Mean fly counts by time in intervention and control balozi in Central Tanzania (West et al 2006 (391). Reprinted from The Lancet, Vol 368, West SK, Emerson PM, Mkocha H, Mchiwa W, Munoz B, Bailey R, Mabey D. Intensive insecticide spraying for fly control after mass antibiotic treatment for trachoma in a hyperendemic setting: a randomised trial, 596–600 © (2006), with permission from Elsevier.)

The E component: environmental improvement

The E component covers a very broad category of potential activities, and in some ways is the most difficult component of the SAFE Strategy to comprehend and define. The WHO has produced several booklets mentioned above that provide more detail in this area, but most field and programmatic work is focused on the provision of latrines, fly control or the provision of water.

Several studies on fly control have been undertaken in The Gambia. In the initial study, two pairs of villages were randomised for one to receive deltamethrim ultra-low-volume spraying to control flies (691). At three months, the number of eye-seeking flies (*Musca sorbens*) had been reduced by 75%, and this was associated with a 75% reduction in the expected seasonal increase in the number of new cases of trachoma. A larger study followed and involved seven triplets of villages randomised to receive fly control, the provision of new latrines, or no additional activities (374). Individuals with intense trachoma were treated with either tetracycline or azithromycin. After six months the number of *M. sorbens* on children's faces had decreased by 88% with fly control and

30% in the villages with new latrines. At six months, the prevalence of trachoma in children in the fly control villages fell from 14% to 7%, in the latrine villages from 11% to 8% and increased in the control villages from 9% to 10%. Subsequently Emerson showed that the installation of a Gambian Improved Household Latrine could dramatically reduce the number of *M. sorbens* (373) and new latrines were usually well received (692).

However, a recent large study in a hyperendemic area in Tanzania did not support the added importance of fly control to azithromycin distribution (391). In a prospective study, 16 neighbourhoods (balozi) were randomised to have intensive fly control for 12 months. Azithromycin treatment was given to all residents in these neighbourhoods. Although intervention significantly reduced fly counts, in the intervention villages, there was no significant difference between groups of villages in either clinical trachoma or infection rates determined by PCR (see Table 9.7). This study strongly suggests that intensive insecticide spraying to reduce flies gave no added benefit over community-based azithromycin treatment (see Figure 9.28).

An Ethiopian study showed that mass

Table 9.7: Baseline characteristics of children in fly spray intervention and control neighbourhoods (balozi) (391)

	Intervention	Control
No. of balozi	8	8
Mean percentage of children surveyed	82	86
Mean percentage of children who are female	52	45
Mean age of sentinel children (years)	3.4	3.5
Mean number of children aged 1–7 years per household	2.0	2.2
Mean percentage of TF, TI, or both	63	68
Mean percentage of chlamydia infection	29	35
Mean percentage receiving azithromycin treatment	84	94
Mean number of flies per board per day	2.3	3.9

TF= trachomatous inflammation (follicular)

TI = trachomatous inflammation (intense)

azithromycin treatment greatly reduced the frequency with which chlamydial DNA could be detected in flies (378). One year after treatment 23% of flies from untreated villages were PCR positive compared to 0.3% in treated villages. There was a strong correlation between the PCR positivity rates in children and flies.

A health education study in Mali used a factorial design and found that weekly health education sessions in addition to topical tetracycline treatment led to a significant reduction in the six month incidence of trachoma: 4.2% versus 7.6% (693). The Cochrane Review on this subject concluded that insecticide spray could significantly reduce trachoma, although the provision of latrines did not (694). They also concluded that health education may be effective in reducing trachoma.

A rather unusual attempt at environmental improvement has occurred recently in Western Australia. Under a program of "shared responsibility agreements" with indigenous communities, the Australian Government committed to provide a petrol pump (gasoline bowser) (695). In exchange, the people in the community agreed to keep their children's faces clean and undertake a range of other environmental activities to reduce trachoma and skin infection (670). After some 18 months, the petrol tank had not been installed, nor had the rate of trachoma dropped. There are no data available on the prevalence of facial cleanliness. Subsequently, the Australian Government has made a renewed commitment to review its approach to trachoma and new guidelines have been released that incorporate a more comprehensive approach to trachoma control (696).

The SAFE Strategy and the next steps

The first reports assessing the effectiveness of implementation of the complete SAFE Strategy with all four components have finally been published. The first was a review of the activities conducted under the sponsorship of the International Trachoma Initiative and was purely concerned with process indicators (697). An evaluation was undertaken in Ethiopia, Ghana, Mali, Morocco, Nepal, Niger, Tanzania and Vietnam. In Morocco, the full SAFE Strategy was being implemented across all endemic areas, but in the other countries only a small proportion of the endemic communities were included.

In most countries, only small numbers of trichiasis surgeries were being performed. There were usually enough trichiasis surgeons, but the output per surgeon was low due to both community and provider barriers. In most instances, the evaluation of surgical outcome was inadequate. The mass distribution of azithromycin was usually well done and coverage exceeded 80% in most areas. The review reported variation in distribution policies regarding the treatment of women and young children.

The impact of a facial cleanliness and health promotion program was much more variable and often led to superficial knowledge rather than behavioural change. Environmental activities were also difficult and required strong linkage with other collaborators such as government agencies and NGOs. Unfortunately, no effort was made to evaluate the impact of these activities on trachoma rates as such.

The three-year evaluation of the implementation of the full SAFE Strategy in southern Sudan showed a much more encouraging picture (680). The progress in four areas was reviewed. Surgical coverage was low in all four areas (0.5% to 6%) and obviously needed further work. Antibiotic coverage was relatively high in three of the four areas with 87% to 94% of houses that reported receiving at least one of three annual doses. These areas also had a high recall of the facial cleanliness messages (72% to 90%). Two areas had reasonable access to water, although latrine ownership was low (3% to 16%) across all four areas (see Table 9.8, Figure 9.29).

The two areas with a good uptake of antibiotic, facial cleanliness and access to water had a marked increase in facial cleanliness and a dramatic reduction in active trachoma (TF). The changes in facial cleanliness were less marked in the other two communities, as were the changes in TF. The prevalence of TI was dramatically reduced in three areas with good antibiotic coverage and facial cleanliness recall.

These results are very encouraging and although this evaluation of an ongoing intervention program lacks the precision of a formal clinical trial, it has given very encouraging results in a real world

Table 9.8: Uptake of SAFE components and trachoma status at baseline and after three years in southern Sudan (680)

	Area 1	Area 2	Area 3	Area 4
Surgery uptake	6%	5%	0.5%	3%
Antibiotic coverage*	35%	92%	94%	87%
Health education*	49%	90%	72%	76%
Water < 30 min*	64%	19%	43%	39%
Latrine*	4%	6%	16%	3%
TF/I+				
Baseline	81%	68%	52%	74%
Three year	73%	43%	4%	6%
Decrease	10%	37%	92%	92%
TI+				
Baseline	55%	59%	21%	40%
Three year	36%	6%	0.5%	0.2%
Decrease	35%	90%	98%	100%
Unclean Face				
Baseline	61%	80%	31%	45%
Three year	55%	67%	4%	28%
Decrease	10%	16%	87%	38%

* Household
+ Children 1–9 years

situation. It will be most interesting to see if these findings can be replicated in other regions.

The full SAFE Strategy was also implemented in an area in southern Zambia (698) and new wells were provided in 26 villages. Roxithromycin was used instead of azithromycin due to differences in cost. Five doses were administered to each person with the intent to treat the entire community. Patients were screened for trichiasis and referred for surgery as required. Health education messages included facial cleanliness and fly control by cleaning villages and penning livestock. Latrines were dug as required. After two years, the prevalence of trachoma in children under the age of 10 had dropped from 55% to 11%. The number of new cases of active trachoma declined markedly. There was no documentation of the uptake of interventions or changes in parameters such as facial cleanliness. Nevertheless, this study also shows an impressive reduction in trachoma prevalence with the implementation of the full SAFE Strategy.

Two studies of the SAFE Strategy have been reported from Central Australia. One by Ewald was a longitudinal study in a single community (699) and the other study by Lansingh compared the impact of A, F and E in one community and A and F in the other (700). In each community surgical services were already available. The first study showed a modest reduction in the prevalence of active trachoma over the course of intervention, changes in environmental conditions were minimal and the number of houses with completely adequate health hardware facilities increased from 0% to 16% (699).

The second study is interesting, although limited in statistical power with only two participating communities (700). In both communities, azithromycin coverage was high and out of a

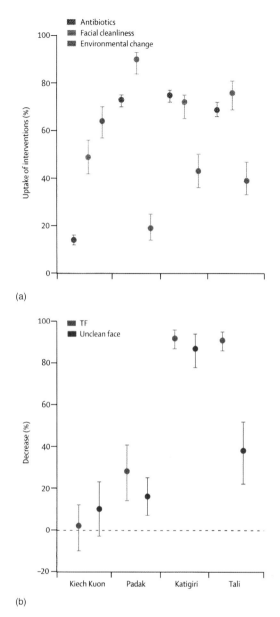

(a)

(b)

Figure 9.29 Outcome of three years of SAFE Strategy intervention in southern Sudan (Ngondi 2006 (680)) (a) uptake of antibiotics, facial cleanliness, and environmental change interventions, and (b) percentage decrease in TF and unclean face in children aged one to nine years in the four intervention areas (reprinted from The Lancet, Vol 368, Ngondi J, Onsarigo A, Matthews F, Reacher M, Brayne C, Baba S, Solomon AW, Zingeser J, Emerson PM. Effect of three years of SAFE (surgery, antibiotics, facial cleanliness and environmental change) Strategy for trachoma control in southern Sudan: a cross sectional study, 589–95, © (2006), with permission from Elsevier).

combined population of 403, only one infant was known not to have been treated. An active health education campaign emphasising facial cleanliness had been instituted in the schools and radio clips, a poster (front cover) and storyboards were developed. Facial cleanliness rates improved dramatically.

In one community, a comprehensive program of environmental improvement was undertaken (700). Sixteen of 22 houses in Community 1 were earmarked for upgrades in areas related to the nine healthy living practices outlined in the National Indigenous Housing Guide. Briefly, these practices include washing people; washing clothes and bedding; removing waste safely; improving nutrition; reducing crowding; reducing negative contact between people and animals, vermin or insects; reducing the negative impact of dust; controlling the temperature of the living environment; and reducing trauma around the house and living environment. Environmental interventions consisted of road sealing; demolition of poorly built or maintained houses, and erection of appropriately designed houses; bi-weekly trash collection; repair of heating/cooling systems; upgrades in sewerage and water lines; installation of rainwater tanks; house yard fences bordering roads, planting of trees, grass, and native plants in areas where wind and dust were prevalent; earthworks and diversions to create micro-catchments and water ponding; and installation of drinking water fountains in the school and health clinic. These measures were intended to reduce the dust and fly population, and promote appropriate water use and disposal. In total, these improvements cost about A$1.25 million.

The rates of active trachoma (TF) dropped in both communities at three months from 48% and 50% to 21% and 24% respectively and increased to 24% and 30% at 12 months. There was no significant difference between the two communities (see Figure 9.30).

Two conclusions can be suggested from these findings. To control trachoma in these areas, more sustained effort is required, possibly treating a larger area to reduce the impact of "migration", retreating every six months and certainly continuing A and F for longer periods. Despite the extensive and expensive efforts to improve E, the environmental improvements made no discernable

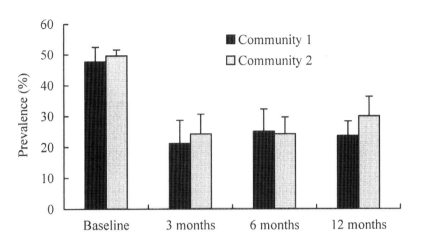

Figure 9.30 Prevalence of TF in children aged <15 years in Aboriginal communities before and after intervention (redrawn from Lansingh 2005 (700)).

difference to the rate of active trachoma over the duration of this study.

In addition to these published reports of the success of the SAFE Strategy, the WHO and the Global Alliance have also reviewed annual reports from countries implementing trachoma control activities. In April 2006, 36 of 46 countries thought to have endemic trachoma had activities underway and in almost half, Ultimate Intervention Goals (UIG) had been set (598). Particularly impressive were the achievements in Morocco (597) where over 10 years, rates of trachoma in children had dropped from in excess of 80% to between 0.2% and 8%. Trichiasis rates in women had also fallen dramatically as a result of a very large and committed program that operated in the five endemic provinces for 10 years. The program started with pilot projects in each province and included all four components of the SAFE Strategy spread to cover endemic areas in each of the provinces. Programs were also implemented for women's literacy, school rehabilitation, road development, income generation and local community development. Although the trachoma program had well-focused national advocacy, it built a decentralised administration with grassroots ownership. In addition to the SAFE strategies, other development programs were implemented for women's literacy, school rehabilitation, road development, income generation and local community development. In just over 10 years, Morocco is now close to achieving the goals of GET 2020 with the elimination of blinding trachoma as a public health problem. Mass

treatment ceased in 2006. Equally impressive progress is being made in Iran, Mali and Oman with the development of large national programs (598). It is proposed that active trachoma may be eliminated as a public health problem from The Gambia, Iran and Oman in 2007; China, Ghana, Myanmar and Nepal in 2010; and Cambodia, Niger, Pakistan and Senegal in 2015.

Interesting insights about the relative cost of the different components of the SAFE Strategy come from Ghana (240). They estimated that the S component would cost some US$600,000, the A component US$850,000, the F component US$800,000 and the E component US$22.5 million. The huge cost for E activities reflects the enormous infrastructure costs in the provision of water and sewerage—10 times more than the others combined! This is similar to the disproportionate cost of E in the Australian study quoted above. With a more precise focus on facial cleanliness rather than the universal provision of new wells and latrines it is quite likely that the resources required for the E component could be substantially reduced. In addition, the provision of these basic services is an essential component of rural development and other partners, both government and non-government organisations, are more likely to assist. This development is clearly linked to Millennium Development Goal 7. Those involved with trachoma control activities need to encourage development agencies to build these activities into their work and prioritise trachoma areas for development activities.

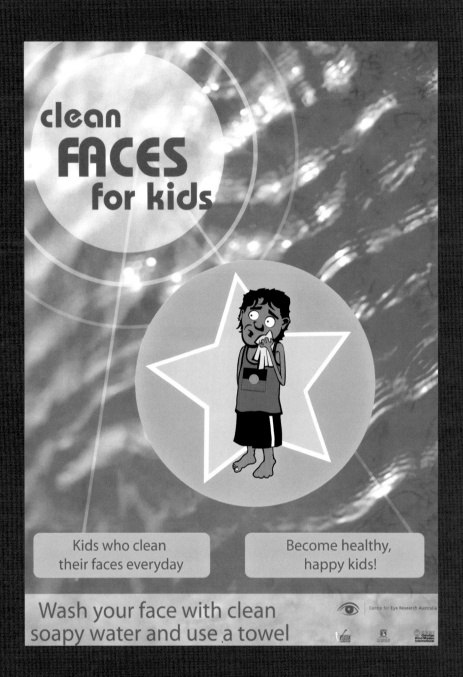

CHAPTER TEN

Will trachoma disappear before we eliminate it?

Trachoma is a public health problem of the highest importance
and too much consideration cannot be given to its control

JOHN McMULLEN, 1913

What is the Problem?

IT IS HARD to tell how many people have trachoma, how many people need treatment and how many people need trichiasis surgery. From time to time the WHO has made estimates on the number of people suffering from active trachoma (33,59,102,107,575,701). Although the best available data are used, there are often large gaps in the data and great variation in data quality. However, as can be seen, there has been a dramatic reduction in the estimated number of people with active trachoma since 1981 when 500 million people were thought to be affected (see Figure 10.1). The most current estimate in 2003 was 84 million (3). There has also been a marked drop in the amount of blindness attributable to trachoma. The 1981 estimate was six to seven million whereas the estimate in 2003 was 1.6 million (3,702).

When assessing the data in 2003, the WHO Scientific Group revised the list of endemic countries to include 56. Several had been excluded as more recent data showed blinding trachoma was no longer a public health problem. To further refine the estimates provincial or district level data were used where possible. For countries for whom data were not available, prevalence data from similar countries were applied to the rural population. The current estimated numbers are shown in Table 10.1 (3). Global data were used also to develop maps of the distribution of trachoma (see Figure 2.7) (62).

Some have noted that each time a WHO Scientific Group reviews the numbers of people with trachoma, the numbers have declined. This has led to the rueful suggestion that if these WHO groups met more often, trachoma could be eliminated quite quickly.

Global Magnitude of Active Trachoma

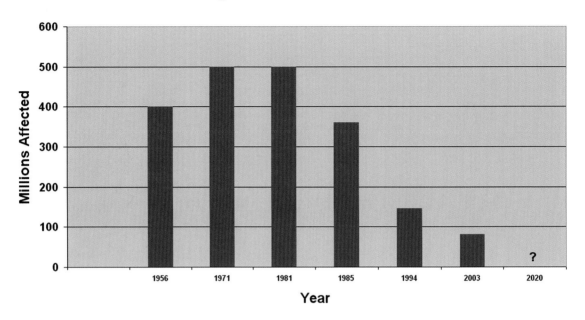

Figure 10.1 Sequence of WHO meetings on trachoma and WHO
estimates of the total number of people with active trachoma since 1956.

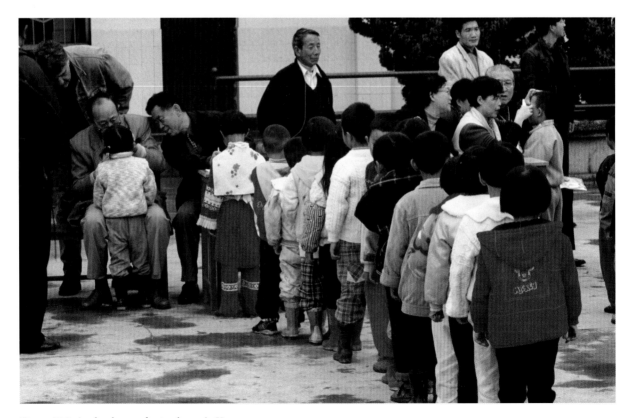

Figure 10.2 A school exam for trachoma in Yunnan
Province (China 1999).

TABLE 10.1: Regional and Global Burden of Trachoma, WHO, 2003 (3)

WHO REGION	Population estimates year 2000 UN Demographic Services	Population living in specifically designated endemic areas	TF/TI cases all ages (% of total)	TT cases all ages (% of total)
AFR	485,784,687	236,202,330	24,559,043 (29)	2,297,247 (30.2)
EMR	420,731,490	175,383,205	9,788,816 (11.5)	1,715,007 (22.5)
SEAR	1,079,726,212	745,002,385	20,791,760 (24.5)	336,517 (4.4)
WPR	1,404,434,386	688,897,001	28,601,516 (33.7)	3,236,310 (42.5)
AMR	181,789,829	268,689	1,066,467 (1.3)	26,952 (0.4)
Total	**3,572,466,604**	**1,845,753,609**	**84,807,602**	**7,612,034**

Data for the two largest countries, China and India, show a high degree of uncertainty. Good quality recent data were not available, and the 2003 estimates were based on some very small recent surveys and historical data. As these countries have such huge populations, even a small change in prevalence makes a great difference in the estimated number of people affected. In China some 27 million people are estimated to have active trachoma, nearly one-third of the world's total. A series of surveys and studies to refine these estimates are underway (see Figure 10.2). It was estimated that 1.14 million people in India had trachoma, although this number also needs to be refined and some have suggested that trachoma may no longer be a problem in India. Informal reports from both countries suggest rates of active trachoma are now quite low and confined to smallish pockets, although scarring and trichiasis remain significant problems especially in China.

The secular trend

Others have drawn attention to the gradual and progressive decrease in the global numbers of people with trachoma, and have recognised this as a "secular trend" associated with a general improvement in living conditions associated with socioeconomic development (703). These non-specific changes led to the disappearance of

trachoma in western Europe and North America by the middle of the 20th century (74,91) (see also chapter two for more detailed discussion). Similar changes have been reported from a number of other areas that have shown rapid development such as Taiwan (94), India (535), Saudi Arabia (704) and Vietnam (334), and from areas with less obvious development such as Papua New Guinea (705), The Gambia (346), Malawi (706) and Nepal (707).

It is worth dwelling for a moment on the factors that may have contributed to this secular trend that has led to a tipping of the balance so that trachoma has slowly disappeared. Obvious factors to consider include the broad range of improvements in domiciliary and urban hygiene; piped water, good sewage systems, garbage collection and fly reduction or protection; the reduction of close contact with animals, whether cattle in a rural context, or horses in an urban setting as they were replaced by cars. Paved roads and dust reduction also contribute and electrification resulted in improved housing. The separation of bedrooms from living and cooking areas, less crowding in bedrooms and less children sharing beds (reduced family size and heating will have both contributed), adequate hot water and indoor bathrooms. Education, especially maternal education with a non-specific emphasis on hygiene, will also have

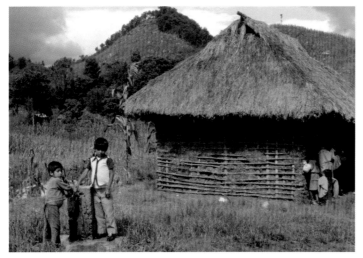

Figure 10.3 The secular trend of decreasing trachoma with socioeconomic development
LEFT piped water in a mountain top village in Chiapas (1985)
BELOW LEFT the arrival of both piped water and electricity in a village in Vietnam (2002)
BELOW RIGHT road building in the mountains of Ethiopia (2007) (courtesy, Tom Lietman).

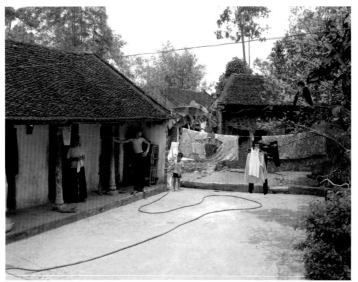

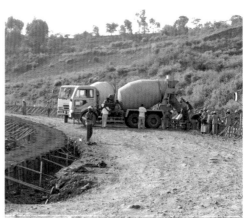

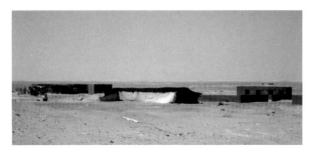

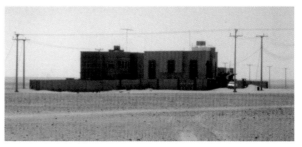

Figure 10.4 The disappearance of trachoma in Saudi Arabia (1990)
ABOVE LEFT Bedouin living in a traditional tent on the outskirts of town
ABOVE RIGHT newly constructed cement block house with reticulated water, electricity, air conditioning
RIGHT Al Sommer examining a recently rehoused Bedouin child. Within two years of rehousing, active trachoma had essentially disappeared.

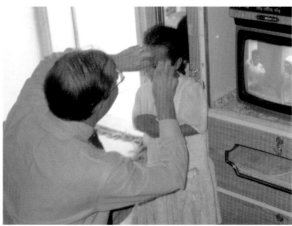

contributed. These potential changes can only have had an effect on trachoma by reducing the ease or frequency of transmission. To my mind, the final common pathway here again revolves around facial cleanliness and factors that influence this (see also chapter six and Figures 10.3, 10.4).

To those changes associated with general socioeconomic development the introduction of antimicrobial agents must be added. In 1949, Lindner wrote "A few years ago trachoma was one of the most serious diseases of the eye. That this is no longer the case is due to the sulfonamides" (560). Their use was credited also with the final elimination of trachoma in both the UK (65) and the USA (6). Others have drawn attention to the effect on trachoma of the widespread use of antibiotics prescribed for other purposes. Lietman and his group in Nepal have demonstrated the annual "background" use of antibiotics with antichlamydial activity is almost equivalent to an annual round of mass treatment with azithromycin (708,709). Computer models suggest that a threshold level of antibiotic use may reduce transmission rates sufficiently for trachoma to eventually disappear (the so-called "Allee effect") (710,711).

Given all this, if we sat and waited long enough, it is most probable that trachoma would eventually disappear on its own as development slowly creeps to the last of the impoverished villages with hyperendemic blinding trachoma. However, as the Alma-Ata Declaration of 1978 says "Gross inequities in health status (are) politically, socially and economically unacceptable" (55). This sentiment was reiterated in the World Health Assembly Resolution on Trachoma in 1998 (585) (see Table 10.2).

More recently Dr Silvio Mariotti, the WHO Co-ordinator of the Global Alliance GET 2020, has pointedly asked "But can the international community afford to wait for the promised economic development while millions more people needlessly become blind from trachoma? The answer is certainly no" (685).

However, even if it were possible to eliminate active trachoma today, there is still the generation of children who currently have active trachoma and their older brothers and sisters, who already have sufficient scarring to put them at high risk of

trichiasis and blindness. Estimates have suggested that the number of people with trichiasis in Egypt may double or even treble over a 20 to 30 year period due to changing demographics (304,309). It is quite clear that even after active trachoma disappears, ongoing surveillance for trichiasis and the provision of corrective surgery will be required for a long time. China and Vietnam are other good examples. Certainly in the 1960s the rates of lacrymal surgery in St Louis were said to be twice those of the rest of the United States because of the residual effects of previous trachoma.

Economic drivers

As early as 1951, economic arguments have been used to promote trachoma control activities. Nataf pointed out that "the control of trachoma and infectious eye disease is relatively inexpensive compared with the benefit derived by the country", although he lacked firm evidence to support this claim (52). Initial estimates of the global burden of trachoma were compromised by uncertainty around estimates of the number of people affected (712,713). Using the 2003 estimates, a more refined analysis suggested that the total costs of trachoma were likely to be US$5.3 billion in 2003 dollars (348). This calculation of productivity loss took into account the impact of blindness and low vision. The presence of trichiasis alone, before it causes vision loss, is also associated with a substantial function limitation and disability that is quantitatively similar to that seen from vision loss itself (714). When trichiasis and vision loss occur together the disability is further increased. If the disability associated with trichiasis was also included, the estimate of total costs of trachoma would increase by another 50% to almost US$8 billion. However, even these estimates may be far too low as they do not fully take into account all the indirect costs and costs attributable to the loss of well-being (or "burden of disease") (715).

Frick points out that countries with blinding endemic trachoma are approximately 1.6 times more likely to be poor, that is, have an annual average value added per agricultural worker of less than US$1000 per year in 1998 compared to countries that did not have trachoma (348). This

TABLE 10.2: World Health Assembly Resolution on Trachoma, WHA 51.11, 1998 (585)

WHA51.11 Global elimination of blinding trachoma

The Fifty-first World Health Assembly,

Recalling resolutions WHA22.29, WHA25.55 and WHA28.54 on the prevention of blindness, and WHA45.10 on disability prevention and rehabilitation;

Aware of previous efforts and progress made in the global fight against infectious eye diseases, in particular trachoma;

Noting that blinding trachoma still constitutes a serious public health problem amongst the poorest populations in 46 endemic countries;

Concerned that there are at present some 146 million active cases of the disease, mainly among children and women and that, in addition, almost six million people are blind or visually disabled as a result of trachoma;

Recognizing the need for sustainable community-based action – including surgery for inturned eyelids, antibiotics use, facial cleanliness and environmental improvement (the SAFE strategy) – for the elimination of blinding trachoma in the remaining endemic countries;

Encouraged by recent progress towards simplified assessment and enhanced management of the disease, including large-scale preventive measures, particularly for vulnerable groups;

Noting with satisfaction the recent establishment of the WHO alliance for the global elimination of trachoma, comprising certain collaborating nongovernmental organizations and foundations and other interested parties

1.CALLS ON Member States:

(1) to apply the new methods for the rapid assessment and mapping of blinding trachoma in the remaining endemic areas;

(2) to implement, as required, the strategy – including surgery for inturned eyelids, antibiotics use, facial cleanliness and environmental improvement (the SAFE strategy) – for the elimination of blinding trachoma;

(3) to collaborate in the WHO alliance for the global elimination of trachoma and its network of interested parties for the global coordination of action and specific support;

(4) to consider all possible intersectoral approaches for community development in endemic areas, particularly for greater access to clean water and basic sanitation for the populations concerned;

2.REQUESTS the Director-General:

(1) to intensify the cooperation needed for the elimination of blinding trachoma with Member States in which the disease is endemic;

(2) further to refine the components of the SAFE strategy for trachoma elimination, particularly through operational research, and by considering potential antibiotic or other treatment schemes for safe large-scale application;

(3) to strengthen interagency collaboration, particularly with UNICEF and the World Bank, for the mobilization of the necessary global support;

(4) to facilitate the mobilization of extrabudgetary funds;

(5) to report on progress, as appropriate, to the Executive Board and the Health Assembly.

(Tenth plenary meeting, 16 May 1998 – Committee A, fourth report)

again emphasises the inverse linkage between a productive economy and the prevalence of blinding trachoma, although it does not indicate cause or effect.

Trichiasis surgery has been shown to be highly cost effective. In Myanmar the surgical correction of trichiasis cost $10 per Handicap Adjusted Life Year (HALY) (716). In The Gambia, trichiasis surgery was associated with a total lifetime productivity gain of US$89 using 1998 dollars (714). Further analysis using international dollars showed trichiasis surgery cost I$13 per Disability Adjusted Life Year (DALY) and if 80% of those with trichiasis were to have corrective surgery the

savings would be 11 million DALY per year (717). Again, these figures are indicative but they do not take into account the full cost of vision loss on the one hand, or long-term efficacy of trichiasis surgery on the other.

Modelling of the cost of azithromycin distribution showed that mass distribution was more cost effective than targeted household treatment (718). The overall cost benefit outcome of the distribution of azithromycin was very dependent on the cost of the drug itself and on the distribution process (348). Frick also modelled the effect of the price of azithromycin on the cost-effectiveness of the distribution program. With azithromycin tablets and suspension priced at the listed value (I$7.50 per pill and I$29.51 for the suspension), mass treatment in Africa would cost I$9.01 per DALY. If azithromycin were available at current generic prices (pills I$0.47 and suspension I$1.84), it would cost I$4.24 per DALY (717). Using the donated drug, treatment became even more cost-effective at I$3.92 per DALY, although the distribution costs remain significant. The mass treatment of 80% of the children with active trachoma would save some 4 million DALY per year (717). A study in Tanzania showed that although two-thirds were prepared to pay at least something for azithromycin, one-third would not (719). This resistance would seriously limit an attempt to fund azithromycin distribution by cost recovery methods.

A model has also been developed to assess the possible usefulness of a vaccine (720). This modelling showed that in hyperendemic areas, even a relatively ineffective vaccine would have considerable economic advantage. However, as we have seen in chapter eight, it may be a bit premature to count too strongly on a vaccine.

What tools do we have?

The SAFE Strategy

The SAFE Strategy concisely brings together the behavioural, medical and surgical elements required to address trachoma. The specific focus on facial cleanliness and environmental barriers coupled with a very potent antibiotic tool give a highly targeted intervention to reduce both the level of infection and pressure of reinfection. This coherent strategy is based on solid evidence from field research and controlled trials (721). It provides an invaluable tool and is a significant advance over previous attempts to control trachoma.

The identification of facial cleanliness as the key component, or critical pathway, through which the environment and socioeconomic conditions impact on trachoma has been a major advance. This enables programs to specifically focus on the clearly defined and achievable goal of ensuring that "every child has a clean face". Similarly, the advent of azithromycin has been a major advance. The

distribution of a single annual (or biennial) oral dose of azithromycin is a realistic goal, whereas the long-term intermittent treatment strategies using topical tetracycline or weeks of oral antibiotics were not. Components F and A are the two major advances in our knowledge and armamentarium for the elimination of trachoma by 2020 (see Figure 10.5).

Some may see this as an oversimplification, but I firmly believe that we need to focus our attention on these two issues and address those environmental and logistic barriers that stop us achieving clean faces and appropriate azithromycin distribution. This is not to say that other factors also may be important in a particular area and will need to be addressed before F and A can be fully achieved.

These powerful tools have been translated into a comprehensive and accessible suite of background teaching and material by the WHO and the partners of the Global Alliance (127,128,583,587, 589,590,722,723). This has made the necessary information and practical technical procedures widely available and accessible to program managers, those in the field and policy makers.

The creation of the Global Alliance for the Elimination of Trachoma (GET 2020) is also a major strength as it brings together the key NGOs, researchers, representatives of national governments and the corporate sector and WHO experts. This group can help endemic countries set

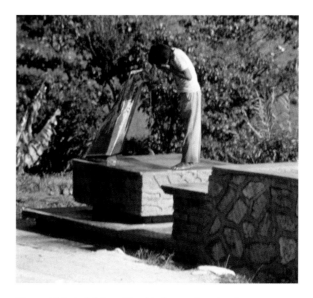

Figure 10.5 A child washing his face at the school tap, Mexico (1985).

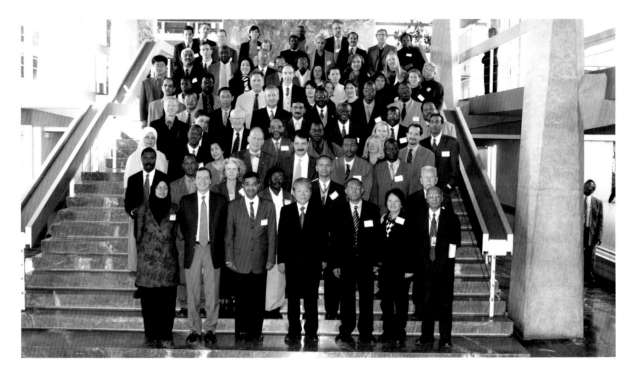

Figure 10.6 Members of the eighth meeting of the WHO Alliance for the Global Elimination of Blinding Trachoma, Geneva 2004.

targets and provide technical assistance, monitor progress or undertake operational research to refine or refocus programmatic activities. These activities have added enormously to the likelihood of the successful elimination of blinding trachoma (see Figure 10.6).

Azithromycin, the International Trachoma Initiative and Pfizer

In 1984 a meeting was held for the Edna McConnell Clark Foundation to review the current knowledge of trachoma (582). Two broad areas were considered: animal models and immuno-pathogenesis, and epidemiologic and field studies. This initiated the interest and support of the Clark Foundation in trachoma research and they became major players in the field. The trachoma activities of the Clark Foundation were guided by their enthusiastic Medical Director, Joe Cook, who had previously studied schistosomiasis in the Caribbean. The Foundation supported much of the epidemiologic research from the late 1980s and the fieldwork undertaken to assess trichiasis surgery, the use of azithromycin and other environmental interventions into the 1990s. They worked closely

with WHO to publish the key SAFE Strategy manuals including *Primary Health Care Level Management of Trachoma* (128), *Achieving Community Support for Trachoma Control* (583) and *Trichiasis Surgery for Trachoma, the Bilamellar Tarsal Rotation Procedure* (587).

In 1998, with the recognition of the usefulness of azithromycin for the treatment of trachoma, Pfizer Inc. initiated a major donation program to provide azithromycin for use in approved trachoma control programs in endemic areas. The Edna McConnell Clark Foundation and Pfizer established the International Trachoma Initiative (ITI). The ITI is a single purpose NGO that was established to achieve the global elimination of blinding trachoma (724,725). Initially the ITI had multiple roles including the ongoing support of research activities continued from the Clark Foundation, the initiation of specific country programs and the co-ordination of the Zithromax (azithromycin) Donation Program. With time, the focus of the ITI has sharpened, as it has progressively expanded the size of its existing national programs and expanded the number of countries in which it worked.

In 2005 the ITI distributed over 16.5 million

doses of azithromycin and supported nearly 78,000 trichiasis operations (726). The ITI has partnered with the national government, the WHO and others in the very successful program in Morocco. It has also taken a lead in countries such as Mali, Sudan, Tanzania and Vietnam and has continued to work very closely with the WHO. The ITI, following the lead of the Clark Foundation, has co-sponsored a number of publications expanding the SAFE Strategy. They include *Implementing the SAFE Strategy for Trachoma Control* (590), the *SAFE Strategy Preventing Trachoma* (589) and *Trachoma Control, A Guide for Program Managers* (127) and *Guidelines for the Rapid Assessment for Blinding Trachoma* (246).

Behind the success of the ITI lies the very impressive Zithromax Donation Program established by Pfizer to distribute azithromycin worldwide for trachoma control (727). It followed the Mectizan Donation Program that provides ivermectin to treat river blindness. Started in 1987, the Mectizan Program was a trailblazing initiative almost two decades ahead of its time. It became a model for public private partnerships (PPP) (728,729,730). With the development of the UN Global Fund, the Millennium Development Goals and the War on Poverty, the value of public private partnerships has been widely recognised and much

appreciated. This method brings the private sector and for-profit corporations together with governments and non-government organisations to improve the health and well-being of targeted communities. Hank McKinnell, President of Pfizer, recognised that most people with trachoma could not afford to buy azithromycin, nor could their national governments afford to purchase it for use in national trachoma control programs. Having already provided azithromycin at no cost for clinical trials and pilot intervention programs in a number of countries, in 2003 McKinnell announced to the United Nations that Pfizer would provide 135 million doses over five years to support the global program (731) (see Figure 10.7).

The engagement and strong commitment of what is now the world's largest pharmaceutical company makes a tremendous difference to the prospects for success of the SAFE Strategy. In 2005 Pfizer indicated that they would continue to provide donated Zithromax to countries with a serious commitment to the elimination of trachoma beyond 2010 (598). In 2006 some 29 million doses of azithromycin were distributed (598) and the ITI had distributed nearly 54 million doses in total (see Table 10.3, Figure 10.8).

One of the problems faced by the GET 2020 program has been the ability to ramp up the

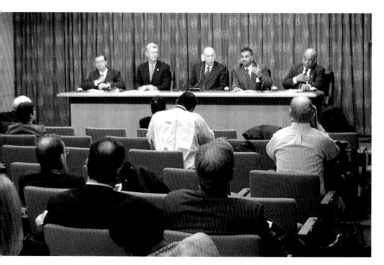

Figure 10.7 The launch of the Zithromax Donation Program at the United Nations building, New York. From left to right, Serge Resnikoff (WHO), Hank McKinnell (Pfizer), Dr Fouad Hammadi (Minister of Health, Morocco), Jacob Kumaresan (ITI), Gourisankar Ghosh, (Water Supply and Sanitation Collaborative Council), November 2003.

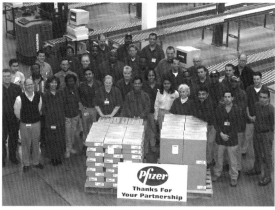

Figure 10.8 A donated shipment of azithromycin ready to leave the Pfizer warehouse. Some countries may need 400 pallets of the drug each year (courtesy, Pfizer).

TABLE 10.3: ITI program progress since inception (as of 31/12/06) (780)

Country	Surgeries	Antibiotics
Ethiopia	76,198	8,497,725
Ghana	3,905	2,258,167
Mali	22,545	11,799,524
Mauritania	961	1,126,471
Morocco	29,905	4,372,459
Nepal	11,302	2,681,176
Niger	26,439	8,506,793
Senegal	1,761	701,627
Sudan	8,052	1,405,352
Tanzania	18,273	10,153,687
Vietnam	77,312	2,054,38
Total	**276,653**	**53,557,362**

ITI facilitates Pfizer Inc's donation of the antibiotic Zithromax®. For the year ended 31 December 2006, the value of such facilitated donations approximated $594.2 million. These goods were recorded at wholesale value on the date of the contribution.

capacity to distribute the donated azithromycin and co-ordinate this with the full implementation of the SAFE Strategy. One constraint is the cost of the distribution of azithromycin including the initial delivery to the country. Treatment for one million people fills about 60 pallets or two truck loads. In 2007 a cargo-carrying 747 aircraft was required to take the annual doses for 6.7 million people in Niger at a transport cost of about US$250,000 (732). Shipping, clearance and storage fees and the considerable cost of donation programs are all borne by Pfizer. The actual in-country distribution costs of road transport and personnel are very significant but vary. Typically they may be around US$0.30 per person. This is still US$300,000 per million people which needs to be found by the government or donors. The costs for S, F and E components are also considerable. Currently the ITI facilitates programs in 12 countries and by 2010 plans to increase its coverage with azithromycin and eliminate blinding trachoma in Morocco, Ghana, Mauritania, Nepal and Vietnam. This significant effort will have helped reduce the

global burden of blinding trachoma by 25%. However, even these ambitious plans would still leave three-quarters of the problem of blinding trachoma unaddressed by 2010. Without additional resources we cannot reach our goal.

The magnitude of the programs that need to be implemented are quite staggering. The Global Alliance reviewed the needs of the 33 worst affected countries and estimated their Ultimate Intervention Goals (597). Over eight million trichiasis operations were required and excluding China, 196 million people needed to be treated with azithromycin. If the suspected levels of endemicity in China were confirmed, an additional 156 million Chinese may also need to be treated (597). However, one can have some optimism when one can see the achievements of other global programs for onchocerciasis, lymphatic filariasis or Vitamin A distribution.

The elimination of trachoma will clearly require the mobilisation of considerable additional resources, increased national government involvement and ownership, the utilisation of global funding sources, the building of PPP and the engagement of civil society to focus on the issue of trachoma. All this needs to be done in a milieu of competition from multiple worthy causes ranging from HIV/AIDS, malaria and TB to the War on Poverty and even the War on Terrorism.

Vision 2020

Vision 2020 is a major global initiative jointly undertaken by the World Health Organization and the International Agency for the Prevention of Blindness (IAPB). Whereas the WHO brings together national governments and technical expertise, the IAPB brings together non-government organisations and professional bodies that work in the field of eye care and prevention of blindness.

Vision 2020: The Right to Sight aims to eliminate avoidable blindness by 2020 (43,57). It has three major areas of activity: disease control, human resource development and infrastructure development. Under disease control five major conditions are addressed: cataract, trachoma, onchocerciasis, childhood blindness and refractive error and low vision. These conditions were selected because of their public health importance and the availability of public health interventions to address them (733). Vision 2020 has endorsed the program set out for the Global Elimination of Trachoma (GET 2020) and is working with members of the Global Alliance to achieve this goal.

A strong link between GET 2020 and Vision 2020 is of great importance. Efforts to increase the recognition of the need to prevent vision loss will help to raise trachoma awareness, its interventions and the need for raising funds. Clearly the timing of the Vision 2020 Initiative and the close links between this initiative and trachoma are an important strength, and increase the likelihood of the ultimate elimination of blinding trachoma, although close and continuing partnership will be required.

Millennium Development Goals and Neglected Tropical Diseases

In addition to the natural linkage with Vision 2020 and prevention of blindness activities, trachoma is also closely linked with a number of other development objectives. Trachoma has obvious ties to programs addressing poverty, women's rights,

children's health or water, and to more specific programs on neglected diseases, Africa or behavioural change.

The Millennium Development Goals (MDG) were adopted by member countries of the United Nations as a strategy to address global disequity by 2015 (734) (see Table 10.4).

Trachoma control has a strong link with Development Goal 7, Target 10 "halve by 2015, the proportion of people without sustainable access to safe drinking water and basic sanitation" (734). Access to an adequate water supply is an obvious prerequisite for facial cleanliness and basic sanitation will also reduce fly density (735).

Development Goal 8, Target 17 "in co-operation with pharmaceutical companies provide access to affordable essential drugs in developing countries" (734) also relates to trachoma. On the one hand it reinforces the importance of the partnership with Pfizer and the Zithromax Donation Program. On the other, there is also the need to establish long-term sustainable supplies of affordable azithromycin that reach trachoma areas in every affected country. This may require more fully developed public private partnerships to ensure the full distribution of azithromycin everywhere it is needed.

In many ways trachoma activities also enable and interact with Goals 2 and 3: "achieve universal primary education" and "promote gender equality and empower women", and ultimately may also contribute to the achievement of Goal 1: "eradicate extreme poverty" (734).

It is vitally important for trachoma control activities to have close co-operation and collaboration with national governments, international organisations and civil societies that are working towards the achievement of the MDGs. It is a powerful way to gain additional collaborators and help focus and prioritise resources to address issues relating to environ-mental and behavioural components of the SAFE Strategy. The close links with Vision 2020 can only further strengthen this intersectorial and collaborative approach (736).

A new program is being developed by WHO and others to address Africa's neglected tropical diseases (737). It too builds on the PPP and the MDGs (729). This program has identified 13 neglected tropical infectious diseases caused by

TABLE 10.4: Millennium Development Goals and Targets (734)

GOAL 1: Eradicate extreme poverty and hunger

Target 1: Reduce by half the proportion of people living on less than a dollar a day.

Target 2: Reduce by half the proportion of people who suffer from hunger.

GOAL 2: Achieve universal primary education

Target 3: Ensure that all boys and girls complete a full course of primary schooling.

GOAL 3: Promote gender equality and empower women

Target 4: Eliminate gender disparity in primary and secondary education preferably by 2005, and at all levels by 2015.

GOAL 4: Reduce child mortality

Target 5: Reduce by two-thirds the mortality rate among children under five.

GOAL 5: Improve maternal health

Target 6: Reduce by three-quarters the maternal mortality ratio.

GOAL 6: Combat HIV/AIDS, malaria and other disease

Target 7: Halt and begin to reverse the spread of HIV/AIDS.

Target 8: Halt and begin to reverse the incidence of malaria and other major diseases.

GOAL 7: Ensure environmental sustainability

Target 9: Integrate the principles of sustainable development into country policies and programmes; reverse loss of environmental resources.

Target 10: Reduce by half the proportion of people without sustainable access to safe drinking water.

Target 11: Achieve significant improvement in lives of at least 100 million slum dwellers, by 2020.

GOAL 8: Develop a global partnership for development

Target 12: Develop further an open trading and financial system that is rule-based, predictable and non-discriminatory, includes commitment to good governance, development and poverty reduction – nationally and internationally.

Target 13: Address the least developed countries' special needs. This includes tariff- and quota-free access for their exports; enhanced debt relief for heavily indebted poor countries; cancellation of official bilateral debt; and more generous official development assistance for countries committed to poverty reduction.

Target 14: Address the special needs of landlocked and small island developing states.

Target 15: Deal comprehensively with developing countries' debt problems through national and international measures to make debt sustainable in the long term.

Target 16: In cooperation with the developing countries, develop decent and productive work for youth.

Target 17: In cooperation with pharmaceutical companies, provide access to affordable essential drugs in developing countries.

Target 18: In cooperation with the private sector, make available the benefits of new technologies – especially information and communication technologies.

protozoa, helminths or bacteria. This program includes trachoma and emphasises that these neglected diseases both occur in poor areas and contribute to poverty (598). These conditions often co-exist and are amenable to rapid impact interventions. It has been calculated that at an annual cost of some US$0.40 per person, a program addressing these diseases could have a major impact on the health and economic well-being of these disadvantaged African populations.

For a typical African country, this may add to only one-tenth the current health budget spent on anti-viral drugs to treat HIV+ people. This may provide another opportunity for trachoma control programs to link and find synergy with other disease control initiatives in those areas where these diseases co-exist. Many of the other "tropical" diseases occur in tropical areas and are associated with water, onchocerciasis (river blindness), schistosomiasis and guinea worm. Thus trachoma is more a disease of the deserts.

What is the likely outcome?

Dominique Negrel has decades of experience of trachoma in West Africa and worked with the WHO. In a report to the International Organization Against Trachoma (53), he outlined the four essentials he considered necessary for the successful elimination of trachoma: knowledge, techniques, resources and political will. He considered the necessary knowledge and resources were already available. They included the simplified grading; knowledge from epidemiologic surveys, targeted rapid assessment and modern geographic information systems; bilamellar tarsal rotation; azithromycin; and the integration of these components into the SAFE Strategy. He regarded these as the trump cards we held in what was "the winning hand to defeat trachoma" (53).

Although these trumps are important they need to be complemented by the other two factors—resources and political will. Through the commitment of Pfizer, the Zithromax Donation Program is a massive resource. The mobilisation by members of the Global Alliance and those involved in Vision 2020 brings additional focus and further resources.

A reflection of the political will that exists includes both the specific WHO Resolution on Trachoma in 1998 (585) (Table 10.2) and the reiteration of support for Vision 2020 by the World Health Assembly in 2006 (738,739). These formally adopted resolutions at the World Health Assembly reflect at least the official commitment of national governments to address the problem of blinding trachoma. A further measure of the commitment of governments of endemic countries

is their ongoing involvement and the reports they provide at annual GET 2020 meetings. In 2006 some 34 countries provided updated reports. Already half the countries had prepared Ultimate Intervention Goals and a number had linked trachoma with the Millennium Development Goals, particularly MDG 7. It would seem that necessary resources and political will are starting to come together with the required knowledge and techniques. Maybe we do have enough trumps.

As we have seen, trachoma disappeared from western Europe and North America in the absence of specific interventions, or in some countries almost despite their small efforts. The relatively limited trachoma interventions conducted in the UK or the USA, for example, cannot be given full credit for the elimination of trachoma in these countries, although they were continued until no more cases of trachoma could be detected. A similar situation probably applies to the rest of Europe. However, in some other countries, specifically targeted trachoma programs may have been more important in contributing to the disappearance of trachoma, although again socioeconomic development proceeded in parallel. Such countries would include Japan (54), Malta (343), Tunisia (577) and Burma (303). These examples give some cause for optimism that a specific trachoma intervention will lead to the elimination of trachoma, particularly if it is associated with parallel developments in socioeconomic status.

What is the experience with the SAFE Strategy?

Recent reports from the Sudan (680), Zambia (698) and Oman (244) give compelling examples of what may be achievable with the full implementation of the SAFE Strategy. In these reports, rates of active trachoma have been dramatically reduced and in Oman, trachoma has almost been eliminated. However, as Negrel points out, S and A are probably the easiest components of the SAFE Strategy to implement (53). They are both medically directed and lend themselves to be implemented and controlled through "vertical" programs. On the other hand, F and E relate to broader health and development issues. They require "horizontal" implementation and intersectorial co-operation. This makes them more difficult to achieve and much more demanding.

The S component requires scaling up of resources and close attention to the quality of surgery through education and careful post-operative follow-up. The A component needs greatly increased resources to achieve wide distribution and attainment of the UIG in all areas. Long lasting behavioural changes in F will be needed to achieve the sustained elimination of blinding trachoma as a public health problem. Fortunately much of the E component can focus specifically on those barriers that influence facial cleanliness. Mischievously one might even suggest that E could be rebadged from "Environmental Change" to "Education" with the particular focus of facial cleanliness and personal hygiene. Strategic alliances and collaboration with other development programs will be the key to achieve changes in E. We need win/win co-operation with development activities already occurring in endemic areas, and the encouragement of the prioritisation of endemic areas for new activities for development programs.

Ongoing monitoring

Edward Jackson (1856–1942) was the doyen of American ophthalmology. In an editorial in 1925 he listed three principal things to be done to eradicate trachoma: the avoidance of the crowding together of infected and uninfected people; the local treatment of active cases; and most relevant in this context, "prolonged supervision that will not be withdrawn until improvement has been secured … shall continue on the alert for recrudescences and relapses" (78). MacCallan was also of the opinion that "in a trachomatous country it is necessary to evert the lid of every person whom it is desirous to state to be free from trachoma" (4).

The propensity for trachoma to have a massive resurgence after apparently successful interventions has been manifestly demonstrated in countries such as Ethiopia and Sudan. WHO reports show dramatic reductions in the amount of trachoma in the 1970s after control programs using intense antibiotic treatment (740), whereas recent surveys from these areas show the return of disease to extraordinary high prevalences (125,306). Similarly, the WHO program in Morocco led to a significant

reduction in trachoma in the 1960s (139) that had resurged again in the 1980s (245). Similar failures to control trachoma are repeatedly seen in Australian Aboriginal communities (741,742). Intense antibiotic treatment, sometimes coupled with health education and environmental messages, can have a short-term impact, but without sustainable changes including having children with clean faces, trachoma will return. The WHO is developing a process for the monitoring of the success of trachoma control programs and the certification of the elimination of blinding trachoma (240).

The first step was to create Ultimate Intervention Goals (UIG) (3) (see Table 10.5). The UIG were created to indicate the final targets that need to be achieved by each intervention to eliminate blinding trachoma. These are dynamic numbers based on the current best estimates of the burden of disease. The UIG were derived from definitions used to establish blinding trachoma as a public health problem and were aimed at an 80% reduction below this threshold prevalence. Operationally, Annual Intervention Objectives (AIO) have been established to build UIGs (see Figure 10.9).

The threshold prevalence for TT was set at 1% or greater in the population aged 15 years and above. This gave a UIG of one case of TT per 1000 of the total population. The threshold recommended for community-wide intervention with A, F and E components for active trachoma was set at a community prevalence of TF of 10%, or higher, in children aged one to nine years. Mass treatment with azithromycin should continue until the community prevalence of TF drops to less than 5% when family-based intervention is recommended. The operational target for A and F was to achieve at least 80% coverage of the community with azithromycin distribution and 80% of children with clean faces.

Monitoring of the E component depended on education, environmental sustainability and poverty alleviation which were all closely linked to Millennium Development Goals. For this reason, the monitoring of E should follow the MDG framework for measuring development.

In the final instance, prevalences that define this target are set at the "community level". The community was defined as "the minimum group of individuals for which mass trachoma control can

TABLE 10.5: Ultimate Intervention Goals for trachoma (3)

Criteria for initiating a trachoma control program.	Denominator is initially district and later community	Guidelines for when trachoma as a blinding disease is being controlled (UIG)
TF 10% or more	1–9 year old population	TF less than 5%
TT 1% or more	15 year and over population	TT less than 0.2%
Trachoma is a blinding disease	Total population	Less than 1 new case of corneal opacity due to trachoma / 10,000 pop.

be implemented, for example, a defined group of households, one village, or a group of neighbouring villages" (3). Operationally, this may translate into groups of 1000 to 5000 people.

The elimination of blinding trachoma

If one is to claim that trachoma has been eliminated one has to be sure that it has. In international health this means "certification". The process of defining the certification of the elimination of blinding trachoma has been initiated, although it has not yet been completed (240). The actual certification will be a complex procedure and many technical issues need to be addressed within the

WHO. An informal working group identified three possible categories of countries. These include Category A, endemic trachoma in at least one district with a prevalence of TF greater than 5%, or TT greater than one per 1000 (current priority countries); Category B, an ongoing problem with TT, but in whom TF was now less than 5% (e.g. United Arab Emirates or Saudi Arabia); Category C, no recent history of TF or TT, although trachoma may have been a problem in the past (e.g. United Kingdom, France and Italy).

It had been suggested that to receive certification a country would need to demonstrate that it had maintained TF at less than 5% for at least three

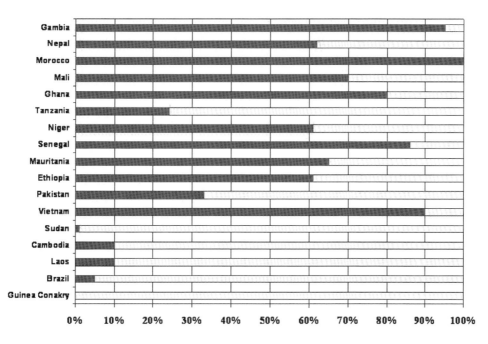

Figure 10.9 Percentage of Annual Intervention Objectives achieved in 2006 by 17 countries providing coverage data to WHO (GET 2020 2007, Cairo © 2007 WHO, reproduced with permission).

17 countries w. coverage data

consecutive years, that it had developed the ongoing capacity and systems to handle incident cases of TT, and that trachoma surveillance and control activities had been incorporated into the ongoing public health systems. Such a process would require targeted prevalence surveys conducted three years after the cessation of mass antibiotic distribution. The cost and complexity of this certification process was recognised as a major impediment and therefore much more work is needed in this area.

To summarise the current position, we seem to have the right tools and many of the resources and the expression of political will that are needed to actually eliminate blinding trachoma. However, the methods of showing that we have actually achieved this goal are still to be developed. At this stage, one could reasonably state:

> We may therefore venture to conclude on a note of reasonable optimism and at the same time express a hope for the future. In many parts of the world, the most widespread world scourge has been or is reported to be overcome. Efficient methods of therapy are already in use and other still more effective ones may be expected in the near future. If the national campaigns already underway are continued and co-ordinated and meet with vigorous international support, our century may perhaps witness the disappearance of trachoma (59).

How much further advanced are we now than they were in 1949, and which century are we talking about?

Trachoma in Australia

It is anomalous that Australia should be the only developed country listed by the WHO as having endemic blinding trachoma (3,62). Some have suggested that the way things are going Australia may be the last country to have trachoma. As we will see, the health and hygiene of Europeans living in Australia showed parallel changes to those in western Europe and North America and trachoma disappeared from Australia's coastal towns and cities 100 years ago. However, trachoma still flourishes in Aboriginal communities in outback Australia.

The past

It is unclear when trachoma first reached Australia. One obvious suggestion is that the European migrants who came to Australia in the 1800s brought trachoma with them from Europe (743). Certainly in the second half of the 19th century conditions in the urban slums or outback shacks of Australia were conducive to trachoma. It is possible that as Europeans moved into outback areas they took trachoma with them as well as measles, syphilis and smallpox, all of which spread to Aboriginal people. Others have suggested that trachoma was introduced to Aboriginal people in northern Australia by Malay traders, and elsewhere by Afghan and Chinese labourers who also came to Australia in the 19th century (744).

The first often quoted European description of Aboriginal people was written in 1688 by William Dampier (1651–1715) when he landed on the west coast of Western Australia:

> Their eyelids are always half-closed, to keep the files out of their eyes; they being so troublesome here, that no fanning will keep them off, they will creep into one's nostrils and mouth too, if the lips are not shut very close: so that from their infancy being thus annoyed with these insects, (the Aborigines) do never open their eyes as other people; and therefore they cannot see far, unless they hold up their heads, as if they were looking somewhat over them (745).

This commentary shows that eye-seeking flies were common in Australia, but does not necessarily indicate the presence of trachoma, and it also belies the subsequent finding that Aboriginal people have the world's best visual acuity vastly superior to Europeans (746).

If trachoma were prevalent in Aboriginal communities, it is likely it would have had a devastating impact in a non-literate society where good vision was essential for navigation, hunting and the passing on of Aboriginal lore and law—all vital for individual and cultural survival. To my knowledge there are no Aboriginal stories about widespread blindness and Aboriginal culture and custom relies on the active involvement of the elderly, not their marginalisation due to failing vision.

However, two interesting studies have suggested

the presence of trachoma before European colonisation of Australia. A study of Aboriginal skulls dating back to 14,000 BP show abnormal changes in the lacrimal fossa of the orbits indicative of chronic dacryoadenitis (747). Chronic dacryoadenitis can be associated with trachoma and these changes have been interpreted to indicate the presence of trachoma in these ancient Aboriginal remains.

In the 1950s and 1960s, extensive efforts were made to remove the remaining family groups of nomadic Aboriginal people from the Western Desert. This had become the target area for rockets fired from the Woomera Rocket Range. In 1957 trachoma was found to be frequent in one group of 42 people (748). In 1964, another group of 88 "desert Aborigines" believed never to have had previous direct contact with Europeans had their eyes examined; half showed signs of trachoma, four had secondary conjunctivitis and another had entropion (749). Two elders were totally blind and another had a phthisical eye. Although it is possible these groups may have acquired European-derived infections indirectly following contact with other groups of Aboriginal people, these desert people certainly had not lived in the squalor of fringe settlements nor had they adopted a European lifestyle.

In white urban Australia, trachoma was a major problem in the last half of the 19th century and led to the foundation in 1866 of what became the Royal Victorian Eye and Ear Hospital. In 1888 in Melbourne "trachoma was easily the most common (eye) disease met with, and occupied most of the time and anxiety of the oculist" (31). However, by 1909 Sir James Barrett (1862–1945), Chief Surgeon at the Eye and Ear Hospital, commented on the marked decrease in cases of trachoma (750). He noted that most cases came from the Goulburn Valley and northern Victoria.

Trachoma was known as "sandy blight" throughout Australia. Ophthalmia had been an integral part of the mythology of the exploration of outback Australia. In 1872, the explorer John Forrest (1847–1914) was temporarily blinded in north western Western Australia and he named the low mountain ridge where he was camping Ophthalmia Range (see Figure 10.10). A road that blazes straight across the desert in Western Australia, the Gunbarrel Highway, has only one intersection, Sandy Blight Junction. However, by the 1920s, even in rural Australia, trachoma was disappearing as most Australians moved into proper housing with separate beds, running water and adequate sewerage and rubbish removal.

By the 1940s trachoma had almost disappeared from Europeans living in south eastern Australia, although blindness from trachoma was the fourth most common cause and accounted for 4% to 6% of the registered blind (31, 751). However, occasional cases of blindness from trachoma were still seen and in 1976, the first corneal graft I

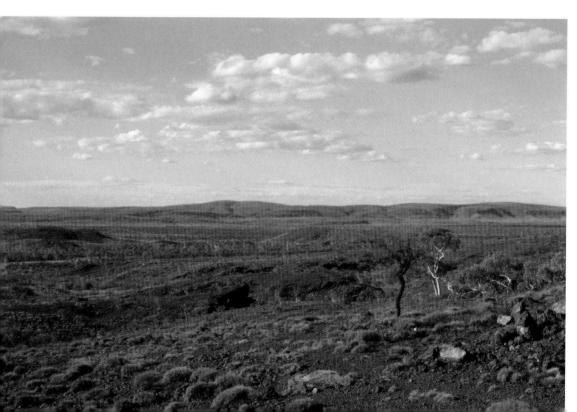

Figure 10.10 The Ophthalmia Range in the Pilbara region of Western Australia.

performed as a trainee was on an elderly man from north western Victoria who was blind from trachoma.

Little information is available about trachoma in Aboriginal people before the 1940s. A German missionary doctor, Erhardt Eylmann, found trachoma and blindness to be present in Aboriginal people in Central Australia and in 1911, trachoma was considered "prevalent" in Western Australia and Queensland (748). A small survey in 1934 reported a 20% prevalence of trachoma amongst Aboriginal people on the east coast of Queensland (743). In the 1920s and 1930s many Aboriginal people in outback Australia were brought into settlements or missions and supervised under a very paternalistic regime. Others lived on extensive cattle properties or stations and worked from time to time as stockmen or domestic help. Although many still lived semi-traditional lives, their diet changed to white flour and white sugar. Trachoma was reported to be present in Aboriginal people living on a number of missions in Central Australia before the start of the Second World War (748,752). One report gave an overall prevalence of 91% for trachoma (753). The rate of blindness was reported to be 7.9% and drew attention to poor hygiene, dust and flies.

Father Frank Flynn (1906–96), an Australian-born London-trained ophthalmologist turned Catholic priest worked as an army chaplain in Darwin in 1941 (see Figure 10.11). He was the first to systematically assess the frequent occurrence of trachoma among indigenous people in the Northern Territory, and their welfare became his life's work. Starting in 1942 and continuing after the war he surveyed a number of communities in Central Australia and found trachoma to be very common: "At the age of two or three years a very high percentage of children already show obvious signs"(383). Trichiasis and corneal opacity and the development of blindness were common in older people (752). Further studies were undertaken across the Northern Territory. Flynn used a combination of the MacCallan Classification and a severity "index" borrowed from Ida Mann. Unfortunately, no age-specific rates for trachoma were provided, but some 20% to 30% of the total population had active trachoma and the presence of chlamydia was confirmed by Giemsa cytology.

Flynn noted that trachoma tended to be more severe and cause more blindness in the central desert regions and was less severe in northerly coastal regions. He initiated campaigns with the systemic distribution of sulphas combined with topical tetracycline ointment and non-specific health education.

After World War Two, Dame Ida Mann, a remarkable English ophthalmologist with whom Frank Flynn had worked in London before the war, moved to Perth. She subsequently conducted extraordinary trips throughout the outback, examining and treating many Aboriginal people with trachoma (382) (see Figure 10.12). She found active trachoma in 45% of children under the age of one year and 80% of Aboriginal children aged one to nine years (754). Trichiasis was present in 20% of those over the age of 60, and two-thirds had corneal scarring. She organised sporadic treatment with oral sulphas in outback Western Australia.

Further studies were undertaken in South Australia that confirmed a high prevalence of both active and cicatricial trachoma (755). This group also confirmed the presence of chlamydia by Giemsa stain and made the first chlamydial isolates in Australia. An attempt to culture chlamydia from "fly emulsions" was unsuccessful. Trachoma was a notifiable disease in several Australian states (748). Data from 1954 to 1984 show that nine cases were reported in Victoria, some hundreds of cases were reported each year in Western Australia (until notification stopped in 1964), and very variable numbers were reported from the Northern Territory and South Australia. Trachoma was not notifiable in New South Wales, Queensland or Tasmania. The reported data are so variable they add little useful information, and this is not an uncommon problem with some notifiable diseases.

In the 1960s, Fred Hollows took up his position as Professor of Ophthalmology at the University of New South Wales and became aware of the importance of trachoma in Australia (756). First working with the Gurindji people at Wave Hill in the Northern Territory and then with Aboriginal people living around Bourke in far western New South Wales, he cajoled the federal government and the Royal Australian College of Ophthalmologists into establishing the National Trachoma and Eye

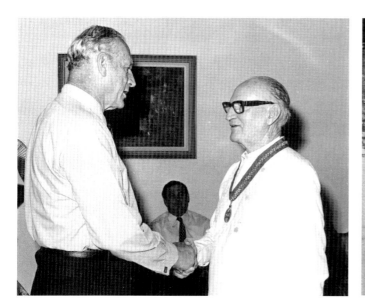

Figure 10.11 Frank Flynn at the time of his investiture as a Companion of the Order of Australia by Administrator John England at Government House in 1995 (NT govt. photographer, Northern Territory Library and Information Service © NTL).

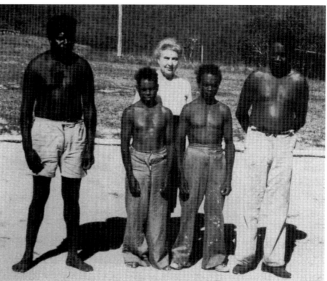

Figure 10.12 Ida Mann during fieldwork in the Torres Strait (382) (From Mann I, Culture, Race, Climate and Eye Disease. 1966. Courtesy of Charles C Thomas Publisher, Ltd; Springfield, Illinois).

Health Program (the "Trachoma Program") (757).

In 1967 a constitutional referendum gave full citizenship to Aboriginal people. The church-run missions were closed and replaced by government funds and control. Indigenous people received the vote, pensions and unemployment benefits and unrestricted access to alcohol.

Between 1976 and 1978 the NTEHP visited every indigenous community in Australia and examined over 62,000 indigenous people and nearly 40,000 others (103) (see Figure 10.13). It gave a clear picture of the number of people affected with trachoma and its distribution. The NTEHP showed the widespread presence of trachoma in Aboriginal Australians throughout rural and outback Australia. This showed a higher prevalence of trachoma in central desert areas, lower prevalences in urban areas, and more settled rural areas in the south-east and coastal areas (103) (see Figure 10.14). The NTEHP also treated nearly 25,000 people for trachoma and established clear guidelines and recommendations of what was needed to be done to eliminate trachoma.

Following the report of the NTEHP, state trachoma committees were organised to supervise the running of ongoing trachoma control activities. Initially these committees were under federal supervision, but later they were devolved to the states with Aboriginal leadership (758). Increasing Aboriginal and community control was sought and many Aboriginal organisations including community-controlled Aboriginal Medical or Health Services were established. Some committees in South Australia, Western Australia, the Northern Territory and Queensland continued into the 1990s and they became increasingly concerned with the provision of visiting specialist eye care and spectacles and trachoma activities were more limited. A meta-analysis of data collected in the Northern Territory over a 40 year period showed more evidence of survey variation than a consistent change in trachoma rates (759).

The present

In 1997 I prepared a report on indigenous eye health for the Commonwealth Government (758). In addition to considering the broad issues relating to ocular health, information was specifically

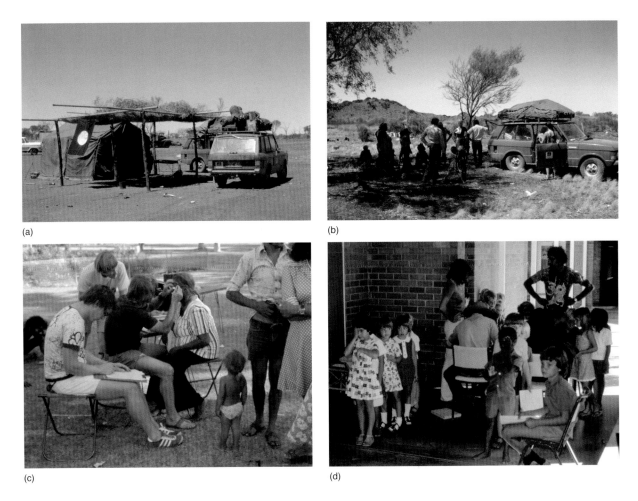

Figure 10.13 The NTEHP examinations (1976–77)

(a) a clinic in makeshift facilities in central Western Australia

(b) examining a group of Aboriginal people beside the road

(c) the author recording data for Fred Hollows as he examines people in a park

(d) schoolchildren having their visual acuity measured prior to trachoma grading.

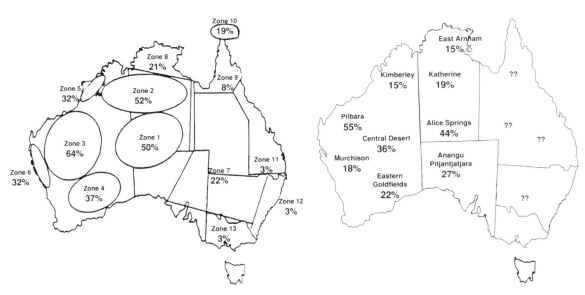

Figure 10.14 The prevalence of follicular trachoma amongst Aboriginal children found by NTEHP 1976 to 1978 and reported between 1989 and 1996 (Taylor 1997; Eye Health in Aboriginal and Torres Strait Islander Communities, Hugh R. Taylor, © 1997 Commonwealth of Australia, reproduced with permission).

collected on trachoma. Trachoma had decreased significantly in some areas; in some of the larger towns and regional centres trachoma had almost disappeared. In other areas, active trachoma was less common, although the elders still had scarred eyelids and trichiasis. However, it was devastating to return to some communities in the Western Desert and Central Australia to find that hyperendemic rates of trachoma had not changed since I first visited those communities with the NTEHP 20 years before. In one community in 1997, 70% of the children had trachoma. I summarised these observations:

> Although the prevalence and intensity of trachoma may have decreased in some areas, other areas show little or no improvement over the last 20 years. Many seem to have disregarded trachoma and current data on active trachoma underestimate the problem as they often come from incomplete cohorts of older children. Information on trichiasis was grossly inadequate and in most areas, cases were not actively sought. An integrated primary health approach was required to manage trachoma. This should combine screening, azithromycin antibiotic treatment, personal hygiene and environmental improvement. This approach has been codified by the World Health Organization in 'SAFE strategy'. It is unconscionable that trachoma remains a blinding disease in Australia (758).

This review recommended that eye care should be delivered to indigenous Australians through a regional public private model. Three specific recommendations were made with regard to trachoma. These related to the development of clinical practice guidelines, the provision of azithromycin treatment through the National Pharmaceutical Benefits Scheme, and the need for further improvements in the regional delivery of housing, infrastructure and the resources to maintain these (758). The Report also recommended the establishment of a national information network to provide a two-way flow of information as a conduit of technical information to those working in the field and to gather central data on both eye care activities (process) and ocular status (outcome).

The most straightforward of these recommendations, the listing of azithromycin, was achieved in 1998 (1). Specialist eye health

guidelines for use in Aboriginal and Torres Strait Islander populations that included a section on the management of trachoma appeared in 2001 (760). These guidelines advocated the use of the WHO Simplified Grading, the implementation of the SAFE Strategy including the bilamellar tarsal rotation procedure, mass distribution of azithromycin and emphasis on facial cleanliness. They also recommended the collection of a basic set of health information reiterating the prior recommendation.

Sporadic reports suggest fluctuating rates of ongoing trachoma in Aboriginal communities. For example, one report used data collected over 24 years by three surveys each using different grading systems (307). It showed a possible decrease in active trachoma in two to nine year olds from about 50% to 30% in these communities. A report of school screening between 1999 and 2003 suggested only 15% of children had active trachoma (761). However, a population-based examination in some of the same communities in 2000 showed a point prevalence of active trachoma in children aged one to 10 years to be 49% (311). Moreover, over a one year period up to 79% of the children had TF on at least one occasion. These differences that highlight the vagaries of sample selection are further reinforced by another report using data collected over 12 years (762).

A population-based report from 11 communities in the Pilbara showed TF rates in children under the age of five ranged from about 12% to almost 100% (763). The prevalence of trachoma was lowest in communities closer to the coast. This report also stressed that 40% of Aboriginal people lacked access to a shower, toilet or washing machine and that heated water was almost universally absent. A measure of the appalling standards of ocular "promiscuity" and hygiene prevailing in these communities was an outbreak of non-sexually transmitted gonococcal conjunctivitis that infected people from north western Australia through the Northern Territory and into South Australia (764).

Reports of trichiasis were also sporadic, but prevalences are still remarkably high despite the presence of ophthalmic surgical services. In the Kimberley, the overall regional prevalence in those over the age of 50 was 2.8%, although in some communities trichiasis rates ranged up to 11% (765). Another report from Central Australia showed that 8% over the age of 40 had trichiasis (766). In South Australia, rates of trachoma of 1.3% have been recently reported (340). Visiting ophthalmologists provide periodic eye care to those in remote areas (767). People seen with cataract, trichiasis or diabetic retinopathy who need treatment are usually transferred to a regional or state centre for surgery. This means that trichiasis can be surgically corrected if detected, but trichiasis is not systematically sought. In Adelaide, rates of lid surgery in Aboriginal people are six times higher than in non-Aboriginal people (768) and most lid surgery in Aboriginal people was for trichiasis.

A recent population-based survey in one community in Central Australia found the rate of TF to be 55% in children aged one to nine years (341). In adults over 40, 74% had TS, 11% had TT and 5% had CO. Bilateral blindness was found in 2% of adults over 40, and 40% was due to trachoma.

Antibiotic treatment programs for trachoma were also rather sporadic and most focused on individual interventions. Some programs had implemented targeted treatment of children with azithromycin, although the impact of this intervention was quite limited (310,742,769).

A trachoma control program has operated in the Kimberley for 15 years (742,770) treating schoolchildren with trachoma and some family members. And yet the overall prevalence of 23% active trachoma in 2005 had not changed from 1991! (742). Data for 2005 were available for 32 of 38 schools; 18 had prevalences greater than 20% and only four had no trachoma. These data show that despite good intentions and efforts, the ineffectiveness of inappropriately directed azithromycin treatment was compounded by the failure to implement other components of the SAFE Strategy (see Figure 10.15). They stand in stark contrast to the concurrent reports from the Sudan (680) or Zambia (698) (see Figure 10.9).

Two short-term programs in Central Australia have tried to implement the full SAFE Strategy (699,700). Trichiasis control activities had been implemented previously. Antibiotic coverage was relatively limited in the first study and a real advance in the improvement of the E component was not made (699). The proportion of houses with completely adequate facilities increased from 0 to 16% (see Figure 10.16). However, the other study showed no added benefit from a significant and comprehensive effort of environmental improvement over and above that obtained from A and F (700). Both of these studies show that for a sustained reduction in trachoma a more sustained effort would be required. They also suggested that in hyperendemic areas treatment every six months may be preferable. Further, given the high mobility of many Aboriginal people, regional-based interventions would be preferable rather than focusing on the treatment of single communities. They also highlight the abysmal state of health hardware in many of these communities. A much bigger investment in time and effort is therefore required.

Interestingly, a dramatic reduction in skin infections and otitis media was reported following the building of swimming pools in two Aboriginal communities (771). Unfortunately no thought was given to assessing trachoma. Swimming pools provide an easy way to wash, but also provide exercise, recreation and a community focal point (see Figure 10.17). A "no school no pool" policy also improved school attendance. This finding generated great interest and may be a way of addressing facial cleanliness, personal hygiene and trachoma. This approach may be more successful than the promise of the installation of petrol pumps (695,772). A study to specifically examine the impact of swimming pools on trachoma rates was attempted but thwarted by prolonged delays in installing pools (341).

In 2004 the report of a review on the implementation of the Aboriginal Eye Health Program was released (767). This review found that despite the presence of several Australian guidelines recommending trachoma control with the SAFE Strategy, these recommendations had not been systematically implemented. They noted that little data had been collected and these data were highly variable in quality and form. Nevertheless, the review recognised that trachoma still occurred at a high prevalence in some communities and the presence of chlamydia was confirmed by PCR. They also found that azithromycin distribution activities had been conducted in some communities for upwards of 10 years without any documented adverse effects. They recognised the high prevalence of trichiasis occurring in some communities, and that many people, including

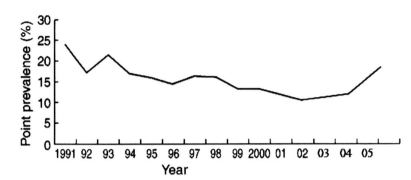

Figure 10.15 Reported prevalence of trachoma in schoolchildren in the Kimberley region, 1991 to 2005 (data redrawn from Johnson GH et al. An evaluation of a SAFE-style trachoma control program in central Australia. MJA 2003; 179:116–7 © 2003, *The Medical Journal of Australia* – reproduced with permission, and Collinson 2006 (742)).

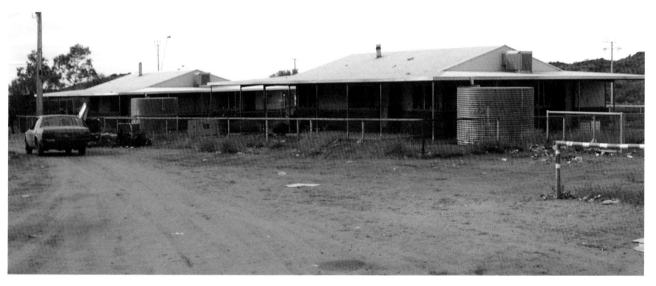

Figure 10.16 Aboriginal housing of reasonable standard in Central Australia. The key to adequate housing is regular and ongoing maintenance and the provision of sufficient houses so that each family has their own functional house.

some ophthalmologists and public health practitioners, did not necessarily give trachoma control activities a high priority.

Their complex report contained some 38 recommendations of which only one related to trachoma:

Trachoma control should be the responsibility of government-run and regional public health units and be organised on a regional basis where population mobility is high. Primary health care services should be involved in the detection and treatment of trachoma under the co-ordination of public health units (767).

The Commonwealth Government acknowledged the need for cross jurisdictional arrangements to address trachoma and for a "… nationally consistent approach to collection and reporting of prevalence data" (773). The government also indicated that trachoma activities could be incorporated into ongoing well-baby and well-adults health checks. It was decided that the Communicable Diseases Network Australia would be the body to co-ordinate Australia's trachoma activities.

Endemic trachoma persists in Aboriginal communities because poor personal and community hygiene permit the frequent spreading

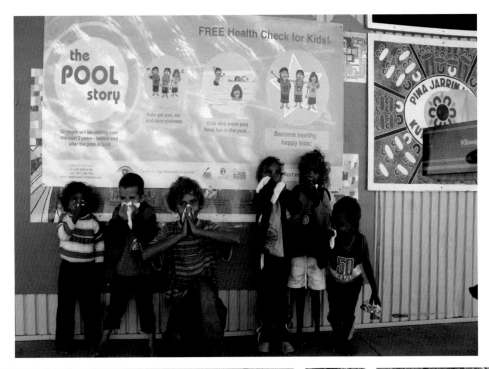

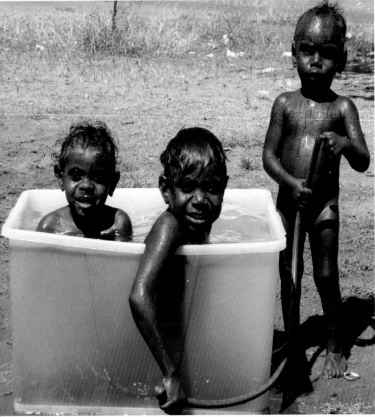

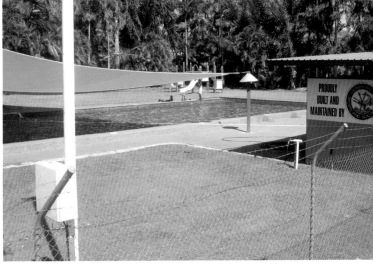

Figure 10.17 Aboriginal children in swimming pools

TOP children demonstrating how they blow their nose as part of facial cleanliness in front of a poster announcing the future construction of a swimming pool (courtesy, Heathcote Wright)

LEFT children in the same community improvising while they wait (courtesy, Heathcote Wright)

ABOVE RIGHT the community club pool in Oenpelli, NT.

TABLE 10.6: Summary of key recommendations from guidelines for the public health management of trachoma, CDNA, 2006 (776)

Recommendation:

Organisation

Trachoma control should be organised and run on a regional basis by regional population health units in conjunction with primary health care services, community representatives and other key stakeholders.

Priority should be given to areas with the highest number or the highest prevalence of active trachoma.

Data should be collected in accordance with the national trachoma dataset.

Surgery

The detection and management of trichiasis should be organised regionally with full stakeholder involvement.

The burden of trichiasis should be quantified in endemic regions.

Where trachoma is or has been endemic, Aboriginal and Torres Strait islander people aged 40-54 years should be screened every two years and those aged 55+ years should be screened annually for trichiasis as part of an adult health check.

Patients with trichiasis should be referred to an ophthalmologist for surgery and then followed up annually.

Antibiotics

The minimum target group for active trachoma screening should be Indigenous children aged 5–9 years living in communities/towns where trachoma is endemic.

Annual screening for active trachoma is recommended until active trachoma prevalence is < 5% for five consecutive years.

All children with active trachoma (TF and/or TI) should be treated with single-dose azithromycin.

If the prevalence is ≥ 10% and there is no obvious clustering, all children aged six months to 14 years and all household contacts should receive single-dose azithromycin

If the prevalence is ≥ 10% and cases are obviously clustered within several households and health staff can easily identify all household contacts of cases, single-dose azithromycin is recommended for all household contacts. Community-wide treatment is not required.

If the prevalence is < 10%, single-dose azithromycin is recommended for all household contacts.

Antibiotic treatment should be completed within two weeks of screening.

In regions where population mobility is high, screening and treatment activities should be completed in as short a timeframe as possible to minimise reinfection and achieve high coverage.

Facial cleanliness

Facial cleanliness in children should be promoted by including regular face-washing as part of a holistic personal hygiene program.

Environmental health

Environmental health, school and health promotion staff should be involved as key stakeholders when regional population health units and primary health care services plan and implement trachoma control activities so that 'F' and 'E' strategies appropriate to individual communities/regions can be implemented.

of infected eye secretion from one child to another (1) (Figure 10.18). If trachoma is to be reduced in Aboriginal communities, the swapping of infected eye secretions must be stopped by improving living conditions (as occurred 100 years ago for Europeans living in Australia). Australians living in urban and rural areas insist on the basic facilities required for healthy living, that is, a house, electricity, clean running water, sewerage, sealed roads and rubbish collection. Reports indicate that half the Aboriginal people in the Northern Territory do not have adequate housing (774,775), and one in six communities do not have potable water. This basic infrastructure is provided by local and state governments to everyone else in Australia. However, when one considers the conditions encountered in the communities of American Indians in the south west of America in the 1960s and how trachoma was subsequently eliminated with a sustained commitment (80), a similar outcome in Australia has to be possible and is sorely needed.

The future

In 2006 the Australian Government took some significant steps in the recognition and prioritisation of trachoma control activities. The most notable was the publication of the long-awaited national guidelines for the public health management of trachoma in Australia (776) (see Table 10.6).

These guidelines establish minimum best practice to be applied throughout Australia for the control of trachoma and provide recommendations to be followed by regional population health units in each state and territory. They advocate the co-ordination of activities with appropriate groups and the strong involvement of the local community. They provide clear guidelines for the implementation of the SAFE Strategy including the distribution of azithromycin. The Australian guidelines have some specific areas of difference from WHO recommendations, particularly with regard to the use of mass community treatment. Nevertheless, they are a strong forward move. The government will also support the development of a national trachoma dataset, monitoring of activities (696) and training of an appropriate workforce.

A study of the barriers in implementing a trachoma control program in northern Australia showed that a successful program needed input from government, regional health networks, local health staff and the community (341). Although input and engagement are required at each level, the key driver for a successful program was seen to be the presence of government policy and priority followed by the commitment of adequate resources for use at the more peripheral levels. Without these, those in the more peripheral levels would either not commit to the program, or become despondent and give up. At the local level, the provision of adequate time and staff to undertake trachoma activities are essential. Data collation and feedback were also important.

A review of the distribution of trachoma in Australia highlighted the variable way in which data had been collected. The reported community prevalence of active trachoma varied from 5% to 50% (741) although others still report active trachoma in 60% or 70% in some schoolchildren (742). The reported prevalence of trichiasis ranges from 1% to 19%.

Overall, these encouraging moves by the Australian Government to address trachoma are matched by other developments in the delivery of Aboriginal health. These include an increased focus on targeted operational research (777), more effective use of Aboriginal health workers (778) and the appropriate use of specialist outreach visits to remote Aboriginal communities as an effective delivery of specialist care (779). The latter is particularly relevant in the provision of trichiasis surgery.

What is really required to eliminate blinding trachoma in Australia is an ongoing political commitment at all levels of government. On a global scale we clearly have the tools and in Australia the resources are available. What is needed to eliminate trachoma as a blinding problem is sustained political will and the commitment to follow through.

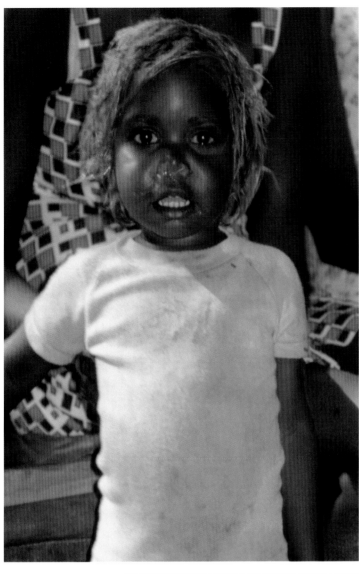

Figure 10.18 Aboriginal children
LEFT 1976
BELOW 2006 (courtesy, Heathcote Wright).

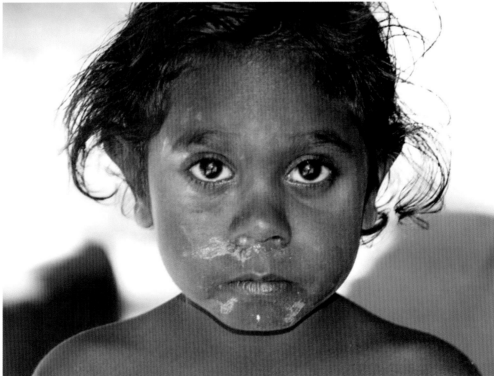

References

1. Taylor HR. Trachoma in Australia. Med J Aust. 2001;175:371–2.
2. Taylor HR. Trachoma. Int Ophthalmol. 1990;14:201–4.
3. World Health Organization. Report of the 2nd Global Scientific Meeting on Trachoma. Geneva, Switzerland: WHO 25–27 August, 2003.
4. MacCallan AF. Trachoma. London: Butterworth & Co. (Publishers) Ltd.; 1936.
5. Stephens RS. Chlamydial Evolution: A Billion Years and Counting. In: Schachter J, Christiansen G, Clarke IN, Hammerschlag MR, Kaltenboeck B, Kuo C-C, et al., editors. Chlamydial Infections. Proceedings of the Tenth International Symposium on Human Chlamydial Infections. June 16–21, 2002. Antalya – Turkey. San Francisco: International Chlamydia Symposium; 2002; 3–12.
6. Siniscal AA. The trachoma story. Public Health Rep. 1955;70:497–507.
7. Duke-Elder S, Wybar KC. System of Ophthalmology Vol II The Anatomy of the Visual System. St Louis: The C.V. Mosby Company; 1961.
8. Chen YZ. Ramble in Chinese ophthalmology, past and present. Chin Med J. 1981;94:1–4.
9. Siebeck R. The Global Distribution of Trachoma 1930–1955. In: Rodenwaldt E, Jusatz HJ, editors. World Atlas of Epidemic Diseases Part III. Hamburg: Falk-Verlag; 1961.
10. Hirschberg J. The History of Ophthalmology, in Eleven Volumes 1: Antiquity. Bonn: JP Wayenborgh Verlag; 1982.
11. Hirschberg J. The History of Ophthalmology in Eleven Volumes. Bonn: JP Wayenborgh Verlag; 1982–1994.
12. Millar MI, Lane SD. Ethno-ophthalmology in the Egyptian Delta: an historical systems approach to ethnomedicine in the Middle East. Soc Sci Med. 1988;26:651–7.
13. <http://en.wikipedia.org/wiki/Book_of_Tobit>, viewed August 2006.
14. Johnson HA. Fish bile and cautery: trachoma treatment in art. J R Soc Med 2005;98:30–32.
15. Boldt J. Trachoma. London: Hodder and Stoughton; 1904.
16. Vetch J. An Account of the Ophthalmia which appeared in England since the Return of the British Army from Egypt. London: Longman, Hurst, Rees & Orme; 1807.
17. Celsus AC. De Medicina (On Medicine) Celsus On Medicine Book VI: Loeb Classical Library 1935.
18. Hirschberg J. The History of Ophthalmology, in Eleven Volumes 2: The Middle Ages; The sixteenth and seventeenth centuries. Bonn: JP Wayenborgh Verlag; 1985.
19. Al-Rifai KMJ. Trachoma through history. Int Ophthalmol. 1988;12:9–14.
20. World Health Organization. Expert Committee on Trachoma. First Report. Geneva: WHO; 1952.
21. Isaacs HD. Medieval Judaeo-Arabic medicine as described in the Cairo Geniza. J R Soc Med. 1990;83:734–7.
22. Talbot D. Trachoma Importe D' Egypte En Italie Des Le XIII Siecle. Rev Int du Trach 1930;7:112–14.
23. Eldredge LM. A thirteenth-century ophthalmologist, Benvenutus Grassus: his treatise and its survival. J R Soc Med. 1998;91:47–52.
24. Cuenod A, Nataf R. Le Trachome. 120, Boulevard Saint-Germain, Paris (VI): Masson et Cie, Editeurs, Libraires de l'Academie de Medecine; 1930.
25. MacCallan AF. Trachoma and its complications in Egypt. Cambridge: Cambridge University Press; 1913.
26. Meyerhof M. A Short History of Ophthalmia during the Egyptian Campaigns of 1798–1807. Br J Ophthalmol. 1932:129–52.
27. Edmonston A. An Account of an Ophthalmia which appeared in the Second Regiment of Argyleshire Fencibles in the months of February, March and April. London; 1802.
28. Feibel RM. John Vetch and the Egyptian ophthalmia. Surv Ophthalmol. 1983;28:128–34.
29. Mackenzie W. A Practical Treatise on the Diseases of the Eye. London: Longman, Rees, Orme, Brown & Green; 1830.
30. Treacher Collins E. Introductory Chapter. In: Trachoma by J. Boldt. London: Hodder and Stoughton; 1904; xi–lii.
31. Barrett J. The Decline of Trachoma in Southern Australia. Trans Ophthalmol Soc Aust. 1941;111:1–7.
32. Wilson RP. Ophthalmia Aegyptiaca. Am J Ophthalmol. 1932;15:397–406.
33. World Health Organization. Expert Committee on Trachoma. Second Report. Geneva: WHO; 1956.

34. Vetch J. III. A Report on the influence of a Moist Atmosphere in aggravating the form, and retarding the cure of the Infectious Ophthalmia, drawn up by desire of Deputy Inspector Ferguson. Edin Med Surg J. 1808;4:151–6.

35. Benedek TG. Gonorrhea and the beginnings of clinical research ethics. Perspect Biol Med. 2005;48:54–73.

36. Taylor HR. Trachoma – the future for a disease of the past. Br J Ophthalmol. 1993;77:66–7.

37. Davidson L. 'Identities Ascertained': British Ophthalmology in the First Half of the Nineteenth Century: Oxford University Press; 1996.

38. Wilde RW. The Organs of Sight and Hearing. Lancet. 1845:431–5.

39. Treacher Collins E. The History & Traditions of the Moorfields Eye Hospital. One Hundred Years of Ophthalmic Discovery & Development. London: H.K. Lewis & Co Ltd; 1929.

40. Sorsby A, Sorsby M. A Short History of Ophthalmology. London, New York: Staples Press; 1948.

41. Duke-Elder S. A Century of International Ophthalmology (1857–1957). London: Henry Kimpton; 1958.

42. <http://www.iapb.org>, viewed September 2006

43. <http://www.v2020.org>, viewed September 2006

44. League of Nations Health Committee. Proceedings of 16th Session. Geneva; 1929.

45. League of Nations Health Organization Report. Geneva; 1931.

46. Mackenzie MD. A study of some of the research work carried out during the past five years on the distribution, etiology, treatment and prophylaxis of trachoma. Epidemiological Report 1935;14:41–78.

47. World Health Organization. Summary Report on the 1st Session of the Joint OIHP-WHO Study Group on Trachoma. Geneva: WHO; 1948. Report No.: WHO/Trachoma/1.

48. World Health Organization. Resolution WHA3.22. Trachoma. In: Third World Health Assembly, 25 May 1950, Geneva:, WHO; 1950.

49. World Health Organization. Expert Committee on Trachoma. Third Report. Geneva: WHO; 1962.

50. World Health Organization. Fourth WHO Scientific Group on Trachoma Research. Report. Geneva: WHO; 1966.

51. Keeney AH. Lessons in trachoma control. Sight Sav Rev. 1962;32:136–41.

52. Nataf R. Organization of Control of Trachoma and Associated Infections in Underdeveloped Countries. Geneva: WHO; 1951. Report No.: WHO/Trachoma/19.

53. Negrel AD. The Winning Hand to Defeat Trachoma. Rev Int Trach. 1999;76e Annee nouvelle serie:71–125.

54. Konyama K. History of Trachoma Control in Asia. Rev Int Trach. 2004–2005;82 Annee nouvelle serie:107–68.

55. World Health Organization. Alma-Ata 1978 Primary Health Care. Report of the International Conference on Primary Health Care, Alma-Ata, USSR, 6–12 September 1978. Geneva: WHO; 1978.

56. World Health Organization. Resolution WHA28.54. Prevention of blindness. Geneva: WHO 28 May 1975.

57. World Health Organization. Global Initiative for the Elimination of Avoidable Blindness. Geneva: WHO; 1997. Report No.: PBL/97.61.

58. Wibaut F. Mappa Mundi Trachomae. XIII Concilium Ophthalmologicum Amsterdam: ICO; 1929.

59. Sidky MM, Freyce MS. World distribution and prevalence of trachoma in recent years. Epidem Vital Stat Rep. 1949;II:230–77.

60. Rodenwaldt E, Jusatz HJ, editors World Atlas of Epidemic Diseases Part III. Hamburg: Falk-Verlag; 1961.

61. Foulds W. Personal communication. 2007.

62. Polack S, Brooker S, Kuper H, Mariotti S, Mabey D, Foster A. Mapping the global distribution of trachoma. Bull World Health Organ. 2005;83:913–19.

63. Wibaut F. Rev Int Trach. 1939;16:155.

64. Sorsby MA. Trachoma in Great Britain. Rev Int Trach. 1939;16:148–55.

65. Sorsby A. The Treatment of Trachoma. With special reference to local sulphonamide therapy. Br J Ophthalmol. 1945;29:98–102.

66. Jones BR. Changing concepts of trachoma and its control. Trans Ophthalmol Soc UK. 1980;100:25–9.

67. Chalmers AK. XXIII – Trachoma. In: Health of Glasgow: Glasgow Corporation; 1930; 415–28.

68. Gradle HS. Trachoma in the United States of America. Rev Int Trach. 1939;16:143–48.

69. Thygeson P. Epidemiologic observations on trachoma in the United States. Invest Ophthalmol. 1963;2:482–89.

70. Hildreth JS. Statement of Cases of Gonorrhoeal and Purulent Ophthalmia treated in Desmarres (U.S. Army) Eye and Ear Hospital, Chicago, Special Report of Treatment Employed. Tran Am Ophth Soc. 1865;1:12–28.

71. McMullen J. Trachoma, its prevalence and control among immigrants. JAMA. 1913;61:1110–13.

72. Markel H. "The Eyes Have It": Trachoma, the Perception of Disease, the United States Public Health Service, and the American Jewish Immigration Experience, 1897–1924. Bull Hist Med. 2000;74:525–60.

73. MacCallan AF. The epidemiology of trachoma. Br J Ophthalmol. 1931;15:369–411.

74. Allen SK, Semba RD. The Trachoma "Menace" in the United States, 1897–1960 – History of Ophthalmology. Surv Ophthalmol. 2002;47: 500–509.

75. Stucky JA. Trachoma among the natives of the mountains of Eastern Kentucky. JAMA. 1913;61:1116–24.

76. Schereschewsky J. Trachoma among the Indians. JAMA. 1913;61:1113–16.

77. Stucky JA. Ophthalmia and trachoma in the mountains of Kentucky. Trans Am Ophthalmol Soc. 1911:321–28.

78. Jackson E. To Eradicate Trachoma. Am J Ophthalmol. 1925;8:497–9.

79. Hoshiwara I, Powers DK, Krutz G. Comprehensive trachoma control program among the southwestern American Indians. XXI Concilium Ophthalmologicum Mexico 1970 Acta. 1970:1935–47.

80. Portney GL, Portney SB. Five-Year Perspective on Trachoma in the San Xavier Papago Indian. Arch Ophthalmol. 1974;92:211–12.

81. Friederich R. Eye disease in the Navajo Indians. Ann Ophthalmol. 1982;14:38–40.

82. Nataf R. Ophtalmologie et microbiologie la prevention de la cecite a l'echelle mondiale. L'ophtalmologie des origines a nos jours. 1973:183–4.

83. Nakajima A, Otake T. Smear cytology of the conjunctival epithelium in trachoma and some other diseases. Rev Int Trach. 1957;4:398–438.

84. Bietti G. Trachoma as a cause of visual impairment and blindness. Rev Int Trach. 1974;51:59–76.

85. Bendz JC. Quelques considerations sur la nature de l'ophthalmie militaire en Danemark. Copenhague; 1858.

86. Raehlmann E. Pathologish-anatomische Untersuchungen ueber die follikulaere Entzuendung der Bindehaut des Auges oder das Trachom. In: Albrecht von Graefe's Archiv fur Ophthalmologie; 1883; 73–166.

87. Hirschberg J. Ueber die koernige Augenentzuendung in Ost-und Westpreussen und ihre Bekampfung; 1897.

88. Greeff CR. Greeff Studien ueber epidemische Augenkrankheiten: Jena; 1898.

89. MacCallan AF. Ophthalmic conditions in the government schools in Egypt and their amelioration. The Ophthalmoscope. 1908;6: 856–863; 947–52.

90. Mann I. Correlation of race and way of life in Australia and the Territory of Papua and New Guinea with incidence and severity of clinical trachoma. Am J Ophthalmol. 1967;63:1302–9.

91. Jones BR. The prevention of blindness from trachoma (Bowman Lecture). Trans Ophthalmol Soc UK. 1975;95:16–33.

92. Nichols RL, Bobb AA, Haddad NA, McComb DE. Immunofluorescent studies of the microbiologic epidemiology of trachoma in Saudi Arabia. Am J Ophthalmol. 1967;63:1372–1408.

93. Güraksin A, Güllüulülu G. Prevalence of trachoma in Eastern Turkey. Int J Epidemiol. 1997;26:436–42.

94. Assaad FA, Maxwell-Lyons F. The use of catalytic models as tools for elucidating the clinical and epidemiological features of trachoma. Bull World Health Organ. 1966;34:341–55.

95. Thygeson P. The Limbus and Cornea in Experimental and Natural Human Trachoma and Inclusion Conjonctivitis. In: Gordon FB, editor. The Biology of the Trachoma Agent. New York: The New York Academy of Sciences; 1962; 201–11.

96. Wilson RP. A short slit lamp study of the corneal vessels in Egyptian trachoma with a discussion of their diagnostic value in doubtful cases. Folio Medica Orientalia. 1932;1:52.

97. Cuenod A, Nataf R. Biomicroscopie de la conjonctive. Paris: Masson et Cie Editeurs; 1934.

98. Herbert H. Trachomatous pannus and associated corneal changes. Trans Ophthalmol Soc UK. 1904;24:67–77.

99. Jui YL. Trachomatous pannus as a tool in the epidemiological study of the disease. XXI Concilium Ophthalmologica Acta, Mexico. 1970:1898–1902.

100. Dawson C. Personal Communication. 2006.

101. Assaad FA, Maxwell-Lyons F. Application of clinical scoring systems to trachoma research. Am J Ophthalmol. 1967;63:1327–56.

102. Tarizzo ML. Field methods for the control of trachoma. Geneva: World Health Organization; 1973.

103. Royal Australian College of Ophthalmologists. The National Trachoma and Eye Health Program of the Royal Australian College of Ophthalmologists. Sydney: Royal Australian College of Ophthalmologists; 1980.

104. Dawson CR, Jones BR, Darougar S. Blinding and non-blinding trachoma: assessment of intensity of upper tarsal inflammatory disease and disabling lesions. Bull World Health Organ. 1975;52:279–82.

105. Jones BR. Laboratory tests for chlamydial infection. Br J Ophthalmol. 1974;58:438–44.

106. Burton MJ, Kinteh F, Jallow O, Sillah A, Bah M, Faye M, et al. A randomised controlled trial of azithromycin following surgery for trachomatous trichiasis in the Gambia. Br J Ophthalmol. 2005;89:1282–8.

107. Dawson CR, Jones BR, Tarizzo ML. Guide to trachoma control. Geneva: World Health Organization; 1981.

108. Taylor HR, Prendergast RA, Dawson CR, Schachter J, Silverstein AM. An animal model of cicatrizing trachoma. Invest Ophthalmol Vis Sci. 1981;21:422–33.

109. Taylor HR, Velasco FM, Munoz EC, Ruvalcaba AM, Greene BM. Trachoma in Chiapas, Mexico. Rev Int Trach Pathol Ocul Trop Subtrop. 1983;60:17–27.

110. Taylor HR, Millan-Velasco F, Sommer A. The ecology of trachoma: an epidemiological study of

trachoma in Southern Mexico. Bull World Health Organ. 1985;63:559–67.

111. Tielsch JM, West KP Jr, Johnson GJ, Tizazu T, Schwab L, Chirambo MC, et al. Trachoma grading: observer trials conducted in Southern Malawi. Br J Ophthalmol. 1987;71:371–4.

112. Thylefors B, Dawson CR, Jones BR, West SK, Taylor HR. A simple system for the assessment of trachoma and its complication. Bull World Health Organ. 1987;65:477–83.

113. Taylor HR, West SK, Katala S, Foster A. Trachoma: evaluation of a new grading scheme in the United Republic of Tanzania. Bull World Health Organ. 1987;65:485–8.

114. West SK, Taylor HR. Reliability of photographs for grading trachoma in field studies. Br J Ophthalmol. 1990;74:12–13.

115. Solomon AW, Bowman RJC, Yorston D, Massae PA, Safari S, Savage B, et al. Operational Evaluation of the Use of Photographs for Grading Active Trachoma. Am J Trop Med Hyg. 2006;74:505–8.

116. Reacher MH, Munoz B, Alghassany A, Daar AS, Elbualy M, Taylor HR. A controlled trial of surgery for trachomatous trichiasis of the upper lid. Arch Ophthalmol. 1992;110:667–74.

117. Melese M, Alemayehu W, Bejiga A, Adamu Y, Worku A. Modified grading system for upper eyelid trachomatous trichiasis. Ophthalmic Epidemiol. 2003;10:75–80.

118. Hosni FA. The cornea and trachoma in developing countries. Experience in one of the Gulf States (Qatar). Rev Int Trach Pathol Ocul Trop Subtrop. 1980;57:107–14.

119. Rapoza PA, West SK, Turner VM, Katala SJ, Muñoz B, Taylor HR. Etiology of corneal opacification in central Tanzania. Int Ophthalmol. 1993;17:47–51.

120. Wilson MC, Keyvan-Larijani E, Millan-Velasco F, Tielsch JM, Taylor HR. The epidemiology of trachoma in Chiapas (Mexico). Rev Int Trach. 1987;64:159–66.

121. Dawson CR. Trachoma and Other Chlamydial Eye Diseases. In: Orfila J, Byrne GI, Chernesky MA, Grayston JT, Jones RB, Ridgway GL, et al., editors. Chlamydial Infections. Proceedings of the Eighth International Symposium on Human Chlamydial Infections, Chateau de Montvillargenne, 602700 Gouvieux – Chantilly, France, 19–24 June, 1994. Bologna – Italy: Societa Editrice Esculapio; 1994; 277–86.

122. West ES, Munoz B, Mkocha H, Holland MJ, Aguirre A, Solomon AW, et al. Mass Treatment and the Effect on the Load of *Chlamydia trachomatis* Infection in a Trachoma-Hyperendemic Community. Invest Ophthalmol Vis Sci. 2005;46:83–7.

123. Katz J, West KP, Khatry SK, LeClerq SC, Pradhan EK, Thapa MD, et al. Prevalence and risk factors for trachoma in Sarlahi district, Nepal. Br J Ophthalmol. 1996;80:1037–41.

124. Bobo LD, Novak N, Munoz B, Hsieh YH, Quinn TC, West S. Severe disease in children with trachoma is associated with persistent Chlamydia trachomatis infection. J Infect Dis. 1997;176:1524–30.

125. Ngondi J, Onsarigo A, Adamu L, Matende I, Baba S, Reacher M, et al. The epidemiology of trachoma in Eastern Equatoria and Upper Nile States, southern Sudan. Bull World Health Organ. 2005;83:1–12.

126. Bailey R, Duong T, Carpenter R, Whittle H, Mabey D. The duration of human ocular *Chlamydia trachomatis* infection is age dependent. Epidemiol Infect. 1999;123:479–86.

127. Solomon AW, Zondervan M, Kuper H, Buchan JC, Mabey DCW, Foster A. Trachoma Control – A Guide for Programme Managers. Geneva: World Health Organization; 2006.

128. World Health Organization. Primary Health Care Level Management of Trachoma. Geneva: WHO; 1993. Report No.: WHO/PBL/93.33.

129. Dawson CR, Marx R, Daghfous T, Juster R, Schachter J. What Clinical Signs are Critical in Evaluating the Impact of Intervention in Trachoma? In: Bowie WR, Caldwell HD, Jones RP, Mardh P-A, Ridgway GL, Schachter J, et al., editors. Chlamydial Infections. Proceedings of the Seventh International Symposium on Human Chlamydial Infections, Harrison Hot Springs, British Columbia, Canada, 24–29 June 1990. Cambridge: Cambridge University Press; 1990; 271–8.

130. Thygeson P, Dawson CR. Trachoma and follicular conjunctivitis in children. Arch Ophthalmol. 1966;75:3–12.

131. Haddad NA, Ballas SK. Seasonal mucopurulent conjunctivitis. Observations on epidemiology in rural areas in summer. Am J Ophthalmol. 1968;65:225–8.

132. Vastine DW, Dawson CR, Daghfous T, Messadi M, Hoshiwara I, Yoneda C, et al. Severe endemic trachoma in Tunisia. 1. Effect of topical chemotherapy on conjunctivitis and ocular bacteria. Br J Ophthalmol. 1974;58:833–42.

133. Yoneda C, Dawson CR, Daghfous T, Hoshiwara I, Jones P, Messadi M, et al. Cytology as a guide to the presence of chlamydial inclusions in Giemsa-stained conjunctival smears in severe endemic trachoma. Br J Ophthalmol. 1975;59:116–24.

134. Dawson CR, Whitcher JP, Lyon C, Schachter J. Response to treatment in ocular chlamydial infections (trachoma and inclusion conjunctivitis): analogies with nongonococcal urethritis. In: Hobson D, Holmes KK, editors. Nongonococcal urethritis and related infections. Washington, DC: American Society for Microbiology; 1977; 135–9.

135. Schachter J, Moncada J, Dawson CR, Sheppard J, Courtright P, Said ME, et al. Nonculture methods

for diagnosing chlamydial infection in; patients with trachoma: a clue to the pathogenesis of the disease? J Infect Dis. 1988;158:1347–52.

136. Chumbley LC, Thomson IM. Epidemiology of trachoma in the West Bank and Gaza Strip. Eye. 1988;1:463–70.

137. Mazloum H, Totten PA, Brooks GF, Dawson CR, Falkow S, James JF, et al. An unusual Neisseria isolated from conjunctival cultures in rural Egypt. J Infect Dis. 1986;154:212–24.

138. Dawson CR, Daghfous T, Messadi M, Hoshiwara I, Schachter J. Severe endemic trachoma in Tunisia. Br J Ophthalmol. 1976;60:245–52.

139. Reinhards J, Weber A, Nizetic B, Kupka K, Maxwell-Lyons F. Studies in the epidemiology and control of seasonal conjunctivitis and trachoma in southern Morocco. Bull World Health Organ. 1968;39:497–545.

140. Wright HR, Keeffe JE, Taylor HR. Trachoma and the Need for a Coordinated Community-Wide response: A Case-Based Study. PLoS Med. 2006;3:186–90.

141. Whitcher JP, Cevallos V. Moraxella, down but not out – the eye bug that won't go away. Br J Ophthalmol. 2006;90:1215–16.

142. Halberstaedter L, von Prowazek S. Uber zelleinschusse parasitarer natur beim trachom. (On cell inclusions of a parasitic nature in trachoma). Arb. K. Gesundh. Amt. 1907;26: 44–7.

143. Nicolle C, Cuenod A, Baizot L. Etude experimentale du trachome. Arch Instit Pasteur de Tunis 1913;4:157–82.

144. Lindner. Zur Atiologie der gonokokkenfreien Urethritis. Wein. klin. Wchnschr. 1910;23:283.

145. Lindner K. Zur Biologie des Einschlussblennorrhoe- (Trachom) Virus. Arch f. Ophth. 1913;84:1.

146. Fritsch H, Hofstatter A, Lindner K. Experimentelle Studien sur Trachomfrage. Arch. f. Ophth. 1910;76:547.

147. Lindner K. Zur Trachomforschung. Zeitschrift fuer Augenheilkunde. 1909;22:547–50.

148. Thygeson P, Hanna L, Dawson C, Zichosch J, Jawetz E. Inoculation of human volunteer with egg-grown inclusion conjunctivitis virus. Am J Ophthalmol. 1962;53:786–95.

149. Thygeson P. Inoculation of the human conjunctiva with trachomatous materials. Am J Ophthalmol. 1933;16:409–11.

150. Thygeson P, Proctor FI, Richards P. Etiologic significance of the elementary body in trachoma. Am J Ophthalmol. 1935;18:811–13.

151. Hanna L. Immunofluorescence in chronic TRIC infections of American Indians and Tunisians: influence of trauma on results of tests. In: Nichols RL, editor. Trachoma and Related Disorders. Amsterdam: Excerpta Medica; 1971; 461–68.

152. World Health Organization. Guide to the laboratory diagnosis of trachoma. Geneva: WHO; 1975.

153. Hardy D, Surman PG, Howarth WH, Path MC. A system of representation of cytologic features of external eye infections with special reference to trachoma. Am J Ophthalmol. 1967;63:1535–37.

154. Noguchi H. The Etiology of Trachoma. J Exp Med. 1928;48:1–53.

155. Robbins AR. Ophthalmologic Review. Role of Bacterium granulosa in trachoma. Arch Ophthalmol. 1935;14:629–40.

156. T'ang FF, Chang HL, Huang YT, Wang KC. Studies on the etiology of trachoma with special reference to isolation of the virus in chick embryo. Chin Med J. 1957;75:429–47.

157. Rake G, Jones HP. Studies on Lymphogranuloma Venereum I. Development of the Agent in the Yolk Sac of the Chicken Embryo. J Exp Med. 1942;75:323–37.

158. Chang HL, Chang E. Achievements in research on trachoma virus and prevention and treatment of trachoma in China. (Contributions at the 301–17). In: GEN: 142, Peking Symposium, 1964; Peking; 301–17.

159. Collier LH, Sowa J, Sowa S. The serum and conjunctival antibody response to trachoma in Gambian children. J Hyg Cambridge. 1972;70:727–40.

160. Macchiavello A. Estudios sobre Tifus Examtematico; III. Un neuvo metodo para tenier Rickettsia. Rev Chil Hyg Med. 1937;1:101–6.

161. Macchiavello A. El virus del tracoma y su cultivo en el saco vitelino del huevo de gallino. Rev Ecuatoriana de Hig y Med Trop Guayaquil. 1944;1:33.

162. Freyche M-J. Some Gaps in the Present Knowledge of the Epidemiology of Trachoma. Geneva: WHO; 1951. Report No.: WHO/Trachoma/6.

163. Macchiavello A. The virus of trachoma and its cultivation in the yolk sac of the hen's egg. Trop Dis Bull. 1948;4:1112–14.

164. Poleff L. Culture des corps du trachoma a la lumiere des acquisition nouvelles. Rev Int Trach. 1948;26:175–6.

165. Stewart FH, Badir G. Experiments on the cultivation of trachoma virus in the chick embryo. J Pathol Bacteriol. 1950;62:457–60.

166. Gordon FB, Quan AL. Isolation of the trachoma agent in cell culture. Proc Soc Exp Biol Med. 1965;118:354–9.

167. Taylor HR, Rapoza PA, Johnson S, Muñoz B, Katala S, Mmbaga BBO, et al. The epidemiology of infection in trachoma. Invest Ophthalmol Vis Sci. 1989;30:1823–33.

168. Solomon AW, Holland MJ, Burton MJ, West SK, Alexander NDE, Aguirre A, et al. Strategies for control of trachoma: observational study with quantitative PCR. Lancet. 2003;362:198–204.

169. Bedson SP. The use of the complement-fixation reaction in the diagnosis of human psittacosis. Lancet. 1935;2:1277–80.

170. Schachter J, Dawson CR. Human Chlamydial Infections. Littleton, Massachusetts: PSG Publishing Company; 1978.

171. Darougar S, editor. The Humoral Immune Response to Chlamydial Infection in Humans. Chicago, Illinois: The University of Chicago; 1985.

172. Wang S-P. A micro immunofluorescence method. Study of antibody response to TRIC organisms in mice. In: Nichols RL, editor. Trachoma and related disorders caused by chlamydial agents. Amsterdam: Excerpta Medica; 1971; 273–88.

173. Wang S-P, Grayston JT. Classification of TRIC and related strains with micro immunofluorescence. In: Nichols RL, editor. Trachoma and related disorders caused by chlamydial agents. Amsterdam: Excerpta Medica; 1971; 305–21.

174. Wang S-P, Grayston JT. Local and systemic antibody response to trachoma eye infection in monkeys. In: Nichols RL, editor. Trachoma and related disorders caused by chlamydial agents. Amsterdam: Excerpta Medica; 1971; 217–32.

175. Dhir SP, Wang S-P, Grayston JT. Type-specific antigens of trachoma organisms. In: Nichols RL, editor. Trachoma and related disorders caused by chlamydial agents. Amsterdam: Excerpta Medica; 1971; 133–41.

176. Wang S-P, Grayston JT, Kuo CC, Alexander ER, Holmes KK. Serodiagnosis of Chlamydia trachomatis infection with the micro immunofluorescence test. In: Hobson D, Holmes KK, editors. Nongonococcal urethritis and related infections. Washington DC: American Society for Microbiology; 1977; 237–48.

177. Nichols RL, Von Fritzinger K, McComb DE. Epidemiological data derived from immunotyping of 338 trachoma strains isolated from children in Saudi Arabia. In: Trachoma and related disorders caused by chlamydial agents. Amsterdam: Excerpta Medica; 1971; 337–57.

178. Grayston JT, Yeh LJ, Wang SP, Kuo C-C, Beasley RP, Gale JL. Pathogenesis of ocular Chlamydia trachomatis infections in humans. In: Hobson D, Holmes KK, editors. Nongonococcal urethritis and related infections. Washington DC: American Society for Microbiology; 1977; 113–25.

179. Caldwell HD, Kromhout J, Schachter J. Purification and partial characterization of the major outer membrane protein of Chlamydia trachomatis. Infect Immun. 1981;31:1161–76.

180. Wang S-P, Kuo C-C, Barnes RC, Stephens RS, Grayston JT. Immunotyping of Chlamydia trachomatis with monoclonal antibodies. J Infect Dis. 1985;152:791–800.

181. Wang S-P, Grayston JT. Micro Immunofluorescence Antibody Responses in *Chlamydia trachomatis* Infection, a Review. In: Mardh PA, Holmes KK, Oriel JD, Piot P, Schachter J, editors. Chlamydial Infections. Proceedings of the 5th International Symposium on Human Chlamydial Infections; 1982; Lund (Sweden): Elsevier Biomedical Press; 1982; 301–16.

182. Nichols RL, McComb DE. Immunofluorescent studies with trachoma and related antigens. J Immunol. 1962;89:545.

183. Nichols RL, McComb DE, Haddad N, Murray ES. Studies on trachoma. II. Comparison of fluorescent antibody, Giemsa, and egg isolation methods for detection of trachoma virus in human conjunctival scrapings. Am J Trop Med Hyg. 1963;12:223–9.

184. Jawetz E, Hanna L, Dawson C, Wood R, Briones O. Subclinical infections with TRIC agents. Am J Ophthalmol. 1967;63:1413–24.

185. Schachter J, Hanna L, Tarizzo ML, Dawson CR. Relative efficacy of different methods of laboratory diagnosis in chronic trachoma in the United States. In: Nichols RL, editor. Trachoma and related disorders caused by chlamydial agents. Amsterdam: Excerpta Medica; 1971; 469–75.

186. Caldwell HD. Structural Analysis of the Major Outer Membrane Protein of *Chlamydia* Spp. In: Mardh PA, Holmes KK, Oriel JD, Piot P, Schachter J, editors. Chlamydial Infections. Proceedings of the 5th International Symposium on Human Chlamydial Infections, Lund (Sweden): Elsevier Biomedical Press; 1982; 45–50.

187. Tam MR, Stephens RS, Kuo C-C, Holmes KK, Stamm WE, Nowinski RC. Use of monoclonal antibodies to Chlamydia trachomatis as immunodiagnostic reagents. In: Mardh P-A, Holmes KK, Oriel JD, Piot P, Schachter J, editors. Chlamydial infections. Amsterdam: Elsevier Biomedical Press; 1982; 317–20.

188. Ridgway GL. The Laboratory Diagnosis of Chlamydial Infection. In: Oriel D, Ridgway G, Schachter J, Taylor-Robinson D, Ward M, editors. Chlamydial Infections. Proceedings of the Sixth International Symposium on Human Chlamydial Infections, Sanderstead, Surrey, 15–21 June 1986. Cambridge: Cambridge University Press; 1986; 539–49.

189. Taylor HR, Argawala N, Johnson SL. Detection of experimental Chlamydia trachomatis eye infection in conjunctival smears and in tissue culture by use of fluorescein-conjugated monoclonal antibody. J Clin Microbiol. 1984;20:391–5.

190. Taylor HR, Fitch CP, Murillo-Lopez F, Rapoza P. The diagnosis and treatment of chlamydial conjunctivitis. Int Ophthalmol. 1988;12:95–9.

191. Wilson MC, Millan-Velasco F, Tielsch JM, Taylor HR. Direct-smear fluorescent antibody cytology as a field diagnostic tool for trachoma. Arch Ophthalmol. 1986;104:688–90.

192. Rapoza PA, Quinn TC, Kiessling LA, Green WR, Taylor HR. Assessment of neonatal conjunctivitis with a direct immunofluorescent monoclonal antibody stain for Chlamydia. JAMA. 1986;255:3369–73.

193. Fitch CP, Rapoza PA, Owens S, Murillo-Lopez F, Johnson RA, Quinn TC, et al. Epidemiology and diagnosis of acute conjunctivitis at an inner city hospital. Ophthalmology. 1989;96:1215–20.

194. Rapoza PA, Quinn TC, Terry AC, Gottsch JD, Kiessling LA, Taylor HR. A systematic approach to the diagnosis and treatment of chronic conjunctivitis. Am J Ophthalmol. 1990;109: 138–42.

195. Taylor HR, Siler JA, Mkocha HA, Muñoz B, Velez V, DeJong L, et al. The microbiology of endemic trachoma – a longitudinal study. J Clin Microbiol. 1991;29:1593–95.

196. Solomon AW, Peeling RW, Foster A, Mabey DCW. Diagnosis and Assessment of Trachoma. Clin Microbiol Rev. 2004;17:982–1011.

197. Goldschmidt P, Afghani T, Nadeem M, Ali-Khan W, Chaumeil C, de Barbeyrac B. Clinical and microbiological diagnosis of trachoma in children living in rural areas in the district of Attock, Punjab, Pakistan. Ophthalmic Epidemiol. 2006;13:335–42.

198. Caldwell HD, Schachter J. Immunoassay for detecting Chlamydia trachomatis major outer membrane protein. J Clin Microbiol. 1983;18: 539–45.

199. Evans RT, Taylor-Robinson D. Development and evaluation of an enzyme-linked immunosorbent assay (ELISA), using chlamydial group antigen to detect antibodies to Chlamydia trachomatis. J Clin Pathol. 1982;35:1122–8.

200. Stamm WE. Laboratory Diagnosis of Chlamydial Infection. In: Bowie WR, Caldwell HD, Jones RP, Mardh P, Ridgway GL, Schachter J, et al., editors. Chlamydial Infections. Proceedings of the Seventh International Symposium on Human Chlamydial Infections, Harrison Hot Springs, British Columbia, Canada, 24–29 June 1990. Cambridge: Cambridge University Press; 1990; 459–70.

201. Schachter J. Diagnosis of Human Chlamydial Infections. In: Stephens RS, Byrne GI, Christiansen G, Clarke IN, Grayston TG, Rank RG, et al., editors. Chlamydial Infections. Proceedings of the Ninth International Symposium on Human Chlamydial Infection, Napa, California, USA, June 21–26, 1998. San Francisco, CA 94110, USA: International Chlamydia Symposium; 1998; 577–86.

202. Ward M, Bailey R, Lesley A, Kajbaf M, Robertson J, Mabey D. Persisting inapparent chlamydial infection in a trachoma endemic community in The Gambia. Scand J Infect Dis. 1990;69:137–48.

203. Bailey RL, Arullendran P, Whittle HC, Mabey DW. Randomised controlled trial of single-dose azithromycin in treatment of trachoma. Lancet. 1993;342:453–56.

204. Schachter J. Diagnosis of Chlamydia trachomatis Infection. In: Orfila J, Byrne GI, Cherensky MA, Grayston JT, Jones RB, Ridgway GL, et al., editors.

Chlamydial Infections. Proceedings of the Eighth International Symposium on Human Chlamydial Infections, Chateau de Montvillargenne, 602700 Gouvieux – Chantilly, France, 19–24 June, 1994. Bologna – Italy: Societa Editrice Esculapio; 1994; 293–302.

205. Michel CEC, Solomon AW, Magbanua JPV, Massae PA, Huang L, Mosha J, et al. Field evaluation of rapid point-of-care assay for targeting antibiotic treatment for trachoma control: a comparative study. Lancet. 2006;367:1585–90.

206. Taylor HR, Wright HR. Dip-stick test for trachoma contol programmes. Lancet. 2006;367:1553–54.

207. Hyypia T, Jalava A, Larsen SH, Terho P, Hukkanen V. Detection of Chlamydia trachomatis in clinical specimens by nucleic acid spot hybridization. J Gen Microbiol. 1985;131:975–8.

208. Kahane S, Sarov I. Detection of Chlamydia by DNA hybridization with a Native Chlamydial Plasmid Probe. In: Oriel D, Ridgway G, Schachter J, Taylor-Robinson D, Ward M, editors. Chlamydial Infections. Proceedings of the Sixth International Symposium on Human Chlamydial Infections, Sanderstead, Surrey, 15–21 June 1986. Cambridge: Cambridge University Press; 1986; 574–7.

209. Horn JE, Hammer ML, Falkow S, Quinn TC. Detection of Chlamydia trachomatis in tissue culture and cervical scrapings by in situ DNA hybridization. J Infect Dis. 1986;153:1155–9.

210. Holland SM, Hudson AP, Bobo L, Whittum-Hudson J, Viscidi RP, Quinn TC, et al. Demonstration of chlamydial RNA and DNA during a culture-negative state. Infect Immun. 1992;60:2040–47.

211. Dean D, Pant CR, O'Hanley P. Improved sensitivity of a modified polymerase chain reaction amplified DNA probe in comparison with serial tissue culture passage for detection of Chlamydia trachomatis in conjunctival specimens from Nepal. Diagn Microbiol Infect Dis. 1989;12:133–7.

212. Mahony JB, Luinstra KE, Sellars JW, Cherensky MA. Comparison of Polymerase Chain Reaction (PCR), Enzyme Immunoassay and Culture for the Diagnosis of C. trachomatis Infections in Symptomatic and Asymptomatic Males and Females. In: Bowie WR, Caldwell HD, Jones RP, Mardh P, Ridgway GL, Schachter J, et al., editors. Chlamydial Infections. Proceedings of the Seventh International Symposium on Human Chlamydial Infections, Harrison Hot Springs, British Columbia, Canada, 24–29 June 1990. Cambridge: Cambridge University Press; 1990; 487–90.

213. Quinn TC, Bobo L, Holland SM, Gaydos CA, Hook E, Viscidi RP. Diagnosis of Chlamydia trachomatis Cervical Infections by Polymerase Chain Reaction. In: Bowie WR, Caldwell HD, Jones RP, Mardh P, Ridgway GL, Schachter J, et al., editors. Chlamydial Infections. Proceedings of the Seventh International Symposium on Human

Chlamydial Infections, Harrison Hot Springs, British Columbia, Canada, 24–29 June 1990. Cambridge: Cambridge University Press; 1990; 491–4.

214. Ossewaarde JM, Rieffe M, Buisman NJF, van Loon AM. Diagnosis of Chlamydia trachomatis Conjunctivitis by Polymerase Chain Reaction and Detection of Secretory Immunoglobulin A. In: Bowie WR, Caldwell HD, Jones RP, Mardh P, Ridgway GL, Schachter J, et al., editors. Chlamydial Infections. Proceedings of the Seventh International Symposium on Human Chlamydial Infections, Harrison Hot Springs, British Columbia, Canada, 24–29 June 1990. Cambridge: Cambridge University Press; 1990; 495–8.

215. Frost EH, Deslandes S, Bourgaux-Ramoisy D. Typing Chlamydia Isolates with the Polymerase Chain Reaction. In: Bowie WR, Caldwell HD, Jones RP, Mardh P, Ridgway GL, Schachter J, et al., editors. Chlamydial Infections. Proceedings of the Seventh International Symposium on Human Chlamydial Infections, Harrison Hot Springs, British Columbia, Canada, 24–29 June 1990. Cambridge: Cambridge University Press; 1990; 499–502.

216. Bobo L, Munoz B, Viscidi R, Quinn T, Nkocha H, West S. Diagnosis of Chlamydia trachomatis eye infection in Tanzania by polymerase chain reaction/enzyme immunoassay. Lancet. 1991;338:847–50.

217. Chidambaram JD, Alemayehu W, Melese M, Lakew T, Yi E, House J, et al. Effect of a single mass antibiotic distribution on the prevalence of infectious trachoma. JAMA. 2006;295:1142–6.

218. Yang JL, Schachter J, Moncada J, Habte D, Zerihun M, House JI, et al. Comparison of an rRNA-based and DNA-based nucleic acid amplification test for the detection of Chlamydia trachomatis in trachoma. Br J Ophthalmol. 2007;91:293–5.

219. Goldschmidt P. Microbiological confirmation of the clinical diagnosis of trachoma using amplification of Chlamydial DNA (PCR). In: WHO Trachoma Scientific Informal Workshop 2005; Geneva, Switzerland.

220. Bailey RL, Hayes L, Pickett M, Whittle HC, Ward ME, Mabey DCW. Molecular epidemiology of trachoma in a Gambian village. Br J Ophthalmol. 1994;78:813–17.

221. Schachter J, West S, Mabey D, Dawson CR, Bobo L, Bailey R, et al. Azithromycin in control of trachoma. Lancet. 1999;354:630–5.

222. Apfalter P, Reischl U, Hammerschlag MR. In-house nucleic acid amplification assays in research: how much quality control is needed before one can rely upon the results? J Clin Microbiol. 2005;43: 5835–41.

223. Schachter J. Diagnostics. In: Cherensky MA, Caldwell H, Christiansen G, Clarke IN, Kaltenboeck B, Knirsch C, et al., editors.

Chlamydial Infections. Proceedings of the Eleventh International Symposium on Human Chlamydial Infections, Niagara-on-the-Lake, Ontario, Canada, June 18–23, 2006. San Francisco, CA 94110, USA: International Chlamydia Symposium; 2006; 435–44.

224. Baral K, Osaki S, Shreshta B, Panta CR, Boulter A, Pang F, et al. Reliability of clinical diagnosis in identifying infectious trachoma in a low-prevalence area of Nepal. Bull World Health Organ. 1999;77:461–6.

225. Schachter J, Moncada J. Nucleic Acid Amplification Tests to Diagnose Chlamydia trachomatis Genital Infection…The Glass is More Than Half Full. In: Schachter J, Christiansen G, Clarke IN, Hammerschlag MR, Kaltenboeck B, Kuo C-C, et al., editors. Chamydial Infections. Proceedings of the Tenth International Symposium on Human Chlamydial Infections, June 16–21, 2002, Antalya – Turkey. San Francisco, CA 94110, USA: International Chlamydia Symposium; 2002; 379–88.

226. Solomon AW, Holland MJ, Alexander NDE, Massae PA, Aguirrre A, Natividad-Sancho A, et al. Mass treatment with single-dose azithromycin for trachoma. N Engl J Med. 2004;351:1962–71.

227. Burton MJ, Holland MJ, Faal N, Aryee EAN, Alexander NDE, Bah M, et al. Which members of a community need antibiotics to control trachoma? Conjunctival Chlamydial trachomatis infection load in Gambian villages. Invest Ophthalmol Vis Sci. 2003;44:4215–22.

228. Burton MJ, Holland MJ, Jeffries D, Mabey DCW, Bailey RL. Conjuntival chlamydial 16S ribosomal RNA expression in trachoma: is chlamydial metabolic activity required for disease to develop? Clin Infect Dis. 2006;42:463–70.

229. Taylor HR, Velez V. Clearance of chlamydial elementary bodies from the conjunctival sac. Invest Ophthalmol Vis Sci. 1987;28:1199–201.

230. Davies PO, Ridgway GL. The role of polymerase chain reaction and ligase chain reaction for the detection of Chlamydia trachomatis. Int J STD and AIDS. 1997;8:731–8.

231. Diamant J, Benis R, Schacther J, Moncada J, Pang F, Jha HC, et al. Pooling of Chlamydia laboratory tests to determine the prevalence of ocular chlamydia trachomatis infection. Ophthalmic Epidemiol. 2001;8:109–17.

232. Lietman TM, Dawson CR, Osaki SY, Zegans ME. Clinically active trachoma versus actual Chlamydial infection. Med J Aust. 2000;172:93–4.

233. Miller K, Schmidt G, Alemayehu W, Yi E, Cevallos V, Donnellan C, et al. How reliable is the clinical exam in detecting ocular chlamydial infection. Ophthalmic Epidemiol. 2004;11:255–62.

234. Wright HR, Taylor HR. Clinical examination and laboratory tests for estimation of trachoma prevalence in a remote setting: what are they really telling us? Lancet Infect Dis. 2005;5:313–20.

235. Thein J, Zhao P, Liu H, Xu J, Jha HC, Miao Y, et al. Does clinical diagnosis indicate ocular chlamydial infection in areas with a low prevalence of trachoma? Ophthalmic Epidemiol. 2002;9:263–9.

236. Bird M, Dawson CR, Schachter JS, Miao Y, Shama A, Osman A, et al. Does the diagnosis of trachoma adequately identify ocular chlamydial infection in trachoma-endemic areas? J Infect Dis. 2003;187:1669–73.

237. Kuper H, Solomon AW, Buchan J, Zondervan M, A F, Mabney D. A critical review of the SAFE strategy for the prevention of blinding trachoma. Lancet Infect Dis. 2003;3:372–81.

238. Burton MJ, Holland MJ, Makalo P, Aryee EAN, Alexander NDE, Sillah A, et al. Re-emergence of *Chlamydia trachomatis* infection afer mass antibiotic treatment of a trachoma-endemic Gambian community: a longitudinal study. Lancet. 2005;365:1321–8.

239. Taylor HR, Rapoza PA, West S, Johnson S, Muñoz B, Katala S, et al. The epidemiology of infection in trachoma. Invest Ophthalmol Vis Sci. 1989;30:1823–33.

240. World Health Organization. Report of the Ninth Meeting of the WHO Alliance for the Global Elimination of Blinding Trachoma. Geneva: WHO 21–23 March 2005. Report No.: WHO/PBD/GET/05.1.

241. Taylor HR, West SK, Mmbaga BBO, Katala SJ, Turner V, Lynch M, et al. Hygiene factors and increased risk of trachoma in Central Tanzania. Arch Ophthalmol. 1989;107:1821–5.

242. Schemann J-F, Sacko D, Malvy D, Momo G, Traore L, Bore O, et al. Risk factors for trachoma in Mali. Int J Epidemiol. 2002;31:194–201.

243. Mesfin MM, de la Camera J, Tareke IG, Amanual G, Araya T, Kedir AM. A community-based trachoma survey: prevalence and risk factors in the Tigray region of Northern Ethiopia. Ophthalmic Epidemiol. 2006;13:173–81.

244. Khandekar R, Mohamed AJ, Raisi AL, Kurup P, Shah S, Dirir MH, et al. Prevalence and distribution of active trachoma in children of less than five years of age in trachoma endemic regions of Oman in 2005. Ophthalmic Epidemiol. 2006;13:167–72.

245. Négrel AD, Khazraji YC, Akalay O. Le trachome dans la province de Ouarzazate, Maroc. Bull l'Organis Mondiale Sante. 1992;70:451–6.

246. Negrel AD, Taylor HR, West S. Guidelines for the Rapid Assessment for Blinding Trachoma. Geneva: World Health Organization; 2001. Report No.: WHO/PBD/GET/00.8.

247. Myatt M, Limburg H, Minassian D, Katyola D. Field trial of applicability of lot quality assurance sampling method for rapid assessment of prevalence of active trachoma. Bull World Health Organ. 2003;81: 885–7.

248. World Health Organization. Report of the First Meeting of the WHO Alliance for the Global Elimination of Trachoma. Geneva, Switzerland: WHO 30 June – 1 July 1997. Report No.: WHO/PBL/GET/97.1.

249. Limburg H, Bah M, Johnson GJ. Trial of the trachoma rapid assessment methodology in the Gambia. Ophthalmic Epidemiol. 2001;8:73–85.

250. Paxton A. Rapid assessment of trachoma prevalence – Singida, Tanzania. A study to compare assessment methods. Ophthalmic Epidemiol. 2001;8:87–96.

251. Rabiu MM, Alhassan MB, Abiose A. Trial of Trachoma Rapid Assessment in a subdistrict of northen Nigeria. Ophthalmic Epidemiol. 2001;8:263–72.

252. Myatt M, Mai NP, Quynh NQ, Nga NH, Tai HH, Long NH, et al. Using lot quality-assurance sampling and area sampling to identify priority areas for trachoma control: Viet Nam. WHO Bulletin OMS. 2005;83:756–63.

253. Faye M, Kuper H, Dineen BP, Bailey R. Rapid assessment for prioritisation of trachoma control at community level in one district of the Kaolack Region, Senegal. Trans R Soc Trop Med Hyg. 2006;100:149–7.

254. Ngondi J, Ole-Sempele F, Onsarigo A, Matende I, Baba S, Reacher M, et al. Prevalence and Causes of Blindness and Low Vision in Southern Sudan. PLoS Med. 2006;3:2416–23.

255. Kuper H, Gilbert C. Blindness in Sudan: Is It Time to Scrutinise Survey Methods? PLoS Med. 2006;3:2192–93.

256. Alexander ND, Solomon AW, Holland MJ, Bailey RL, West SK, Shao JF, et al. An index of community ocular Chlamydia trachomatis load for control of trachoma. Trans R Soc Trop Med Hyg. 2005;99:175–7.

257. World Health Organization. Future Approaches to Trachoma Control – Report of a Global Scientific Meeting. Geneva: WHO 17–20 June 1996. Report No.: WHO/PBL/96.56.

258. Solomon AW, Foster A, Mabey DCW. Clinical examination versus *Chlamydia trachomatis* assays to guide antibiotic use in trachoma control programmes. Lancet Infect Dis. 2006;6:5–6.

259. Everett KDE, Bush RM, Andersen AA. Emended description of the order Chlamydiales, proposal of Parachlamydiaceae fam. nov. and Simkaniaceae fam. nov., each containing one monotypic genus, revised taxonomy of the family chlamydiaceae, including a new genus and five new species, and standards for the identification of organisms. Int J Syst Bacteriol. 1999;49:415–40.

260. Kaltenboeck B. Recent Advances in the Knowledge of Animal Chlamydial Infections. In: Chernesky M, Caldwell H, Christiansen G, Clarke IN, Kaltenboeck B, Knirsch C, et al., editors. Chlamydial Infections. Proceedings of the Eleventh International Symposium on Human Chlamydial Infections, Niagara-on-the-Lake, Ontario, Canada,

June 18–23, 2006. San Francisco, CA 94110, USA: International Chlamydia Symposium; 2006; 399–408.

261. Bodetti TJ, Viggers K, Warren K, Swan R, Conaghty S, Sims C, et al. Wide range of Chlamydiales types detected in native Australian mammals. Vet Microbiol. 2003;96:177–87.

262. Weigler BJ, Girjes AA, White NA, Kunst ND, Carrick FN, Lavin MF. Aspects of the epidemiology of Chlamydia psittaci infection in a population of koalas (Phascolarctos cinereus) in southeastern Queensland, Australia. J Wildl Dis. 1988;24:282–91.

263. Bedson SP, Bland JOW. A morphological study of psittacosis virus, with a description of a developmental cycle. Br J Exp Pathol. 1932;13:461–6.

264. Patton DL, Chan KY, CKuo CC, Cosgrove YT, Langley L. In vitro growth of Chlamydia trachomatis in conjunctival and corneal epithelium. Invest Ophthalmol Vis Sci. 1988;29:1087–95.

265. Byrne GI, Merkert TP. Persistence of Chlamydia in gamma interferon treated T24 cells. Abstracts of the Annual Meeting for the American Society of Microbiology. 1988:D-13.

266. Hackstadt T. The Cell Biology of Chlamydia-Host Interactions. In: Chernesky M, Caldwell H, Christiansen G, Clarke IN, Kaltenboeck B, Knirsch C, et al., editors. Chlamydial Infections. Proceedings of the Eleventh International Symposium on Human Chlamydial Infections, Niagara-on-the-Lake, Ontario, Canada, June 18–23, 2006. San Francisco, CA 94110, USA: International Chlamydia Symposium; 2006; 135–44.

267. Hatch TP. Structures of Chlamydia. In: Chernesky M, Caldwell H, Christiansen G, Clarke IN, Kaltenboeck B, Knirsch C, et al., editors. Chlamydial Infections. Proceedings of the Eleventh International Symposium on Human Chlamydial Infections, Niagara-on-the-Lake, Ontario, Canada, June 18–23, 2006. San Francisco, CA 94110, USA: International Chlamydia Symposium; 2006; 123–31.

268. Clarke IN. The Molecular Biology of Chlamydiae. In: Chernesky M, Caldwell H, Christiansen G, Clarke IN, Kaltenboeck B, Knirsch C, et al., editors. Chlamydial Infections. Proceedings of the Eleventh International Symposium on Human Chlamydial Infections, Niagara-on-the-Lake, Ontario, Canada, June 18–23, 2006. San Francisco, CA 94110, USA: International Chlamydia Symposium; 2006; 271–80.

269. Byrne GI, Moulder JW. Parasite-specified phagocytosis of Chlamydia psittaci and Chlamydia trachomatis by L and HeLa cells. Infect Immun. 1978;19:598–606.

270. Belland RJ, Zhong G, Crane DD, Hogan D, Sturdevant D, Sharma J, et al. Genomic transcriptional profiling of the developmental cycle of Chlamydia trachomatis. Proc Nat Acad Sci USA. 2003;100:8478–83.

271. Nicholson TL, Olinger L, Chong K, Schoolnik G, Stephens RS. Global stage-specific gene regulation during the developmental cycle of Chlamydia trachomatis. J Bacteriol. 2003;185:3179–89.

272. Stephens RS, Kalman S, Lammel C, Fan J, Marathe R, Aravind L, et al. Genome sequence of an obligate intracellular pathogen of human: Chlamydia trachomatis. Science. 1998;282:754–9.

273. Caldwell HD. Chlamydial Genomics. In: Chernesky M, Caldwell H, Christiansen G, Clarke IN, Kaltenboeck B, Knirsch C, et al., editors. Chlamydial Infections. Proceedings of the Eleventh International Symposium on Human Chlamydial Infections, Niagara-on-the-Lake, Ontario, Canada, June 18–23, 2006. San Francisco, CA 94110, USA: International Chlamydial Symposium; 2006; 3 12.

274. Bain DL, Lietman T, Rasmussen S, Kalman S, Fan J, Lammel C, et al. Chlamydial Genovar Distribution after Communitywide Antibiotic Treatment. J Infect Dis. 2001;184:1581–88.

275. Zhang J, Lietman TM, Olinger L, Miao Y, Stephens RS. Genetic diversity of chlamydia trachomatis and the prevalence of trachoma. Pediatr Infect Dis J. 2004;23:2057–60.

276. Gomes JP, Bruno WJ, Nunes A, Santos N, Florindo C, Borrego MJ, et al. Evolution of *Chlamydia trachomatis* diversity occurs by widespread interstrain recombination involving hotspots. Genome Res. 2007;17:50–60.

277. Talbot D. Le trachome dans les ecoles du groupe d'oasis de gabes (Sud-Tunisien). Rev Int Trach. 1930;7:143–52.

278. Winkler PG. A morbidity survey on trachoma and other communicable eye diseases in the district of Hebron, Jordan, 1960. Bull World Health Organ. 1963;28:417–36.

279. Treharne JD. Chlamydia trachomatis: serological diagnosis. Infection. 1982;10:25–31.

280. Courtright P, Sheppard J, Lane S, Sadek A, Schachter J, Dawson CR. Latrine ownership as a protective factor in inflammatory trachoma in Egypt. Br J Ophthalmol. 1991;75:322–5.

281. Ostler HB, Thygeson P. Trachoma in American Samoa. Trans Pacific Coast Oto-Ophthalmol Soc. 1972:199–219.

282. Ballard RC, Fehler HG, Fotheringham P, Sutter EE, Treharne JD. Trachoma in South Africa. Soc Sci Med. 1983;17:1755–65.

283. Polack SR, Solomon AW, Alexander ND, Massae PA, Safari S, Shao JF, et al. The household distribution of trachoma in a Tanzanian village: an application of GIS to the study of trachoma. Trans R Soc Trop Med Hyg. 2005;99:218–25.

284. Bailey R, Osmond C, Mabey DCW, Whittle HC, Ward ME. Analysis of the household distribution of trachoma in a Gambian village using a Monte Carlo simulation procedure. Int J Epidemiol. 1989;18:944–51.

285. Luna EJA, Medina NH, Oliveira MB, De Barros OMD, Vranjac A, Melles HHB, et al. Epidemiology of trachoma in Bebedouro State of Sao Paulo, Brazil: Prevalence and risk factors. Int J Epidemiol. 1992;21:169–77.

286. Assaad FA, Sundaresan T, Maxwell-Lyons F. The household pattern of trachoma in Taiwan. Bull World Health Organ. 1971;44:605–15.

287. Grayston JT, Gale JL, Yeh JL, Yang CY. Pathogenesis and immunology of trachoma. Trans Assoc Am Physicians. 1972;85:203–11.

288. Grayston JT, Wang S. New knowledge of Chlamydiae and the diseases they cause. J Infect Dis. 1975;132:87–105.

289. Taylor CE, Gulati PV, Harinarain J. Eye Infections in a Punjab village. Am J Trop Med Hyg. 1958;7:42–50.

290. Barenfanger J. Studies on the role of the family unit in the transmission of trachoma. Am J Trop Med Hyg. 1975;24:509–15.

291. Haddad NA. Trachoma in Lebanon: observations on epidemiology in rural areas. Am J Trop Med Hyg. 1965;14:652–55.

292. Bailey R, Osmond C, Mabey DCW, Ward ME. Household Clustering of Trachoma in the Gambia. In: Oriel D, Ridgway G, Schachter J, Taylor-Robinson D, Ward M, editors. Chlamydial Infections. Proceedings of the Sixth International Symposium on Human Chlamydial Infections, Sanderstead, Surrey, 15–21 June 1986. Cambridge: Cambridge University Press; 1986; 145–8.

293. Mabey DCW, Bailey RL, Ward ME, Whittle HC. A longitudinal study of trachoma in a Gambian village: implications concerning the pathogenesis of chlamydial infection. Epidemiol Infect. 1992;108:343–51.

294. Katz J, Zeger SL, Tielsch JM. Village and household clustering of xerophthalmia and trachoma. Int J Epidemiol. 1988;17:867–9.

295. West S, Muñoz B, Turner VM, Mmbaga BBO, Taylor HR. The epidemiology of trachoma in central Tanzania. Int J Epidemiol. 1991;20:1088–92.

296. Treharne JD. The microbial epidemiology of trachoma. Int Ophthalmol. 1988;12:25–9.

297. Taylor HR, Siler JA, Mkocha HA, Muñoz B, West S. The natural history of endemic trachoma: a longitudinal study. Am J Trop Med Hyg. 1992;46:552–9.

298. West SK, Munoz B, Mkocha H, Holland MJ, Aguirre A, Solomon AW, et al. Infection with Chlamydia trachomatis after mass treatment of a trachoma hyperendemic community in Tanzania: a longitudinal study. Lancet. 2005;366:1296–1300.

299. Broman AT, Shum K, Munoz B, Duncan DD, West SK. Spatial clustering of ocular chlamydial infection over time following treatment, among households in a village in Tanzania. Invest Ophthalmol Vis Sci. 2006;47:99–104.

300. Ministry of Public Health. Fourteenth Report of the Memorial Ophthalmic Laboratory 1939–1944. Giza, Cairo: Ministry of Public Health; 1945.

301. Sowa S, Sowa J, Collier LH, Blyth WA. Trachoma and allied infections in a Gambian village. Spec Rep Ser Med Res Council (GB) 1965;308:1–88.

302. Radovanovic M, Lal M. Final report on trachoma control pilot project in India. WHO Project: India 101. 1956–59. SEA/TRACH 1986;10:1–75.

303. Lay K, Kyaw TA, Gyi K, Tarizzo ML, Assaad FA. Trachoma control in Burma. Rev Int Trach Pathol Ocul Trop Subtrop. 1976;53:119–56.

304. Courtright P, Sheppard J, Schachter J, Said ME, Dawson CR. Trachoma and blindness in the Nile Delta: current patterns and projections for the future in the rural Egyptian population. Br J Ophthalmol. 1989;73:536–40.

305. Schwab L, Kagame K. Blindness in Africa: Zimbabwe schools for the blind survey. Br J Ophthalmol. 1993;77:410–12.

306. Cumberland P, Hailu G, Todd J. Active trachoma in children aged three to nine years in rural communities in Ethiopia: prevalence, indicators and risk factors. Trans R Soc Trop Med Hyg. 2005;99:120–7.

307. Stocks NP, Hiller JE, Newland H, McGilchrist CA. Trends in the prevalence of trachoma, South Australia, 1976 to 1990. Aust N Z J Public Health. 1996;20:375–81.

308. Salim AR, Sheikh HA. Trachoma in the Sudan. Br J Ophthalmol. 1975;59:600–4.

309. Schachter J, Dawson CR. The epidemiology of trachoma predicts more blindness in the future. Scand J Infect Dis. 1990;69:55–62.

310. Laming AC, Currie BJ, DiFrancesco M, Taylor HR, Matthews JD. A targeted, single-dose azithromycin strategy for trachoma. Med J Aust. 2000;172:163–6.

311. Lansingh VC, Weih LM, Keeffe JE, Taylor HR. Assessment of trachoma prevalence in a mobile population in Central Australia. Ophthalmic Epidemiol. 2001;8:97–108.

312. Woolridge RL, Grayston JT, Perrin EB, Yang CY, Cheng KH, Chang IH. Natural history of trachoma in Taiwan school children. Am J Ophthalmol. 1967;63:287–94.

313. Detels R, Alexander ER, Dhir SP. Trachoma in Punjabi Indians in British Columbia: a prevalence study with comparisons to India. Am J Epidemiol. 1966;84:81–91.

314. Dhir SP, Detels R, Alexander ER. The role of environmental factors in cataract, pterygium, and trachoma. Am J Ophthalmol. 1967;64:128–35.

315. Grayston JT. Symposium on trachoma. Biology of the virus. Invest Ophthalmol. 1963;2:460–70.

316. Grayston JT, Wang S-P, Yeh L-J, Kuo C-C. Importance of Reinfection in the Pathogenesis of Trachoma. In: Cook JA, Taylor HR, editors. Reviews of Infectious Diseases, Infectious Causes of Blindness: Trachoma and Onchocerciasis. Chicago:

The University of Chicago Press, Illinois 60637; 1985; 717–25.

317. Grayston JT. Chairman's report and discussion. In: Hobson D, Holmes KK, editors. Nongonococcal urethritis. Washington, D.C: American Society for Microbiology; 1977; 159–64.

318. Hollows FC. Trachoma down the track. Med J Aust. 1989;151:182–3.

319. Holland MJ, Faal N, Sarr I, Joof H, Laye M, Cameron E, et al. The frequency of Chlamydia trachomatis major outer membrane protein-specific CD8+T Lymphocytes in active trachoma is associated with current ocular infection. Infect Immun. 2006;74:1565–72.

320. Natividad A, Wilson J, Koch O, Holland MJ, Rockett K, Faal N, et al. Risk of trachomatous scarring and trichiasis in Gambians varies with SNP haplotypes at the interferon-gamma and interleukin-10 loci. Genes Immun. 2005;6:332–40.

321. West SK, Munoz B, Lynch M, Kayongoya A, Mmbaga BBO, Taylor HR. Risk factors for constant, severe trachoma in preschool children in Kongwa, Tanzania. Am J Epidemiol. 1996;143:73–8.

322. West SK, Munoz B, Mkocha H, Hsieh YH, Lynch MC. Progression of active trachoma to scarring in a cohort of Tanzanian children. Ophthalmic Epidemiol. 2001;8:137–44.

323. Smith A, Munoz B, Hsieh YH, Bobo L, Mkocha H, West S. OmpA genotypic evidence for persistent ocular Chlamydia trachomatis infection in Tanzanian village women. Ophthalmic Epidemiol. 2001;8:127–35.

324. Reinhards J. Current aspects and epidemiological problems of trachoma. Aspects actuels et problemes de l'epidemiologie du trachome. Rev Int Trach Pathol Ocul Trop Subtrop. 1969;47:211–95.

325. Malaty R, Zaki S, Said ME, Vastine DW, Dawson CR, Schachter J. Extraocular infections in children in areas with endemic trachoma. J Infect Dis. 1981;143:853.

326. West S, Munoz B, Bobo L, Quinn TC, Mkocha H, Lynch M, et al. Nonocular chlamydia infection and risk of ocular reinfection after mass treatment in a trachoma hyperendemic area. Invest Ophthal Vis Sci. 1993;34:3194–98.

327. Solomon A, Mabey D, Holland M, Alexander N, Aguirre A, Massae P, et al. Quantification of Nasal *Chlamydial trachomatis* Infection in a Trachoma Endemic Area of Tanzania. In: Schacher J, Christiansen G, Clarke IN, Hammerschlag MR, Kaltenboeck B, Kuo C-C, et al., editors. Chlamydial Infections. Proceedings of the Tenth International Symposium on Human Chlamydial Infections, June 16–21, 2002, Antalya – Turkey. San Francisco, CA 94110: International Chlamydia Symposium; 2002; 527–30.

328. Gower EW, Solomon AW, Burton MJ, Aguirre A, Munoz B, Bailey R, et al. Chlamydial positivity of nasal discharge at baseline is associated with ocular chlamydial positivity 2 months following azithromycin treatment. Invest Ophthalmol Vis Sci. 2006;47:4767–71.

329. Ismail SO, Ahmed HJ, Jama MA, Omer K, Omer FM, Brundin M, et al. Syphilis, gonorrhea and genital chlamydial infection in a Somali village. Genitourin Med. 1990;66:70–5.

330. Brunham RC, Laga M, Simonsen JN, Cameron DW, Peeling R, McDowell J, et al. The prevalence of Chlamydia trachomatis infection among mothers of children with trachoma. Am J Epidemiol. 1990;132:946–52.

331. Kupka K, Nizetic B, Reinhards J. Sampling studies on the epidemiology and control of trachoma in southern Morocco. Bull World Health Organ. 1968;39:547–66.

332. Ko K, Kyaw TA. Socio-economic factors in trachoma. Union Burma J Life Sci. 1968;1:365–9.

333. West S, Nguyen MP, Mkocha H, Holdsworth G, Ngirwamungu E, Kilima P, et al. Gender equity and trichiasis surgery in the Vietnam and Tanzania national trachoma control programmes. Br J Ophthalmol. 2004;88:1368–71.

334. Khandekar R, Nga NH, Mai P. Blinding trachoma in the northern provinces of Vietnam – a cross sectional survey. Ophthalmic Epidemiol. 2006;13:183–9.

335. Faal H, Minassian D, Sowa S, Foster A. National survey of blindness and low vision in The Gambia: results. Br J Ophthalmol. 1989;73:82–7.

336. Congdon N, West S, Vitale S, Katala S, Mmbago BBO. Exposure to children and risk of active trachoma in Tanzanian women. Am J Epidemiol. 1993;137:366–72.

337. Turner VM, West SK, Muñoz B, Katala SJ, Taylor HR, Halsey N, et al. Risk factors for trichiasis in women in Kongwa, Tanzania: a case-control study. Int J Epidemiol. 1993;22:341–7.

338. West SK, Rapoza P, Muñoz B, Katala S, Taylor HR. Epidemiology of ocular chlamydial infection in a trachoma-hyperendemic area. J Infect Dis. 1991;163:752–6.

339. Laga M, Nzanze H, Brunham RC, Maitha G, D'Costa LJD, Plummer FA, et al. Epidemiology of ophthalmia neonatorum in Kenya. Lancet. 1986;2:1145–9.

340. Durkin SR, Casson R, Newland HS, Selva D. Prevalence of trachoma and diabetes-related eye disease among a cohort of adult Aboriginal patients screened over the period 1999–2004 in remote South Australia. Clin Experiment Ophthalmol. 2006;34:329–34.

341. Wright H. Trachoma is still a significant public health concern: evaluation of the SAFE Strategy and the barriers to its implementation in Australia [PhD]. Melbourne: University of Melbourne; 2007.

342. Marshall CL. The relationship between trachoma and piped water in a developing area. Arch Environ Health. 1968;17:215–20.

343. Damato FJ. The fight against trachoma in the Island of Malta. Br J Ophthalmol. 1961; 45:71–4.

344. Bobb AA, Nichols RL. Influence of environment on clinical trachoma in Saudi Arabia. Am J Ophthalmol. 1969;67:235–43.

345. Al Faran M. Low prevalence of trachoma in the South Western part of Saudi Arabia, results of a population-based study. Int Ophthalmol. 1995;18:379–82.

346. Dolin PJ, Faal H, Johnson GJ, Minassian D, Sowa S, Day S, et al. Reduction of trachoma in a sub-Saharan village in absence of a disease control programme. Lancet. 1997;349:1511–12.

347. Schwab L, Whitfield R Jr, Ross-Degnan D, Steinkuller P, Swartwood J, Study Survey Group. The epidemiology of trachoma in rural Kenya. Variation in prevalence with lifestyle and environment. Ophthalmology. 1995;102:475–582.

348. Frick KD, Hanson CL, Jacobson GA. Global Burden of Trachoma and Economics of the Disease. Am J Trop Med Hyg. 2003;69:1–10.

349. Assaad FA, Maxwell-Lyons F, Sundaresan T. Use of local variations in trachoma endemicity in Taiwan to elucidate some of the clinical and epidemiological aspects of the disease. Bull World Health Organ. 1968;39:567–86.

350. Mann I. The Bowman Lecture: Climate, Culture and Eye Disease. Trans Ophth Soc UK. 1961;31:261–83.

351. T'ang FF, Huang YT, Chang HL, Wang KC. Isolation of trachoma virus in chick embryo. J Hyg Epidemiol Microbiol Immunol. 1957;109:1–13.

352. Sowa S, Sowa J. Investigation of neonatal conjunctivitis in the Gambia. Lancet. 1968;2:243–7.

353. Dawson CR. Review of eye infections with Chlamydia trachomatis. In: Mardh P-A, Holmes KK, Oriel JD, Piot P, Schachter J, editors. Chlamydial Infections. Proceedings of the Fifth International Symposium on Human Chlamydial Infections, Lund (Sweden). Amsterdam: Elsevier Biomedical Press; 1982; 71–81.

354. Resnikoff S, Cornand G. Malnutrition et trachome:etude des correlations sur le plan epidemiologique. Rev Int Trach Pathol Ocul Trop Subtrop Sante Publique. 1987:75–87.

355. Lietman TM, Dhital SP, Dean D. Conjunctival impression cytology for vitamin A deficiency in the presence of infectious trachoma. Br J Ophthalmol. 1998;82:1139–42.

356. West KP Jr, Tielsch JM, Keyvan-Larijani E, Katz J, Chirambo MC, Taylor HR. Trachoma and malnutrition. Invest Ophthalmol Vis Sci. 1987;28 (suppl):146.

357. Tedesco LR. Trachoma and environment in the Northern Territory of Australia. Soc Sci Med. 1980;14D:111–17.

358. Assaad FA, Maxwell-Lyons F, Sundaresan T. Use of local variations in trachoma endemicity in depicting

359. Cobb JC, Dawson CR. Trachoma among southwestern Indians. JAMA. 1961;175:151–2.

360. Sahlu T, Larson C. The prevalence and environmental risk factors for moderate and severe trachoma in southern Ethiopia. J Trop Med Hyg. 1992;95:36–41.

361. Tielsch JM, West KP Jr, Katz J, Keyvan-Larijani E, Tizazu T, Schwab L, et al. The epidemiology of trachoma in southern Malawi. Am J Trop Med Hyg. 1988;38:393–9.

362. Polack S, Kuper H, Solomon AW, Massae P, Abuelo C, Cameron E, et al. The relationship between prevalence of active trachoma, water availability and its use in a Tanzanian village. Trans R Soc Trop Med Hyg. 2006;100:1075–83.

363. Kok PW. The epidemiology of trachoma blindness in Southern Africa. Soc Sci Med. 1983;17:1709–13.

364. Bailey R, Downes B, Downes R, Mabey D. Trachoma and water use; a case control study in a Gambian village. Trans R Soc Trop Med Hyg. 1991;85:824–8.

365. Cooper RL, Coid D, Constable IJ. Trachoma: 1985 update in Western Australia. Aust N Z J Ophthalmol. 1986;14:319–23.

366. Prost A, Negrel AD. Water, trachoma and conjunctivitis. Bull World Health Organ. 1989;67:9–18.

367. West S, Lynch M, Turner V, Muñoz B, Rapoza P, Mmbaga BBO, et al. Water availability and trachoma. Bull World Health Organ. 1989; 67:71–5.

368. McCauley AP, Lynch M, Pounds MB, West S. Changing water-use patterns in a water-poor area: lessons for a trachoma intervention project. Soc Sci Med. 1990;31:1233–8.

369. Cairncross S. Trachoma and Water. Community Eye Health. 1999;12:58–9.

370. Cairncross S, Cliff JL. Water use and health in Mueda, Mozambique. Trans R Soc Trop Med Hyg. 1987;81:51–4.

371. Al Arab GE, Tawfik N, El Gendy R, Anwar W, Courtright P. The burden of trachoma in the rural Nile Delta of Egypt: a survey of Menofiya governorate. Br J Ophthalmol. 2001;85:1406–10.

372. Schemann JF, Guinot C, Ilboudo L, Momo G, Ko B, Sanfo O, et al. Trachoma, flies and environmental factors in Burkina Faso. Trans R Soc Trop Med Hyg. 2003;97:63–8.

373. Emerson PM, Simms VM, Makalo P, Bailey RL. Household pit latrines as a potential source of the fly Musca sorbens – a one year longitudinal study from The Gambia. Trop Med Int Health. 2005;10:706–9.

374. Emerson PM, Lindsay SW, Alexander N, Bah M, Dibba S, Faal HB, et al. Role of flies and provision of latrines in trachoma control: cluster-randomised controlled trial. Lancet. 2004;363:1093–8.

interplay between socio-economic conditions and disease. Bull World Health Organ. 1969;41:181–94.

375. Forsey T, Darougar S. Transmission of Chlamydiae by the housefly. Br J Ophthalmol. 1981;65:147–50.

376. Emerson PM, Bailey RL, Mahdi OS, Walraven GE, Lindsay SW. Transmission ecology of the fly Musca sorbens a putative vector for trachoma. Trans R Soc Trop Med Hyg. 2000;94:28–32.

377. Miller K, Pakpour N, Yi E, Melese M, Alemayehu W, Bird M, et al. Pesky trachoma suspect finally caught. Br J Ophthalmol. 2004;88:750–1.

378. Lee S, Alemayehu W, Melese M, Lakew T, Lee D, Yi E, et al. Chlamydia on children and flies after mass antibiotic treatment for trachoma. Am J Trop Med Hyg. 2007;76:129–31.

379. Weir JM, Wasif IM, Hassan FR, Attia SDH, Kader M. An evaluation of health and sanitation in Egyptian villages. Egyptian Pub Health Assoc. 1952;27:55–122.

380. Maxwell Lyons F, Abdin G. The effect of fly control on the epidemic spread of acute ophthalmia. Bull Egypt Ophthalmol Soc. 1952;45:81–8.

381. Ponghis G. Quelques observations sur le role de la mouche dans la transmission des conjonctivites saisonnieres dans le Sud-Marocain. Bull World Health Organ. 1957;16:1013–27.

382. Mann I. Culture, Race, Climate and Eye Disease. Springfield; Illinois, USA: Charles C Thomas; 1966.

383. Flynn F. Trachoma among natives of the Northern Territory of Australia. Med J Aust. 1957;11:269–77.

384. da Cruz L, Dadour IR, McAllister IL, Jackson A, Issacs T. Seasonal variation in trachoma and bush flies in north Western Australian communities. Clin Experiment Ophthalmol. 2002;30:80–3.

385. Taylor HR. Flies and trachoma. Clin Experiment Ophthalmol. 2002;30:65.

386. Taylor HR. A simple method for assessment of association between synanthropic flies and trachoma. Am J Trop Med Hyg. 1988;38:623–27.

387. Greenberg B. Flies and human disease. In: Flies and Disease. Princeton: Princeton University Press; 1973; 214–23.

388. Taylor HR. Trachoma research: laboratory and epidemiologic aspects. Int Rev Trach. 1987:23–58.

389. Brechner RJ, West S, Lynch M. Trachoma and flies. Individual vs environmental risk factors. Arch Ophthalmol. 1992;110:687–98.

390. De Sole G. Impact of cattle on the prevalence and severity of trachoma. Br J Ophthalmol. 1987;71:873–6.

391. West SK, Emerson PM, Mkocha H, Mchiwa W, Munoz B, Bailey R, et al. Intensive insecticide spraying for fly control after mass antibiotic treatment for trachoma in a hyperendemic setting: a randomised trial. Lancet. 2006;368:596–600.

392. West S, Congdon N, Katala S, Mele L. Facial cleanliness and risk of trachoma in families. Arch Ophthalmol. 1991;109:855–7.

393. West S, Muñoz B, Lynch M, Kayongoya A, Chilangwa Z, Mmbaga BBO, et al. Impact of face-washing on trachoma in Kongwa Tanzania. Lancet. 1995;345:155–8.

394. Abdou A, Nassirou B, Kadri B, Moussa F, Munoz BE, Opong E, et al. Prevalence and risk factors for trachoma and ocular chlamydia trachomatis infection in Niger. Br J Ophthalmol. 2007; 91:13–17.

395. Abu El-Asrar AM, Van den Oord JJ, Geboes K, Missotten L, Emarah MH, Desmet V. Immunopathology of trachomatous conjunctivitis. Br J Ophthalmol. 1989;73:276–82.

396. Patton DL, Taylor HR. The histopathology of experimental trachoma: ultrastructural changes in the conjunctival epithelium. J Infect Dis. 1986;153:870–8.

397. Verin P, Gendre P, Comte P. Nouvelle classification du trachome (clinique, histologique et ultrastructurale.). Rev Int Trach. 1987;64:115–21.

398. Harrison HR, Boyce WT, Wang S-P, Gibb GN, Cox JE, Alexander ER. Infection with Chlamydia trachomatis immunotype J associated with trachoma in children in an area previously endemic for trachoma. J Infect Dis. 1985;151:1034–6.

399. Mabey DCW, Bailey RL, Dunn D, Jones D, Williams JHD, Whittle HC, et al. Expression of MHC class II antigens by conjunctival epithelial cells in trachoma: Implications concerning the pathogenesis of blinding disease. J Clin Pathol. 1991;44:285–9.

400. Abu El-Asrar AM, Al-Kharashi SA, Missotten L, Geboes K. Expression of growth factors in the conjunctiva from patients with active trachoma. Eye. 2006;20:362–9.

401. Abu El-Asrar AM, Geboes K, Tabbara KF, al-Kharashi SA, Missotten L, Desmet V. Immunopathogenesis of conjunctival scarring in trachoma. Eye. 1998;12:453–60.

402. Rasmussen SJ, Eckmann L, Quayle AJ, Shen L, Zhang Y-X, Anderson DJ, et al. Secretion of proinflammatory cytokines by epithelial cells in response to Chlamydia infection suggests a central role for epithelial cells in chlamydial pathogenesis. J Clin Invest. 1997;99:77–87.

403. Whittum-Hudson JA, Taylor HR. Antichlamydial specificity of conjunctival lymphocytes during experimental ocular infection. Infect Immun. 1989;57:2977–83.

404. Burd EM, Tabbara KF, Nast AM, Taylor PB. Conjunctival lymphocyte subsets in trachoma. Int Ophthalmol. 1988;12:47–53.

405. Whittum-Hudson JA, Taylor HR, Farazdaghi M, Prendergast RA. Immunohistochemical study of the local inflammatory response to chlamydial ocular infection. Invest Ophthalmol Vis Sci. 1986; 27:64–9.

406. Al-Rajhi AA, Hidayat A, Nasr A, Al-Faran M. The histopathology and the mechanism of entropion in patients with trachoma. Ophthalmology. 1993;100:1293–6.

407. Reacher MH, Pe'er J, Rapoza PA, Whittum-Hudson JA, Taylor HR. T cells and trachoma. Their role in cicatricial disease. Ophthalmology. 1991;98:334–41.

408. Blodi BA, Byrne KA, Tabbara KF. Goblet cell population among patients with inactive trachoma. Int Opthalmol. 1988;12:41–5.

409. Abu El-Asrar AM, Geboes K, al-Kharashi SA, Tabbara KF, Missotten L. Collagen content and types in trachomatous conjunctivitis. Eye. 1998;12:735–9.

410. Abu El-Asrar AM, Geboes K, Al-Kharashi SA, Al-Mosallam AA, Tabbara KF, Al-Rajhi AA, et al. An immunohistochemical study of collagens in trachoma and vernal keratoconjunctivitis. Eye. 1998;12:1000–6.

411. Abu El-Asrar AM, Geboes K, Al-Kharashi SA, Al-Mosallam AA, Missotten L, Paemen L, et al. Expression of gelatinase B in trachomatous conjunctivitis. Br J Ophthalmol. 2000;84:85–91.

412. Duke-Elder S. System of Ophthalmology Vol VIII Diseases of the Outer Eye Part I: Henry Kimpton, London; 1965.

413. Tabbara KF, Bobb AA. Lacrimal system complications in trachoma. Ophthalmology. 1980;87:298–301.

414. Tabbara KF. Trachoma: Immuno-histo-pathology. In: Coscas G, Cornand G, editors. Revue internationale du Trachome et de Pathologie Oculaire Tropicale et Subtropicale et de Sante Publique, Annes 2000/2001/2002. Cedex: Groupe Liaisons S.A.; 2003; 17–65.

415. Rice CD, Kersten RC. Absence of Chlamydia in trachomatous lacrimal sacs. Am J Ophthalmol. 1988;105:203–6.

416. Whitcher JP, Dawson CR, Messadi M, Daghfous T, ben Abdullah N, Triki F, et al. Severe endemic trachoma in Tunisia: changes in ocular bacterial pathogens in children treated by the intermittent antibiotic regimen. Int Rev Trach. 1974;51:49–58.

417. Silverstein AM. The immunologic modulation of infectious disease pathogenesis. Invest Ophthalmol. 1974;13:560–74.

418. Brunham RC, Peeling RW. Chlamydia trachomatis antigens: role in immunity and pathogenesis. Infect Agents Dis. 1994;3:218–33.

419. Thygeson P, Crocker TT. Observations on experimental trachoma and inclusion conjunctivitis. Am J Ophthalmol. 1956;42:76–84.

420. Darougar S, Monnickendam MA, El-Sheikh H, Treharne JD, Woodland RM, Jones BR. Animal models for the study of chlamydial infections of the eye and genital tract. In: Hobson D, Holmes KK, editors. Nongonococcal urethritis and related infections. Washington DC: American Society for Microbiology; 1977; 186–98.

421. Taylor-Robinson D. The Role of Animal Models in Chlamydial Research. In: Oriel D, Ridgway G, Schachter J, Taylor-Robinson D, Ward M, editors.

Chlamydial Infections. Proceedings of the Sixth International Symposium on Human Chlamydial Infections, Sanderstead, Surrey 15–21 June 1986. Cambridge: Cambridge University Press; 1986; 355–66.

422. Patton DL. Experimental Systems. In: Bowie WR, Caldwell HD, Jones RP, Mardh P-A, Ridgway GL, Schachter J, et al., editors. Chlamydial Infections. Proceedings of the Seventh International Symposium on Human Chlamydial Infections, Harrison Hot Springs, British Colombia, Canada, 24–29 June 1990. Cambridge: Cambridge University Press; 1990; 223–31.

423. Tuffrey M. The use of animal models to study human chlamydial diseases. In: Orfila J, Byrne GI, Chernesky MA, Grayston JT, Jones RB, Ridgway GL, et al., editors. Chlamydial Infections. Proceedings of the Eighth International Symposium on Human Chlamydial Infections, Chateau de Montvillargenne, 602700 Gouvieux – Chantilly, France, 19–24 June 1994. Bologna – Italy: Societa Editrice Esculapio; 1994; 513–24.

424. Taylor HR. Ocular models of chlamydial infection. Rev Infect Dis. 1985;7:737–40.

425. Nelson DE, Virok DP, Wood H, Roshick C, Johnson RM, Whitmire WM, et al. Chlamydia IFN-γ immune evasion is linked to host infection tropism. Proc Nat Acad Sci USA. 2005;102: 10658–63.

426. Caldwell HD, Wood H, Crane D, Jones RB, Mabey D, Maclean I, et al. Polymorphisms in Chlamydia trachomatis tryptohan synthase genes differentiate between genital and ocular isolates. J Clin Invest. 2003;111:1757–69.

427. Hvid M, Sventrup HF, Fedder J, Christiansen G, Birkelund S. Circulating Antibodies Against *Chlamydia trachomatis* Major Outer Membrane Protein (MOMP) and its Relationship to Tubal Infertility Factor. In: Chernesky M, Caldwell H, Christiansen G, Clarke IN, Kaltenboeck B, Knirsch C, et al., editors. Chlamydial Infections. Proceedings of the Eleventh International Symposium on Human Chlamydial Infections, Niagara-on-the-Lake, Ontario, Canada, June 19–23 2006. San Francisco, CA 94110, USA: International Chlamydia Symposium; 2006; 607–10.

428. Wang S-P, Grayston JT, Alexander ER. Trachoma vaccine studies in monkeys. Am J Ophthalmol. 1967;63:1615–30.

429. Patton DL, Kuo C-C, Wang S-P, Brenner RM, Sternfeld MD, Morse SA. Chlamydial salpingitis in subcutaneous fimbrial transplants in monkeys. In: Oriel D, Ridgway G, Schachter J, Taylor-Robinson D, Ward M, editors. Chlamydial Infections. Proceedings of the Sixth International Symposium on Human Chlamydial Infections, Sanderstead, Surrey, 15–21 June 1986. Cambridge: Cambridge University Press; 1986; 367–70.

430. Mordhorst CH. Quantitation of the infectivity for cynomolgus monkeys of egg-grown inclusion conjunctivitis virus. Am J Ophthalmol. 1962;53:780–6.

431. Jawetz E, Rose L, Hanna L, Thygeson P. Experimental inclusion and conjunctivitis in man. JAMA. 1965;194:620–632.

432. Dawson CR, Jawetz E, Hanna L, Rose L, Wood TR, P. T. Experimental inclusion conjunctivitis in man. II. Partial resistance to reinfection. Am J Epidemiol. 1966;84:411–25.

433. Bell SD, Fraser CEO. Experimental trachoma in owl monkeys. Am J Trop Med Hyg. 1969;18: 568–72.

434. Taylor HR, Prendergast RA, Dawson CR, Schachter J, Silverstein AM. Animal model of trachoma: III. The necessity of repeated exposure to live chlamydia. Chlamydial Infections. 1982: 387–90.

435. Thygeson P, Dawson C, Hanna L, Jawetz E, Okumoto M. Observations on experimental trachoma in monkeys produced by strains of viruses propagated in yolk sac. Am J Ophthalmol. 1960;50:907–18.

436. Mordhorst CH. Experimental infections and immunogenicity of TRIC agents in monkeys. Am J Ophthalmol. 1967;63:1603–15.

437. Wang S-P, Grayston JT. Pannus with experimental trachoma and inclusion conjunctivitis agent infection of Taiwan monkeys. Am J Ophthalmol. 1967;63:1133–45.

438. Hanna L, Thygeson P, Jawetz E, Dawson C. Elementary-body virus isolated from clinical trachoma in California. Science. 1959;130:1339.

439. Murray ES, Fraser CEO, Peters JH, McComb DE, Nichols RL. The owl monkey as an experimental primate model for conjunctival trachoma infection. In: Nichols RL, editor. Trachoma and related disorders. Amsterdam: Excerpta Medica; 1971; 386–95.

440. Collier LH, Blythe WA. Immunogenicity of experimental trachoma vaccines in baboons. I. Experimental methods, and preliminary tests with vaccines prepared in chick embryos and in HeLa cells. J Hyg Cambridge. 1966;64:513–28.

441. Dawson CR, Jawetz E, Thygeson P, Hanna L. Trachoma viruses isolated in the United States. 4. Infectivity and immunogenicity for monkeys. Proc Soc Exp Biol Med. 1961;106:898–902.

442. Taylor HR, Johnson SL, Prendergast RA, Schachter J, Dawson CR, Silverstein AM. An animal model of trachoma II. The importance of repeated reinfection. Invest Ophthalmol Vis Sci. 1982;23:507–19.

443. Caldwell HD, Stewart S, Johnson S, Taylor H. Tear and serum antibody response to Chlamydia trachomatis antigens during acute chlamydial conjunctivitis in monkeys as determined by immunoblotting. Infect Immun. 1987;55:93–8.

444. Pal S, Pu Z, Huneke RB, Taylor HR, Whittum-Hudson JA. Chlamydia-specific lymphocytes in conjunctiva during ocular infection: Limiting dilution analysis. Reg Immunol. 1991;3:171–6.

445. Taylor HR. Development of immunity to ocular chlamydial infection. Am J Trop Med Hyg. 1990;42:358–64.

446. Taylor HR, Agarwala N, Johnson SL. Detection of experimental Chlamydia trachomatis eye infection in conjunctival smears and in tissue culture by the use of fluorescein-conjugated monoclonal antibody. J Clin Microbiol. 1984;20:391–5.

447. Young E, Schachter J, Prendergast RA, Taylor HR. The effect of cyclosporine in chlamydial eye infection. Curr Eye Res. 1987;6:683–9.

448. Cosgrove PA, Patton DL, Kuo C-C, Wang S-P, Lindquist TD. Experimentally induced ocular Chlamydial infection in infant pig-tailed macaques. Invest Ophthalmol Vis Sci. 1989;30:995–1003.

449. Thygeson P. The etiology of inclusion blennorrhea. Am J Ophthalmol. 1934;17:1019.

450. Patton DL, Cosgrove PA, Grutzmacher RD, Kuo CC, Wang SP. Experimental Trachoma in Subcutaneous Conjunctival Autografts in Macaques. Invest Ophthalmol Vis Sci. 1987;28:1575–82.

451. Wolner-Hanssen P, Patton DL, Holmes KK. Protective immunity in pig-tailed macaques after cervical infection with Chlamydial trachomatis. Sex Trans Dis. 1991;18:21–5.

452. Tsutsui J, Furusawa T, Tsuji S, Takeda S. Development of immunity by repeated infection to trachoma. Arch Ophthalmol. 1957;57:577–84.

453. Chang HL, Chin HY, Wang KC. Experimental trachoma in human volunteers produced by cultured virus. Chin Med J. 1960;80:214–21.

454. Tarizzo ML, Nataf R, Nabil B. Experimental inoculation of thirteen volunteers with agent isolated from inclusion conjunctivitis. Am J Opthalmol. 1967;63:1120–28.

455. Dawson CR, Wood TR, Rose L, Hanna L, Thygeson P. Experimental inclusion conjunctivitis in man. III. Keratitis and other complications. Arch Ophthalmol. 1967;78:341–9.

456. Banks JR, Driesen GV, Stark E. Chlamydia trachomatis in smears from eyes, ears, and throats of children with chronic otitis media. (letter). Lancet. 1985;2:278.

457. Mitsui Y, Higai H, T. K. Free toxic substance of trachoma virus. Arch Ophthalmol. 1962;68:651–3.

458. Hanna L, Jawetz E, Dawson CR, Thygeson P. Long-term clinical, microbiological, and immunological observations of a volunteer repeatedly infected with Chlamydia trachomatis. J Clin Microbiol. 1982;16:895–900.

459. Gale JL, Wang S-P, Grayston JT. Chronic trachoma in two Taiwan monkeys ten years after infection. In: Nichols RL, editor. In: Trachoma and related disorders. Amsterdam: Excerpta Medica; 1971; 489–93.

460. Taylor HR, Kolarczyk RA. Inclusion conjunctivitis or trachoma? The role of reinfection. In: Henkind P, editor. Acta: XXIV International Congress of Ophthalmology: J.B. Lippincott Company, 1983; 203–6.

461. Dawson CR, Mordhorst CH, Thygeson P. Infection of Rhesus and Cynomolgus monkeys with egg-grown virus of trachoma and inclusion conjunctivitis. Ann NY Acad Sci. 1962;98:167–76.

462. Taylor HR, Johnson SL, Schachter J, Prendergast RA. An animal model of trachoma: IV. The failure of local immunosuppression to reveal inapparent infection. Invest Ophthalmol Vis Sci. 1983;24: 647–50.

463. Caldwell HD, Perry LJ. Neutralization of Chlamydia trachomatis infectivity with antibodies to the major outer membrane protein. Infect Immun. 1982;38:745–54.

464. Peeling RW, Brunham RC. Neutralization of Chlamydia trachomatis: kinetics and stoichiometry. Infect Immun. 1991;59:2624–30.

465. Zhang Y-X, Stewart S, Joseph T, Taylor HR, Caldwell HD. Protective monoclonal antibodies recognize epitopes located on the major outer membrane protein of Chlamydia trachomatis. J Immunol. 1987;138:575–81.

466. Watkins NG, Hadlow WJ, Moos AB, Caldwell HD. Ocular delayed hypersensitivity: a pathogenic mechanism of chlamydial conjunctivitis in guinea pigs. Proc Nat Acad Sci USA. 1986;83:7480–4.

467. Taylor HR, Schachter J, Caldwell HD. The stimulus for conjunctival inflammation in trachoma. Chlamydial Infections. 1986:167–70.

468. Taylor HR, Johnson SL, Schachter J, Caldwell HD, Prendergast RA. Pathogenesis of trachoma: the stimulus for inflammation. J Immunol. 1987;138:3023–7.

469. Taylor HR, Maclean IW, Brunham RC, Pal S, Whittum-Hudson J. Chlamydial heat shock proteins and trachoma. Infect Immun. 1990;58:3061–3.

470. Morrison RP, Belland RJ, Lyng K, Caldwell HD. Chlamydial disease pathogenesis. The 57 kD chlamydial hypersensitivity antigen is a stress response protein. J Exp Med. 1989;170:1271–83.

471. Lichtenwalner AB, Patton DL, Van Voorhis WC, Cosgrove Sweeney YT, Kuo C-C. Heat shock protein 60 is the major antigen which stimulates delayed-type hypersensitivity reaction in the macaque model of Chlamydia trachomatis salpingitis. Infect Immun. 2004;72:1159–61.

472. Holland MJ, Conway DJ, Blanchard TJ, Mahdi OMS, Bailey RL. Synthetic peptides based on Chlamydia trachomatis antigens identify cytotoxic T lymphocyte responses in subjects from a trachoma-endemic populations. Clin Exp Immunol. 1997;107:44–9.

473. Ramsey KH. Alternative Mechanisms of Pathogenesis. In: Bavoil PM, Wyrick PB, editors. Chlamydia. Genomics and Pathogenesis. Norfolk, UK: Horizon Bioscience; 2006; 435–73.

474. Rank RG, Dascher C, Bowlin AK, Bavoil PM. Systemic immunization with Hsp60 alters the development of chlamydial ocular disease. Invest Ophthalmol Vis Sci. 1995;36:1344–51.

475. Witkin SS, Jeremias J, Toth M, Ledger WJ. Cell-mediated immune response to the recombinant 57–kDa heat-shock protein of Chlamydia trachomatis in women with salpingitis. J Infect Dis. 1993;167:1379–83.

476. Cohen CR, Koochesfahani KM, Meier AS, Shen C, Karunakaran K, Ondondo B, et al. Immunoepidemiologic profile of Chlamydia trachomatis infection: importance of heat-shock protein 60 and interferon-γ. J Infect Dis. 2005;192:591–9.

477. Kinnunen AH, Surcel HM, Lehtinen M, Karhukorpi J, Tiitinen A, Halttunen M, et al. HLA DQ alleles and interleukin-10 polymorphism associated with Chlamydia trachomatis-related tubal factor infertility: a case-contol study. Hum Reprod. 2002;17:2073–8.

478. Lehtinen M, Paavonen J. Heat-Shock Proteins in the Immunopathogenesis of Chlamydial Pelvic Inflammatory Disease. In: Orfila J, Byrne GI, Chernesky MA, Grayston JT, Jones RB, Ridgway GL, et al., editors. Chlamydial Infections. Proceedings of the Eighth International Symposium on Human Chlamydial Infections, Chateau de Montvillargenne, 602700 Gouvieux – Chantilly, France 19–24 June 1994. Bologna – Italy: Societa Editrice Esculapio; 1994; 599–610.

479. La Verda D, Kalayoglu MV, Byrne GI. Chlamydial Heat Shock Proteins and Disease Pathology: New Paradigms for Old Problems. Infect Dis Obstet Gynecol. 1999;7:64–71.

480. Bulut Y, Faure E, Thomas L, Karahashi H, Michelsen KS, Equils O, et al. Chlamydial Heat Shock Protein 60 Activates macrophages and Endothelial Cells Through Toll-Like Receptor 4 and MD2 in a MyD88–Dependent Pathway. J Immunol. 2002;168:1435–40.

481. Bailey RL, Holland MJ, Whittle HC, Mabey DCW. Subjects recovering from human ocular chlamydial infections have enhanced lymphoproliferative responses to chlamydial antigens compared with those of persistently diseased controls. Infect Immun. 1995;63:389–92.

482. Holland MJ, Bailey RL, Conway DJ, Culley F, Miranpuri G, Byrne GI, et al. T helper type-1 (Th1)/Th2 profiles of peripheral blood mononuclear cells (PBMC); responses to antigens of Chlamydia trachomatis in subjects with severe trachomatous scarring. Clin Exp Immunol. 1996;105:429–35.

483. Peeling RW, Bailey RL, Conway DJ, Holland MJ, Campbell AE, Jallow O, et al. Antibody Response to the 60–kDa Chlamydial Heat-Shock Protein Is

Associated with Scarring Trachoma. J Infect Dis. 1998;177:256–9.

484. Karunakaran KP, Noguchi Y, Read TD, Cherkasov A, Kwee J, Shen C, et al. Molecular Analysis of the Multiple GroEL Proteins of Chlamydiae. J Bacteriol. 2003;185:1958–66.

485. Beatty WL, Morrison RP, GI. B. Immunoelectron-microscopic quantitation of differential levels of chlamydial proteins in a cell culture model of persistent Chlamydia trachomatis infection. Infect Immun. 1994;62:4059–62.

486. Karunakaran KP, Chen L, Shen C, Brunham RC. Do the Multiple Chaperonin Proteins of Chlamydiae Form Hetero-Oligomeric Assembly? In: Cherensky MA, Caldwell H, Christiansen G, Clarke IN, Kaltenboeck B, Knirsch C, et al., editors. Chlamydial Infections. Proceedings of the Eleventh International Symposium on Human Chlamydial Infections, Niagara-on-the-Lake, Ontario, Canada, June 18–23, 2006. San Francisco, CA 94110, USA: International Chlamydia Symposium; 2006; 229–32.

487. Gerard HC, Whittum-Hudson JA, Schumacher HR, Hudson AP. Differential expression of three Chlamydia trachomatis hsp60–encoding genes in active vs. persistent infections. Microb Pathog. 2004;36:35–9.

488. Bavoil PM, Wyrick PB, editors. Chlamydia: Genomics and Pathogenesis. Norfolk, UK: Horizon Bioscience; 2006.

489. Byrne GI, Lehmann LK, Landry GJ. Induction of tryptophan catabolism is the mechanism for gamma-interferon-mediated inhibition of intracellular Chlamydia psittaci replication in T24 cells. Infect Immun. 1986;53:347–51.

490. Puck A, Liappis N, Hildenbrand G. Ion exchange column chromatographic investigation of free amino acids in tears of healthy adults. Ophthalmic Res. 1984;16: 248–84.

491. ChenZhuo L, Murube J, Latorre A, del Rio RM. Different Concentrations of Amino Acids in Tears of Normal and Human Dry Eyes. In: Sullivan D et al, editor. Lacrimal Gland, Tear Film, and Dry Eye Syndromes 3: Kluwer Academic/Plenum Publishers; 2002; 617–21.

492. Byrne GI. Immunity to Chlamydia. In: Stephens RS, Byrne GI, Christiansen G, Clarke IN, Grayston JT, Rank RG, et al., editors. Chlamydial Infections. Proceedings of the Ninth International Symposium on Human Chlamydial Infection, Napa, California, USA, June 21–26, 1998. San Francisco, CA 94110, USA: International Chlamydia Symposium; 1998; 365–74.

493. Wynn TA. Fibrotic Disease and the T_H1/T_H2 Paradigm. Nat Rev Immunol. 2004;4:583–94.

494. Bobo L, Novak N, Mkocha H, Vitale S, West S, Quinn TC. Evidence of a Predominant Proinflammatory Conjunctival Cytokine Response in Individuals with Trachoma. Infect Immun. 1996;64:3273–9.

495. Burton MJ, Bailey RL, Jeffries D, Mabey DCW, Holland MJ. Cytokine and Fibrogenic Gene Expression in the Conjunctivas of Subjects from a Gambian Community Where Trachoma Is Endemic. Infect Immun. 2004;72:7352–6.

496. Burton MJ, Bowman RJC, Faal H, Aryee EAN, Ikumapayi UN, Alexander NDE, et al. Long term outcome of trichiasis surgery in the Gambia. Br J Ophthalmol. 2005;89:575–9.

497. Mozzato-Chamay N, Mahdi OSM, Jallow O, Mabey DCW, Bailey RL, Conway DJ. Polymorphisms in Candidate Genes and Risk of Scarring Trachoma in a *Chlamydia trachomatis* –Endemic Population. J Infect Dis. 2000;182:1545–8.

498. Natividad A, Holland MJ, Rockett KA, Joof HM, Mabey DCW, Bailey RL, et al. Clinical Consequences of Allelic Variation in the *Cis*-Regulation of *IL10* during Active Trachomatous Disease in Humans. In: Cherensky MA, Caldwell H, Christiansen G, Clarke IN, Kaltenboeck B, Knirsch C, et al., editors. Chlamydial Infections. Proceedings of the Eleventh International Symposium on Human Chlamydial Infections, Niagara-on-the-Lake, Ontario, Canada, June18–23, 2006. San Francisco, CA 94110, USA: International Chlamydia Symposium; 2006; 555–8.

499. Penttila T, Haveri A, Tammiruusu A, Vuola JM, Lahesmaa R, Puolakkainen M. Enhanced Clearance but Severe Inflammation during Pulmonary *Chlamydia pneumoniae* infection in IL-10 Knockout Mice. In: Cherensky MA, Caldwell H, Christiansen G, Clarke IN, Kaltenboeck B, Knirsch C, et al., editors. Chlamydial Infections. proceedings of the Eleventh International Symposium on Human Chlamydial Infections, Niagara-on-the-Lake, Ontario, Canada, June 18–23, 2006. San Francisco, CA 94110, USA: International Chlamydia Symposium; 2006; 535–8.

500. Faal N, Bailey RL, Sarr I, Joof H, Mabey DCW, Holland MJ. Temporal cytokine gene expression patterns in subjects with trachoma identify distinct conjuntival responses associated with infection. Clin Experiment Ophthalmol. 2005;142:347–53.

501. Tan M. Regulation of Gene Expression. In: Bavoil PM, Wyrick PB, editors. Chlamydia. Genomics and Pathogenesis. Norfolk, UK: Horizon Bioscience; 2006; 103–31.

502. Borel N, Summersgill JT, Mukhopadhyay S, Kaiser C, Nufer L, Miller RD, et al. Persistent *Chlamydophila Pneumoniae* in Human Coronary Atherosclerotic Tissue: Tissue Microarray Analysis and Ultrstructural Study. In: Cherensky MA, Caldwell H, Christiansen G, Clarke IN, Kaltenboeck B, Knirsch C, et al., editors. Chlamydial Infections. Proceedings of the Eleventh International Symposium on Human Chlamydial Infections, Niagara-on-the-Lake, Ontario, Canada, June 18–23, 2006. San Francisco, CA 94110, USA: International Chlamydia Symposium; 2006; 567–70.

503. Faal N, Bailey R, Joof H, Sarr I, Laye M, Jeffries D, et al. Conjunctival Expression of IFN-γ, IDO, IL-10, and FOXP3 in Gambian Children during Trachoma Episodes. In: Cherensky MA, Caldwell H, Christiansen G, Clarke IN, Kaltenboeck B, Knirsch C, et al., editors. Chlamydial Infections. Proceedings of the Eleventh International Symposium on Human Chlamydial Infections, Niagara-on-the-Lake, Ontario, Canada, June 18–23, 2006. San Francisco, CA 94110, USA: International Chlamydia Symposium; 2006; 381–4.

504. Gervassi AL, Probst P, Stamm WE, Marrazzo J, Grabstein KH, Alderson MR. Functional characterization of Class Ia- and Non-Class Ia-restricted Chlamydia-reactive CD8+ T cell responses in humans. J Immunol. 2003;171:4278–86.

505. Conway DJ, Holland MJ, Campbell AE, Bailey RL, Krausa P, Peeling RW, et al. HLA class I and II polymorphisms and trachomatous scarring in a *Chlamydia trachomatis* – endemic population. J Infect Dis. 1996;174:643–6.

506. Peeling RW, Bailey RL, Conway DJ, Holland MJ, Dillon E, Campbell AE, et al. Antibody response to the chlamydial heat stock protein 60 (CHSP60) is associated with scarring trachoma. Chlamydia Trachomatis. 1997;73.

507. White AG, Bogh J, Leheny W, Kuchipudi P, Varghese M, Al Riyami H, et al. HLA antigens in Omanis with blinding trachoma: markers for disease susceptibility and resistance. Br J Ophthalmol. 1997;81:431–4.

508. Bowman RJC, Faal H, Adegbola R, Foster A, Johnson GJ, Bailey RL. Longitudinal study of trachomatous trichiasis in the Gambia. Br J Ophthalmol. 2002;86:339–43.

509. Burton MJ, Bowman RJC, Faal H, Aryee EAN, Ikumapayi UN, Alexander NDE, et al. The long-term natural history of trachomatous trichiasis in the Gambia. Invest Ophthalmol Vis Sci. 2006;47:847–52.

510. Munoz B, West S. Trachoma: The Forgotten Cause of Blindness. Epidemiol Rev. 1997;19:205–17.

511. Munoz B, Bobo L, Mkocha H, Lynch M, Hsieh Y-H, West S. Incidence of trichiasis in a cohort of women with and without scarring. Int J Epidemiol. 1999;28:1167–71.

512. Bowman RJC, Jatta B, Cham B, Bailey R, Faal H, Myatt M, et al. Natural history of trachomatous scarring in The Gambia. Results of a 12–year longitudinal follow-up. Am J Ophthalmol. 2001;108:2219–24.

513. Melese M, West ES, Alemayehu W, Munoz B, Worku A, Gaydos CA, et al. Characteristics of trichiasis patients presenting for surgery in rural Ethiopia. Br J Ophthalmol. 2005;89:1084–8.

514. Cevallos V, Donnellan C, Zhou Z, Yi E H, Melese M, Alemayehu W, et al. Conjunctival Flora in Patients with Trichiasis Due to Trachoma. In: Association for Research in Vision and Ophthalmology 2005; Fort Lauderdale, Florida, USA.

515. Burton MJ, Adegbola RA, Kinteh F, Ikumapayi UN, Foster A, Mabey DCW, et al. Bacterial Infection and Gene Expression in Cicatricial Trachoma in The Gambia. In: Eleventh Meeting of the WHO Alliance for the Global Elimination of Trachoma by 2020; Eastern Mediterranean Regional Office, Cairo, Egypt, 2007.

516. Gambhir M, Basanez M-G, Grassly NC. A Mathematical Model of Trachoma Infection and Disease. In: Chernesky M, Caldwell H, Christiansen G, Clarke IN, Kaltenboeck B, Knirsch C, et al., editors. Chlamydial Infections. Proceedings of the Eleventh International Symposium on Human Chlamydial Infections, Niagara-on-the-Lake, Ontario, Canada, June 18–23, 2006. San Francisco, CA 94110, USA: International Chlamydia Symposium; 2006; 341–4.

517. Bell TA, Stamm WE, Wang S-P, Kuo CC, Holmes KK, Grayston T. Chronic *Chlamydia trachomatis* infections in infants. JAMA. 1992;267:400–2.

518. Dean D, Suchland RJ, Stamm WE. Apparent Long-Term Persistence of *Chlamydia trachomatis* Cervical Infections – Analysis by OMP1 Genotyping. In: Stephens RS, Byrne GI, Christiansen G, Clarke IN, Grayston JT, Rank RG, et al., editors. Chlamydia Infections. Proceedings of the Ninth International Symposium on Human Chlamydial Infections, Napa, California, USA, June 21–26, 1998. San Francisco, CA 94110, USA: International Chlamydia Symposium; 1998; 31–4.

519. Molano M, Meijer JLM, Weiderpass E, Arslan A, Posso H, Franceschi S, et al. The Natural Course of Chlamydia trachomatis Infection in Asymptomatic Colombian Women: A 5 year Follow-Up Study. J Infect Dis. 2005;191:907–16.

520. Golden MR, Whittington WLH, Handsfield HH, Hughes JP, Stamm WE, Hogben M, et al. Effect of expedited treatment of sex partners on recurrent or persistent gonorrhea or chlamydial infection. N Eng J Med. 2005;352:676–85.

521. Gerard HC, Branigan PJ, Schumacher HR, Hudson AP. Synovial chlamydia trachomatis in patients with reactive arthritis/Reiter's syndrome are viable but show aberrant gene expression. J Rheumatol. 1998;25:610–12.

522. Gerard HC, Schumacher HR, El-Gabalawy H, Goldbach-Mansky R, Hudson AP. Chlamydia pneumoniae present in the human synovium are viable and metabolically active. Microb Pathog. 2000;36:17–24.

523. Robman L, Mahdi O, McCarty C, Dimitrov P, Tikellis G, McNeil J, et al. Exposure to *Chlamydia pneumoniae* Infection and Progression of Age-related Macular Degeneration. Am J Epidemiol. 2005;161:1013–9.

524. Robman L, Olaimatu S, Mahdi O, Wang JJ, Burlutsky G, Mitchell P, et al. Exposure to

Chlamydia pneumoniae infection and age-related macular degeneration: The Blue Mountains Eye Study. Invest Ophthalmol Vis Sci. 2007;48:4007–11.

525. Guymer R, Robman L. Chlamydia pneumoniae and age-related macular degeneration: a role in pathogenesis or merely a chance association? Clin Exp Ophthalmol. 2007;35:89–93.

526. Melese M, Chidambaram JD, Alemayehu W, Lee DC, Yi EH, Cevallos V, et al. Feasibility of eliminating ocular chlamydia trachomatis with repeat mass antibiotic treatments. JAMA. 2004;292:721–5.

527. Scott JG. Trachoma in Africa. SA Med J. 1993;83:243–4.

528. Collier LH, Blyth WA. Immunogenicity of experimental trachoma vaccines in baboons. II Experiments with adjuvants and tests of cross protection. J Hyg Camb. 1966;64:529–44.

529. Collier LH, Smith A. Dissemination and immunogenicity of live TRIC agent in baboons after parenteral injection. Am J Ophthalmol. 1967;63:1589–1602.

530. Sowa S, Sowa J, Collier LH, Blyth WA. Trachoma vaccine trials in The Gambia. J Hyg Camb. 1969;67:699–717.

531. Grayston JT, Kim KSW, Alexander ER, Wang S-P. Protective studies in monkeys with trivalent and monovalent trachoma vaccines. In: Nichols RL, editor. Trachoma and related disorders. Amsterdam: Excerpta Medica; 1971; 377–85.

532. Woolridge RL, Grayston JT, Chang H, Yang CY, Cheng KH. Long-term follow-up of the initial (1959–1960) trachoma vaccine field trial on Taiwan. Am J Ophthalmol. 1967;63:1650–3.

533. Woolridge RL, Grayston JT, Chang IH, Cheng KH, Yang CY, Neave C. Field trial of a monovalent and of a bivalent mineral oil adjuvant trachoma vaccine in Taiwan school children. Am J Ophthalmol. 1967;63:1645–50.

534. Dhir SP, Agarwal LP, Detels R, Wang S-P, Grayston JT. Field trial of two bivalent trachoma vaccines in children of Punjab Indian villages. Am J Ophthalmol. 1967;63:1640–4.

535. Clements C, Dhir SP, Grayston JT, Wang S-P. Long term follow-up study of a trachoma vaccine trial in villages in northern India. Am J Ophthalmol. 1979;87:350–3.

536. Grayston JT. Immunization against trachoma. First International Conference on Vaccines Against Viral and Rickettsial Diseases of Man 1967:546–59.

537. McComb DE, Peters JH, Fraser CEO, Murray ES, MacDonald AB, Nichols RL. Resistance to trachoma infection in owl monkeys correlated with antibody status at the outset in an experiment to test the response to topical trachoma antigens. In: Nichols RL, editor. Trachoma and related disorders. Amsterdam: Excerpta Medica; 1971; 396–406.

538. Nichols RL, Bell SD, Haddad NA, Bobb AA. Studies on trachoma. VI. Microbiological

observations in a field trial in Saudi Arabia of bivalent trachoma vaccine at three dosage levels. Am J Trop Med Hyg 1969;18:723–30.

539. Bietti G, Werner GH. Trachoma Prevention and Treatment. Springfield, Illinois: Charles C Thomas; 1967.

540. Woolridge RL, Cheng KH, Chang IH, Yang CY, Hsu TC, Grayston JT. Failure of trachoma treatment with ophthalmic antibiotics and systemic sulfonamides used alone or in combination with trachoma vaccine. Am J Ophthalmol. 1967;63:1557–83.

541. Morrison RP, Caldwell HD. Immunity to murine chlamydial genital infection. Infect Immun. 2002;70:2741–51.

542. Whittum-Hudson JA, An L-L, Saltzman WM, Prendergast RA, Macdonald AB. Oral immunization with an anti-idiotypic antibody to the exoglycolipid antigen protects against experimental Chlamydia trachomatis infection. Nat Med. 1996;2:1116–21.

543. Eko FO, He Q, Brown T, McMillan L, Ifere GO, Ananaba GA, et al. A novel recombinant multisubunit vaccine against chlamydia. J Immunol. 2004;173:3375–82.

544. Darville T. Immunology of Chlamydia trachomatis Infections and Prospects for the Development of a Vaccine. In: Chernesky M, Caldwell H, Christiansen G, Clarke IN, Kaltenboeck B, Knirsch C, et al., editors. Chlamydial Infections. Proceedings of the Eleventh International Symposium on Human Chlamydial Infections, Niagara-on-the-Lake, Canada, June 18–23. San Francisco, CA 94110: International Chlamydia Symposium; 2006:347–56.

545. Morrison SG, Morrison RP. A Predominant role for antibody in acquired immunity to chlamydial genital tract infection. J Immunol. 2005;175:7536–42.

546. Pal S, Peterson EM, de la Maza LM. Vaccination with the Chlamydia trachomatis major outer membrane protein can elicit an immune response as protective as that resulting from inoculation with live bacteria. Infect Immun. 2005;73:8153–60.

547. Igietseme JU, Eko FO, He Q, Bandea C, Lubitz W, Garcia-Sastre A, et al. Delivery of Chlamydia vaccines. Expert Opin Drug Deliv. 2005;2:549–62.

548. Tan C, Spitznagel JK, Shou H-Z, Hsia R-C, Bavoil PM. The Polymorphic Membrane Protein Gene Family of the Chlamydiaceae. In: Bavoil PM, Wyrick PB, editors. Chlamydia. Genomics and Pathogenesis. Norfolk UK: Horizon Bioscience; 2006; 195–218.

549. Crane DD, Carlson JH, Fischer ER, Bavoil P, Hsia RC, Tan C, et al. Chlamydia trachomatis polymorphic membrane protein D is a species-common pan-neutralizing antigen. Proc Nat Acad Sci USA. 2006;103:1894–9.

550. Singh SB, Davis AS, Taylor GA, Deretic V. Human IRGM Induces Autophagy to Eliminate

Intracellular Mycobacteria. Science. 2006;313:1438–41.

551. Byrne G. Personal Communication. 2006.

552. Fields KA, Hackstadt T. The *Chlamydia* Type III Secretion System: Structure and Implications for Pathogenesis. In: Bavioli P, Wyrick PB, editors. Chlamydia. Genomics and Pathogenesis. Norfolk UK: Horizon Bioscience; 2006; 219–33.

553. Campbell LA, Kuo C-C. Interactions of *Chlamydia* with the Host Cells that Mediate Attachment and Uptake. In: Bavoil PM, Wyrick PB, editors. Chlamydia. Genomics and Pathogenesis. Norfolk, UK: Horizon Bioscience; 2006; 505–22.

554. Pulendran B. Tolls and beyond – many roads to vaccine immunity. N Eng J Med. 2007;356:1776–8.

555. Taylor HR, Young E, MacDonald B, Schachter J, Prendergast RA. Oral immunization against chlamydial eye infection. Invest Ophthalmol Vis Sci. 1987;28:249–58.

556. Taylor HR, Prendergast RA. Attempted oral immunization with chlamydial lipopolysaccharide subunit vaccine. Invest Ophthalmol Vis Sci. 1987;28:1722–6.

557. Taylor HR, Whittum-Hudson J, Schachter J, Caldwell HD, Prendergast RA. Oral immunization with chlamydial major outer membrane protein (MOMP). Invest Ophthalmol Vis Sci. 1988;29:1847–53.

558. Campos M, Pal S, O'Brien TP, Taylor HR, Prendergast RA, Whittum-Hudson JA. A chlamydial major outer membrane protein extract as a trachoma vaccine candidate. Invest Ophthalmol Vis Sci. 1995;36:1477–91.

559. Taylor HR, Stephens RS, Whittum-Hudson JA, Prendergast RA. Initial evaluation of trachoma subunit vaccines. Invest Ophthalmol Vis Sci. 1989;30 (suppl):381.

560. Lindner K. Trachoma. In: Berens C, editor. The Eye and Its Diseases. Second ed. Philadelphia: W. B. Saunders Company; 1949; 399–413.

561. Portney GL, Hoshiwara I. Prevalence of trachoma among southwestern American Indian Tribe. Am J Ophthalmol. 1970;70:843–8.

562. Turner FB. Trachoma in the Northern Territory, 1946–1986. Med J Aust. 1989;151:727.

563. Elphinstone JJ. Health of the Kimberley natives. Appendix XVI: Report of Commission of Public Health WA, Perth; 1963.

564. Alimuddin M. Incidence and treatment of trachoma in Pakistan. Br J Ophthalmol. 1958;42:360–6.

565. Scott JG. Mass treatment of trachoma: field trials of different drugs in 10,033 Bantu children. SA Med J. 1960;83:442–4.

566. Dawson CR, Daghfous T, Messadi M, Hoshiwara I, Vastine DW, Honeda C, et al. Severe endemic trachoma in Tunisia. II. A controlled therapy trial of topically applied chlortetracycline and erythromycin. Arch Ophthalmol. 1974;92: 198–203.

567. Dawson CR, Daghfous T, Whitcher J, Messadi M, Hoshiwara T, Triki F, et al. Intermittent trachoma chemotherapy: a controlled trial of topical tetracycline or erythromycin. Bull World Health Organ. 1981;59:91–7.

568. Dawson CR, Elashoff RM, Hanna L, Hoshiwara I, Ostler HB. The evaluation of a controlled trachoma therapy trial with oral tetracycline. In: Nichols RL, editor. Trachoma and related disorders. Amsterdam: Excerpta Medica; 1971; 545–8.

569. Maitchouk IF. Report on blindness in the Middle East. Regional Office for the Eastern Mediterranean: World Health Organization; 1976.

570. Cerulli L, Cedrone C, Assefa C, Scuderi GL. Evaluation of treatment against trachoma in two regions of Ethiopia. Rev Int Trach Pathol Ocul Trop Subtrop. 1983;60:67–77.

571. Jones BR, Darougar S, Mohsenine H, Poirier RH. Communicable ophthalmia: the blinding scourge of the Middle East. Yesterday, and ? tomorrow. Br J Ophthalmol. 1976;60:492–8.

572. Darougar S, Jones BR, Viswalingam N, Poirier RH, Allami J, Houshmand A, et al. Family-based suppressive intermittent therapy of hyperendemic trachoma with topical oxytetracycline or oral doxycycline. Br J Ophthalmol. 1980;64:291–5.

573. Chumbley LC, Viswalingam ND, Thomson IM, Zeidan MA. Treatment of trachoma in the West Bank. Eye. 1988;2:471–5.

574. Schachter J, Dawson CR. Chlamydial infections, a worldwide problem: epidemiology and implications for trachoma therapy. Sex Trans Dis. 1981;8:167–74.

575. Dawson CR, Schachter J. Strategies for treatment and control of blinding trachoma: cost effectiveness of topical or systemic antibiotics. Rev Infect Dis. 1985;7:768–73.

576. Dawson CR, Hoshiwara I, Daghfous T, Messadi M, Vastine DW, Schachter J. Topical tetracycline and rifampicin therapy of endemic trachoma in Tunisia. Am J Ophthalmol. 1975;79:803–11.

577. Daghfous MT, Romdhane K, Kamoun M, Triki F, Dawson CR, Hoshiwara I. Le trachome en Tunisie apres 20 ans de controle. In: Shimizu K, Oosterhuis JA, editors. International Congress Series No. 450, XXIII Concilium Ophthalmologicum. Amsterdam-Oxford: Excerpta Medica; 1978; 516–22.

578. Hardy D, Surman PG, Howarth WH. The cytology of conjunctival smears from Aboriginal school children at Yalata, South Australia. Am J Ophthalmol. 1967;63:1538–40.

579. Banks JR, Braun P. Trachoma treatment in Aborigines. (Letter). Med J Aust. 1985;142:376.

580. Taylor HR. Report of a workshop: research priorities for trachoma. J Infect Dis. 1985;152: 383–8.

581. Mabey DCW, Downes RM, Downes B, Bailey RL, Dunn DT. The impact of medical services on trachoma in a Gambian village: antibiotics alone

are not the answer. Ann Trop Paediatrics. 1991;11:295–300.

582. Taylor HR. Review of trachoma: an introduction. Rev Infect Dis. 1985;7:711–12.

583. Francis V, Turner V. Achieving Community Support for Trachoma Control. Geneva: World Health Organization; 1993. Report No.: WHO/PBL/93.36.

584. West SK, Bedri A, Thanh TKT, West ES, Mariotti SP. Final Assessment of Trichiasis Surgeons. Geneva: World Health Organization; 2005. Report No.: WHO/PBD/GET/05.2.

585. World Health Organization. WHA51.11 Global elimination of blinding trachoma. Geneva: WHO; 1998.

586. World Health Organization. Report of the Seventh Meeting of the WHO Alliance for the Global Elimination of Trachoma. Geneva: WHO; 2003. Report No.: WHO/PBD/GET04.1.

587. Reacher M, Foster A, Huber J. Trichiasis Surgery for Trachoma – The Bilamellar Tarsal Rotation Procedure. Geneva: World Health Organization; 1993. Report No.: WHO/PBL/93.29.

588 Zithromax. Zithromax in the Control of Blinding Trachoma – A Program Manager's Guide. New York: International Trachoma Initiative; 2002.

589. Mariotti SP, Pruss A. The SAFE Strategy – Preventing trachoma. Geneva: World Health Organization; 2000. Report No.: WHO/PBD/GET/00.7.

590. Emerson P, Frost L, Bailey R, Mabey D. Implementing the SAFE Strategy for Trachoma Control. Geneva: The Carter Centre – International Trachoma Initiative; 2006.

591. World Health Organization. Planning for the Global Elimination of Trachoma (GET). Geneva: WHO 25 & 26 November 1996. Report No.: WHO/PBL/97.60.

592. World Health Organization. Report of the Second Meeting of the WHO Alliance for the Global Elimination of Trachoma. Geneva: WHO 12–14 January 1998. Report No.: WHO/PBL/GET/9.

593. World Health Organization. Report of the Third Meeting of the WHO Alliance for the Global Elimination of Trachoma. Geneva: WHO 19–20 October 1998. Report No.: WHO/PBD/GET/99.3.

594. World Health Organization. Report of the Fourth Meeting of the WHO Alliance for the Global Elimination of Blinding Trachoma. Geneva: WHO 1 & 2 December 1999. Report No.: WHO/PBD/00.9.

595. World Health Organization. Report of the Fifth Meeting of the WHO Alliance for the Global Elimination of Blinding Trachoma. Geneva: WHO 5–7 December 2000. Report No.: WHO/PBD/GET/00.10.

596. World Health Organization. Report of the Sixth Meeting of the WHO Alliance for the Global Elimination of Blinding Trachoma. Geneva: WHO; 2001. Report No.: WHO/PBD/GET/02.1.

597. World Health Organization. Report of the Eighth Meeting of the WHO Alliance for the Global Elimination of Blinding Trachoma. Geneva: WHO 29–30 March 2004. Report No.: WHO/PBD/GET/04.2.

598. World Health Organization. Report of the Tenth Meeting of the WHO Alliance for the Global Elimination of Blinding Trachoma. Geneva: WHO 12 April 2006. Report No.: WHO/PBD/GET/06.1.

599. <http://www.icoph.org/guideintro.html>, viewed June 2006. International Clinical Guidelines Trachoma; 2006.

600. Reacher MH, Taylor HR. The management of trachomatous trichiasis. Rev Int Trach. 1990;67:233–61.

601. Reacher MH, Huber MJE, Canagaratnam R, Alghassany A. A trial of surgery for trichiasis of the upper lid from trachoma. Br J Ophthalmol. 1990;74:109–13.

602. Thanh TTK, Khandekar R, Luong VQ, Courtright P. One year recurrence of trachomatous trichiasis in routinely operated Cuenod Nataf procedure in Vietnam. Br J Ophthalmol. 2004;88:1114–8.

603. Negrel AD, Chami-Khazraji Y, Arrache ML, Ottmani S, Mahjour J. The quality of trichiasis surgery in the kingdom of Morocco. Sante. 2000;10:81–92.

604. West ES, Mkocha H, Munoz B, Mabey D, Foster A, Bailey R, et al. Risk factors for postsurgical trichiasis recurrence in a trachoma-endemic area. Invest Ophthalmol Vis Sci. 2005;46:447–53.

605. West SK, West ES, Alemayehu W, Melese M, Munoz B, Imeru A, et al. Single-dose azithromycin prevents trichiasis recurrence following surgery. Arch Ophthalmol. 2006;124:309–14.

606. Zhang H, Kandel RP, Sharma B, Dean D. Risk factors for recurrence of post-operative trichiasis: implications for trachoma blindness prevention. Arch Ophthalmol. 2004;122:511–16.

607. Zhang H, Kandel RP, Atakari HK, Dean D. Impact of oral azithromycin on recurrence of trachomatous trichiasis in Nepal over 1 year. Br J Ophthalmol. 2006;90:943–8.

608. Bog H, Yorson D, Foster A. Results of community-based eyelid surgery for trichiasis due to trachoma. Br J Ophthalmol. 1993;77:81–3.

609. Alemayehu W, Melese M, Bejiqa A, Worku A, Kebede W, Fantaye D. Surgery for Trichiasis by Ophthalmologists versus Integrated Eye Care Workers: A Randomized Trial. Ophthalmology. 2004;111:578–84.

610. El Toukhy E, Lewallen S, Courtright P. Routine bilamellar tarsal rotation surgery for trachomatous trichiasis: short-term outcome and factors associated with surgical failure. Ophthal Plast Reconstr Surg. 2006;22:109–12.

611. Merbs SL, West SK, West ES. Pattern of recurrence of trachomatous trichiasis after surgery. Ophthalmology. 2005;112:705–9.

612. Yorston D, Mabey D, Hatt S, Burton M. Intervention for trachoma trichiasis. Cochrane Database Syst Rev. 2006;3:CD004008.

613. West ES, Munoz B, Imeru A, Alemayehu W, Melese M, West SK. The association between epilation and corneal opacity among eyes with trachomatous trichiasis. Br J Ophthalmol. 2006;90:171–4.

614. Bowman RJC, Sillah A, van Dehn C, Goode VM, Muquit M, Johnson GJ, et al. Operational comparison of single-dose azithromycin and topical tetracycline for trachoma. Invest Ophthalmol Vis Sci. 2000;41:4074–9.

615. Mahande M, Tharaney M, Kirumbi E, Ngirawamungu E, Geneau R, Tapert L, et al. Uptake of trichiasis surgical services in Tanzania through two village-based approaches. Br J Ophthalmol. 2007;91:139–42.

616. West S, Lynch M, Muñoz B, Katala S, Robin S, Mmbaga BBO. Predicting surgical compliance in a cohort of women with trichiasis. Int Ophthalmol. 1994;18:105–9.

617. Courtright P. Acceptance of surgery for trichiasis among rural Malawian women. East Afr Med J. 1994;71:803–4.

618. Nagpal G, Dhaliwal U, Bhatia MS. Barriers to acceptance of intervention among patients with trachomatous trichiasis or entropion presenting to a teaching hospital. Ophthalmic Epidemiol. 2006;13:53–8.

619. Dhaliwal U, Nagpal G, Bhatia MS. Health-related quality of life in patients with trachomatous trichiasis or entropion. Ophthalmic Epidemiol. 2006;13:59–66.

620. Frick KD, Keuffel EL, Bowman RJ. Epidemiological, demographic, and economic analyses: measurement of the value of trichiasis surgery in The Gambia. Ophthalmic Epidemiol. 2001;8:191–201.

621. Lewallen S, Mahande M, Tharaney M, Katala S, Courtright P. Surgery for trachomatous trichiasis: findings from a survey of trichiasis surgeons in Tanzania. Br J Opthalmol. 2007;91:143–5.

622. Khandekar R, Al-Hadrami K, Sarvanan N, Al Harby S, Mohammed AJ. Recurrence of trachomatous trichiasis 17 years after bilamellar tarsal rotation. Am J Ophthalmol. 2006;141:1087–91.

623. Rees E, Tait IA, Hobson D, Karayiannis P, N. L. Persistence of chlamydial infection after treatment for neonatal conjunctivitis. Arch Dis Child. 1981;56:193–8.

624. Centers for Disease Control and Prevention, Workowski KA, Berman SM. Sexually Transmitted Diseases Treatment Guidelines, 2006. MMWR Recomm Rep 2006;55:1–94.

625. Hoepelman IM, Schneider MME. Azithromycin: the first of the tissue-selective azalides. Int J Antimicrob Agents. 1995;5:145–67.

626. Engel JN. Azithromycin-induced block of elementary body formation in Chlamydia trachomatis. Antimicrob Agents Chemother. 1992;36:2304–9.

627. Patton DL, Wang SK, Kuo CC. The activity of azithromycin on the infectivity of Chlamydia trachomatis in human amniotic cells. J Antimicrob Chemother. 1995;36:951–9.

628. Martin DH, Mroczkowski TF, Dalu ZA, McCarty J, Jones RB, Hopkins SJ, et al. A controlled trial of a single dose of azithromycin for the treatment of chlamydial urethritis and cervicitis. N Engl J Med. 1992;327:921–5.

629. Pfizer Inc. Zithromax (azithromycin tablets) and (azithromycin for oral suspension) 70–5179–00–4. Product Insert 2004;70:1–32.

630. Karcioglu ZA, El-Yazigi A, Jabak MH, Choudhury AH, Ahmed WS. Pharmacokinetics of azithromycin in trachoma patients. Ophthalmology. 1998;105:658–61.

631. Tabbara KF, Al-Kharashi SA, Al-Mansouri SM, Al-Omar OM, Cooper H, El-Asrar AMA, et al. Ocular levels of azithromycin. Arch Ophthalmol. 1998;116:1625–8.

632. Centers for Disease Control and Prevention, Tiwari T, Murphy TV, Moran J, National Immunization Program, CDC. Recommended antimicrobial agents for the treatment and postexposure prophylaxis of pertussis: 2005 CDC Guidelines. MMWR Recomm Rep. 2005;54:1–16.

633. Sarkar M, Woodland C, Koren G, Einarson ARN. Pregnancy outcome following gestational exposure to azithromycin. BMC Pregnancy Childbirth. 2006;6:18.

634. Lietman T, Fry A. Can we eliminate trachoma? Br J Ophthalmol. 2001;85:385–87.

635. Fry AM, Jha HC, Lietman TM, Chaudhary JSP, Bhatta RC, Elliott J, et al. Adverse and beneficial secondary effects of mass treatment with azithromycin to eliminate blindness due to trachoma in Nepal. Clin Infect Dis. 2002;35: 395–402.

636. Shelby-James TM, Leach AJ, Carapetis JR, Currie BJ, Mathews JD. Impact of single dose azithromycin on group A streptococci in the upper respiratory tract and skin of Aboriginal children. Ped Infect Dis J. 2002;21:375–80.

637. Taylor KI, Taylor HR. Distribution of azithromycin for the treatment of trachoma. Br J Ophthalmol. 1999;83:134–5.

638. Cochereau I, Meddeb-Ouertani A, Khairallah M, Amraoui A, Zaghloul K, Pop M, et al. 3–day treatment with azithromycin 1.5% eye drops versus 7–day treatment with tobramycin 0.3% for purulent bacterial conjunctivitis: multicentre, randomised and controlled trial in adults and children. Br J Ophthalmol. 2007;91:465–9.

639 Goldschmidt P, Che Sarria P, Goepogui A, Sow M, Afghani T, de Barbeyrac B, et al. Clinical and microbiological efficacy of stable solution of azithromycin for the topical treatment of children

with active trachoma. In: Eleventh Meeting of the WHO Alliance for the Global Elimination of Trachoma by 2020; Cairo, Egypt, 2007.

640. Tabbara KF, El-Asrar AM, Al-Omar O, Choudhury AH, Al-Faisal Z. Single-dose azithromycin in the treatment of trachoma. A randomized, controlled study. Ophthalmology. 1996;103:842–6.

641. Dawson CR, Schachter J, Sallam S, Sheta A, Rubinstein RA, Washton H. A comparison of oral azithromycin with topical oxytetracycline/polymyxin for the treatment of trachoma in children. Clin Infect Dis. 1997;24:363–8.

642. Mabey D, Fraser-Hurt N, Powell C. Antibiotics for Trachoma. Cochrane Database Syst Rev. 2005:CD001860.

643. Schachter J, Dawson C, Sallam S, el Manadily N, Schneider E, Moncada J, et al. Follow-up Studies 10 years after community-wide treatment for trachoma in rural Egypt. In: Chernesky M, Caldwell H, Christiansen G, Clarke IN, Kaltenboeck B, Knirsch C, et al., editors. Chlamydial Infections. Proceedings of the Eleventh International Symposium on Human Chlamydial Infections, Niagara-on-the-Lake, Ontario, Canada. San Francisco, CA 94110: International Chlamydia Symposium; 2006; 337–40.

644. Summerskill W. Cochrane Collaboration and the evolution of evidence. Lancet. 2005;366:1760.

645. Wright HR, Keeffe JE, Taylor HR. Elimination of trachoma: are we in danger of being blinded by the randomised controlled trial? Br J Ophthalmol. 2006;90:1139–1340.

646. Shapiro B, Dickersin K, Lietman T. Trachoma, antibiotics and randomised controlled trials. Br J Ophthalmol. 2006;90:1443–4.

647. Harding-Esch E, Solomon A, Massae P, Mabey D. Five year Impact of Mass Azithromycin Treatment on Trachoma in Rombo District, Tanzania. In: Chernesky M, Caldwell H, Christiansen G, Clarke IN, Kaltenboeck B, Knirsch C, et al., editors. Chlamydial Infections. Proceeding of the Eleventh International Symposium on Human Chlamydial Infections, Niagara-on-the-Lake, Ontario, Canada, June 18–23, 2006. San Francisco, CA 94110: International Chlamydia Symposium; 2006; 333–6.

648. Chidambaram JD, Melese M, Alemayehu W, Yi E, Prabriputaloong T, Lee DC, et al. Mass antibiotic treatment and community protection in trachoma control programs. Clin Infect Dis. 2004;39:e95–e97.

649. West SK, Mkocha H, Munoz B, Gaydos C, Wood BJ, Holden J, et al. *Chlamydia trachomatis* Infection and Trachoma in Children Born into a Trachoma-hyperendemic Village after Two Rounds of Mass Treatment: Evidence for Modest Protection. In: Chernesky M, Caldwell H, Christiansen G, Clarke IN, Kaltenboeck B, Knirsch C, et al., editors. Chlamydial Infections. Proceedings of the Eleventh International

Symposium on Human Chlamydial Infections, Niagara-on-the-Lake, Ontario, Canada, June 18–23, 2006. San Francisco, CA 94110: International Chlamydia Symposium; 2006; 329–32.

650. Holm SO, Jha HC, Bhatta RC, Chaudary JSP, Thapa BB, Davis D, et al. Comparison of two azithromycin distribution strategies for controlling trachoma in Nepal. Bull World Health Organ. 2001;79:194–200.

651. Khandekar R, Mohammed AJ. Outcome of azithromycin treatment of active trachoma in Omani schoolchildren. La Revue de Sante de la Mediterranee orientale. 2003;9:1026–33.

652. Somani J, Bhullar VB, Workowski KA, Farshy CE, Black CM. Multiple drug-resistant *Chlamydia trachomatis* associated with clinical treatment failure. J Infect Dis. 2000;181:1421–7.

653. Ridgway GL. Antibiotic Resistance in Human Chlamydial Infection: Should We Be Concerned? In: Schachter J, Christiansen G, Clarke IN, Hammerschlag MR, Kaltenboeck B, Kuo C-C, et al., editors. Chlamydial Infections. Proceedings of the Tenth International Symposium on Human Chlamydial Infections, June 16–21, 2002, Antalya – Turkey. San Francisco, CA94110: International Chlamydia Symposium; 2002; 343–52.

654. Dugan J, Rockey DD, Jones L, Andersen AA. Tetracycline Resistance in *Chlamydia suis* Mediated by Genomic Islands Inserted into the Chlamydial *inv*-Like Gene. Antimicrob Agents Chemother. 2004;48:3989–95.

655. Malhotra-Kumar S, Lammens C, Coenen S, Van Herck K, Goossens H. Effect of azithromycin and clarithromycin therapy on pharyngeal carriage of macrolide-resistant streptococci in healthy volunteers: a randomised, double-blind, placebo-controlled study. Lancet. 2007;369:482–90.

656. Dawson CR, Ostler HB, Hanna L, Hoshiwara I, Jawetz E. Tetracyclines in the treatment of chronic trachoma in American Indians. J Infect Dis. 1971;124:255–63.

657. Adegbola RA, Mulholland EK, Bailey R, Secka O, Sadiq T, Glasgow K, et al. Effect of azithromycin on pharyngeal microflora. Ped Infect Dis J. 1995;14:335–6.

658. Leach AJ, Shelby-James TM, Mayo M, Gratten M, Laming AC, Currie BJ, et al. A prospective study of the impact of community-based azithromycin treatment of trachoma on carriage and resistance of Streptococcus Pneumoniae. Clin Infect Dis. 1997;24:356–62.

659. Chern KC, Shrestha SK, Cevallos V, Dhami HL, Tiwari P, Chern L, et al. Alterations in the conjunctival bacterial flora following a single dose of azitrhomycin in a trachoma endemic area. Br J Ophthalmol. 1999;83:1332–5.

660. Gaynor BD, Halbrook KA, Whicher JP, Holm SO, Jha HC, Chaudhary JSP, et al. Community treatment with azithromycin for trachoma is not

associated with antibiotic resistance in Streptococcus pneumoniae at 1 year. Br J Ophthalmol. 2003;87:147–8.

661. Coleman K, Mein J. Characterising Kimberley invasive pneumococcal infections and vaccine coverage, 2003–2005. Kimberley Population Health Unit Bulletin – January 2006:5.

662. Currie B. The rationale for restricting azithromycin use in the Northern Territory. The Northern Territory Communicable Diseases Bulletin 1996;3:16–17.

663. The Australian Group on Antimicrobial Resistance. Antimicrobial Susceptibility Report on Streptococcus pneumoniae Isolates from the Australian Group on Antimicrobial Resistance (AGAR), 2005 Surveillance Report; 2006.

664. Clinical and Laboratory Standards Institute. Performance Standards for Antimicrobial Susceptibility Testing, Sixteenth Informational Supplement; 2006.

665. Lietman T, Bird M, Farell V, Miao Y, Bhatta R, Jha H, et al. Why is Trachoma Disappearing From Nepal? In: Schachter J, Christiansen G, Clarke IN, Hammerschlag MR, Kaltenboeck B, Kuo C-C, et al., editors. Chlamydial Infections. Proceedings of the Tenth International Symposium on Human Chlamydial Infections, June 16–21, 2002, Antalya – Turkey. San Francisco CA 94110: International Chlamydia Symposium; 2002; 523–6.

666. Brunham RC, Pourbohloul B, Mak S, White R, Rekart ML. The unexpected impact of a Chlamydia trachomatis infection control program on susceptibility to reinfection. J Infect Dis. 2005;192:1836–44.

667. Su H, Morrison R, Messer R, Whitmire W, Hughes S, Caldwell HD. The effect of doxycycline treatment on the development of protective immunity in a murine model of chlamydial genital infection. J Infect Dis. 1999;180:1252–8.

668. Dicker LW, Mosure DJ, Levine WC, Black CM, Berman SM. Impact of Switching Laboratory tests on reported trends in Chlamydia trachomatis infections. Am J Epidemiol. 2000;151:430–5.

669. Atik B, Thanh TTK, Luong VQ, Lagree S, Dean D. Impact of annual targeted treatment on infectious trachoma and susceptibility to Reinfection. JAMA. 2006;296:1488–97.

670. Anderson I. Findings from trachoma study cast doubts on SAFE strategy. Lancet Infect Dis. 2006;6:690.

671. Mabey D, Bailey R, Solomon A, Burton M, Gilbert C, Foster A, et al. Letter to the Editor: Targeted Treatment of Active Trachoma. JAMA. 2007;297:588.

672. Dawson CR, Schachter J. Letter to the Editor: Targeted Treatment of Active Trachoma. JAMA. 2007;297:588–9.

673. Taylor HR, Duke BOL, Muñoz B. The selection of communities for treatment of onchocerciasis with ivermectin. Trop Med Parasitol. 1992;43:267–70.

674. Basilion EV, Kilima PM, Mecaskey JW. Simplification and improvement of height-based azithromycin treatment for paediatric trachoma. Trans R Soc Trop Med Hyg. 2005;99:6–12.

675. WHO Expert Committee on Onchocerciasis Control. Onchocerciasis and Its Control. Report of a WHO Expert Committee on Onchocerciasis Control. Geneva: World Health Organization; 1995.

676. Sutter EE, Ballard RC. Community participation in the control of trachoma in Gazankulu. Soc Sci Med. 1983;17:1813–7.

677. Lynch M, West S, Munoz B, Frick KD, Mkocha H. Azithromycin treatment coverage in Tanzanian children using community volunteers. Ophthalmic Epidemiol. 2003;10:167–75.

678. Solomon AW, Akudibillah J, Abugri P, Hagan M, Foster A, Bailey RL, et al. Pilot study of the use of community volunteers to distribute azithromycin for trachoma control in Ghana. Bull World Health Organ. 2001;79:8–14.

679. Amazigo U, Okeibunor J, Matovu V, Zoure H, Bump J, Seketeli A. Performance of predictors: evaluating sustainability in community-directed treatment projects of the African programme for onchocerciasis control. Soc Sci Med. 2007;64:2070–82.

680. Ngondi J, Onsarigo A, Matthews F, Reacher M, Brayne C, Baba S, et al. Effect of 3 years of SAFE (surgery, antibiotics, facial cleanliness, and environmental change) strategy for trachoma control in southern Sudan: a cross sectional study. Lancet. 2006;368:589–95.

681. Turner A, Islam A, Taylor H. Factors influencing the outcome of azithromycin mass treatment for trachoma. Unpublished 2005.

682. Lietman T, Porco T, Dawson C, Blower S. Global elimination of trachoma: How frequently should we administer mass chemotherapy? Nat Med. 1999;5:572–6.

683. Gaynor BD, Yi E, Lietman T. Rationale for mass antibiotic distribution for trachoma elimination. Int Ophthalmol Clin. 2002;42:85–92.

684. Lee DC, Chidambaram AD, Porco TC, Lietman TM. Seasonal effects in the elimination of trachoma. Am J Trop Med Hyg. 2005;72:468–70.

685. Mariotti SP. New steps toward eliminating blinding trachoma. N Engl J Med. 2004;351:2004–7.

686. Hughes WT. A tribute to toilet paper. Rev Infect Dis. 1988;19:218–22.

687. De Sole G, Martel E. Test of the prevention of blindness health education programme for Ethiopian primary schools. Int Ophthalmol. 1988;11:255–9.

688. Peach HG, Piper SJ, Devanesen D, Dixon B, Jeffries C, Braun P, et al. Northern Territory trachoma control and eye health committee's randomised controlled trial of the effect of eye drops and eye washing on follicular trachoma among aboriginal

children. Annual Report of the Menzies School of Health Research. 1986:74–6.

689. Edwards T, Cumberland P, Hailu G, Todd J. Impact of Health Education on Active Trachoma in Hyperendemic Rural Communities in Ethiopia. Ophthalmology. 2006;113:548–55.

690. McCauley AP. Household decisions among the Gogo people of Tanzania: determining the roles of men, women and the community in implementing a trachoma prevention program. Soc. Sci Med. 1992;34:817–24.

691. Emerson P, Lindsay SW, Walraven GEL, Faal H, Bogh C, Lowe K, et al. Effect of fly control on trachoma and diarrhoea. Lancet. 1999;353: 1401–3.

692. Simms VM, Makalo P, Bailey RL, Emerson PM. Sustainability and acceptability of latrine provision in The Gambia. Trans R Soc Trop Med Hyg. 2005;99:631–7.

693. Resnikoff S, Peyramaure F, Bagayogo CO, Huguet P. Health Education and Antibiotic Therapy in Trachoma Control. Rev Int Trach Pathol Ocul Trop Subtrop Sante Publique. 1995;72:89–98,101–10.

694. Rabiu M, Alhassan M, Ejere H. Environmental sanitary interventions for preventing active trachoma. Cochrane Database System Rev 2005; Issue 2. Art No:CD004003. DOI:10. 1002/14651858. CD004003.pub2.:1–2.

695. Kowal E. Mutual obligation and Indigenous health: thinking through incentives and obligations. Med J Aust. 2006;184:292–3.

696. Mak DB. Better late than never: a national approach to trachoma control. Med J Aust. 2006;184:487–8.

697. Kuper H, Solomon AW, Buchan JC, Zondervan M, Mabey D, Foster A. Participatory evaluations of trachoma control programmes. Trop Med Int Health. 2005;10:764–72.

698. Astle WF, Wiafe B, Ingram AD, Mwanga M, Glassco CB. Trachoma control in southern Zambia – an international team project employing the SAFE strategy. Ophthalmic Epidemiol. 2006;13:227–36.

699. Ewald DP, Hall GV, Franks CC. An evaluation of a SAFE-style trachoma control program in Central Australia. Med J Aust. 2003;178:65–8.

700. Lansingh VC. Primary health care approach to trachoma control in Aboriginal communities in Central Australia [PhD]. Melbourne: University of Melbourne; 2005.

701. Thylefors B, Négrel A-D, Pararajasegaram R, Dadzie KY. Global data on blindness. Bull World Health Organ. 1995;73:115–21.

702. Resnikoff S, Pascolini D, Etya'ale D, Kocur I, Pararajasegaram R, Pokharel GP, et al. Global data on visual impairment in the year 2002. Bull World Health Organ. 2004;82:844–51.

703. Melese M, Gaynor B, Yi E, Whitcher JP, Lietman T. What more is there to learn about trachoma? Br J Ophthalmol. 2003;87:521–2.

704. Tabbara KF, Al-Omar OM. Trachoma in Saudi Arabia. Ophthalmic Epidemiol. 1997;4:127–40.

705. Dethlefs R. The trachoma status and blindness rates of selected areas of Papua New Guinea in 1979–80. Aust J Ophthalmol. 1982;10:13–18.

706. Hoechsmann A, Metcalfe N, Kanjaloti S, Godia H, Mtambo O, Chipeta T, et al. Reduction of trachoma in the absence of antibiotic treatment: Evidence from a population-based survey in Malawi. Ophthalmic Epidemiol. 2001;8:145–53.

707. Jha H, Chaudary JS, Bhatta R, Miao Y, Osaki-Holm S, Gaynor B, et al. Disappearance of trachoma from Western Nepal. (Brief Report). Clin Infect Dis. 2002;35:765–8.

708. Schiedler V, Bhatta RC, Miao Y, Bird M, Jha H, Chaudary JSP, et al. Pattern of antibiotic use in a trachomaendemic region of Nepal: implications for mass azithromycin distribution. Ophthalmic Epidemiol. 2003;10:31–6.

709. Chidambaram AD, Bird M, Schiedler V, Fry AM, Porco T, Bhatta RC, et al. Trachoma decline and widespread use of antimicrobial drugs. Emerging Infect Dis. 2004;10:1895–9.

710. Gaynor BD, Miao Y, Cevallos V, Jha H, Chaudary JS, Bhatta R, et al. Eliminating trachoma in areas with limited disease. Emerging Infect Dis. 2003;9:596–8.

711. Chidambaram JD, Lee DC, Porco TC, Lietman TM. Mass antibiotics for trachoma and the Allee effect. Lancet Infect Dis. 2005;5:194–6.

712. Ranson MK, Evans TG. The global burden of trachomatous visual impairment: I. Assessing prevalence. Int Ophthalmol. 1995–1996;19: 261–70.

713. Evans TG, Ranson MK. The global burden of trachomatous visual impairment: II. Assessing burden. Int Ophthalmol. 1995–1996;19:271–80.

714. Frick KD, Melia M, Buhrmann RB, West SK. Trichiasis and disability in a trachoma-endemic area of Tanzania. Arch Ophthalmol. 2001;119:1839–44.

715. Taylor HR, Keeffe JE, Vu HTV. Clear Insight: the Economic Impact and Cost of Vision Loss in Australia. Melbourne: Centre for Eye Research Australia; 2004.

716. Evans TG, Ranson MK, Kyaw TA, Ko CK. Cost effectiveness and cost utility of preventing trachomatous visual impairment: lessons from 30 years of trachoma control in Burma. Br J Ophthalmol. 1996;80:880–9.

717. Baltussen RM, Sylla M, Frick KD, Mariotti SP. Cost-effectiveness of trachoma control in seven world regions. Ophthalmic Epidemiol. 2005:91–101.

718. Frick KD, Lietman TM, Holm SO, Jha HC, Chaudary JSP, Bhatta RC. Cost-effectiveness of trachoma control measures: comparing targeted household treatment and mass treatment of children. Bull World Health Organ. 2001;79: 201–7.

719. Frick KD, Lynch M, West S, Munoz B, Mkocha HA. Household willingness to pay for azithromycin treatment for trachoma control in the United Republic of Tanzania. Bull World Health Organ. 2003;81:101–7.

720. Frick KD, Colchero MA, Dean D. Modeling the economic net benefit of a potential vaccination program against ocular infection with Chlamydia trachomatis. Vaccine. 2004;22:689–96.

721. Bailey R, Lietman T. The SAFE strategy for the elimination of trachoma by 2020: will it work? Bull World Health Organ. 2001;79:233–6.

722. Wellcome Trust. Topics in International Health – Trachoma 2nd Edition: A guide to trachoma and the SAFE strategy, May 2005.

723. <http://www.cartercenter.org>, viewed September 2006.

724. Kumaresan JA, Mecaskey JW. The global elimination of blinding trachoma: progress and promise. Am J Trop Med Hyg. 2003;69:24–8.

725. <http://www.trachoma.org>. International Trachoma Initiative, viewed September 2006.

726. International Trachoma Initiative. 2005 Annual Report; 2005.

727. <http://www.pfizer.com/pfizer/history/1998.jsp>. Exploring Our History.1951–1999.1998– Trachoma; 2006, viewed September 2006.

728. Reich MR. Public-private partnerships for public health. Nature. 2000;6:617–20.

729. Molyneux DH, Nantulya V. Public-private partnerships in blindness prevention: reaching beyond the eye. Eye. 2005;19:1050–6.

730. Omura S, Crump A. The life and times of ivermectin – a success story. Nat Rev Microbiol. 2004;2:984–989.

731. Knirsch C, Mecaskey J, Chami-Khazraji Y, Kilima P, West S, Cook J. Trachoma Elimination and a Public Private Partnership: The International Trachoma Initiative (ITI). In: Schachter J, Christiansen G, Clarke IN, Hammerschlag MR, Kaltenboeck B, Kuo C-C, et al., editors. Chlamydial Infections. Proceedings of the Tenth International Symposium on Human Chlamydial Infections, June 16–21, 2002, Antalya – Turkey. San Francisco, CA 94110: International Chlamydia Symposium; 2002; 485–94.

732. Selingsen R. Personal Communication. 2007.

733. WHO. State of the World's Sight: VISION 2020: the Right to Sight: 1999–2005. Geneva: World Health Organization; 2005.

734. <http://www.un.org/milleniumgoals>. UN Millennium Goals; 2005, viewed September 2006.

735. Rheingans R, Dreibelbis R, Freeman MC. Beyond the Millennium Development Goals: Public health challenges in water and sanitation. Global Public Health. 2006;1:31–48.

736. Carrin M. The Millennium Development Goals and Vision 2020. IAPB News. 2005.

737. Molyneux DH, Hotez PJ, Fenwick A. rapid-impact how a policy of integrated control for Africa's neglected tropical diseases could benefit the poor. PLoS Med. 2005;2:1–13.

738. World Health Organization. Resolution of the World Health Assembly on the Elimination of Avoidable Blindness Resolution. World Health Assembly 2003;WHA56.26.

739. WHO. Resolution of the World Health Assembly on prevention of avoidable blindness and visual impairment. Geneva: <http://www.who.int/blindness/publications/WHA_EB/en/index.html>; 2006, viewed September 2006.

740. Maitchouk IF. Report on trachoma control in the eastern Mediterranean region (evaluation). Regional Office for the Eastern Mediterranean: World Health Organization; 1976.

741. Mak DB, O'Neill LM, Herceg A, McFarlane H. Prevalence and control of trachoma in Australia, 1997–2004. Comm Dis Intell. 2006;30:236–47.

742. Collinson H, Mein J, Coleman K. Trachoma Control Program 2005. Kimberley Population Health Unit Bulletin. 2006:8–9.

743. Ryan H. Trachoma in Australia. XXI Concilium Ophthalmologicum, Mexico 1970:1944–7.

744. Mann I. Probable origins of trachoma in Australia. Bull World Health Organ 1956;16:1165.

745. Dampier W. Dampier's Voyages. London: E. Grant Richards; 1906.

746. Taylor HR. Racial variation in visual acuity and refractive error. Invest Ophthalmol Vis Sci. 1978;17 (suppl):113.

747. Webb SG. Prehistoric eye disease (trachoma?) in Australian Aborigines. Am J Physical Anthropol. 1990;81:91–100.

748. Webb RC. Personal Communication. 2001.

749. Elphinstone JJ. The health of Australian Aborigines with no previous association with Europeans. Med J Aust. 1971:293–301.

750. Barrett JW, Orr WF. Trachoma in the State of Victoria. Intercolonial Medical Journal 1909;September 20:450–5.

751. Anderson JR. Blindness in private practice. Med J Aust. 1939:680–8.

752. Webb RC. Medical practice in Central Northern Territory. Med J Aust. 1957:460–3.

753. Schneider M. A sociological study of the Aborigines in the Northern Territory and their eye disease. Med J Aust 1946:99–104.

754. Mann I, Rountree P. Geographic ophthalmology. A report on a recent survey of Australian Aborigines with an addendum on bacteriology. Am J Ophthalmol. 1968;66:1020–34.

755. Moore MC, Howarth WH, Wilson KJ, Derrington AW, Surman PG. Clinical and laboratory assessment of trachoma in South Australia. Med J Aust. 1965:441–6.

756. Hollows F, Corris P. Fred Hollows. An Autobiography. Balmain, NSW: Kerr Publishing Pty Ltd; 1992.

757. Hollows FC. The National Trachoma and Eye Health Program. Aust J Ophthalmol. 1977;5: 151–4.

758. Taylor HR. Eye Health in Aboriginal and Torres Strait Islander Communities. Canberra: Commonwealth of Australia; 1997.

759. Meredith SJ, Peach DG, Devanesen D. Trachoma in the Northern Territory of Australia, 1940–1986. Med J Aust. 1989;151:190–6.

760. Office for Aboriginal and Torres Strait Islander Health. Specialist Eye Health Guidelines for use in Aboriginal and Torres Strait Islander Populations. Canberra: Commonwealth of Australia; 2001.

761. Durkin SR, Casson RJ, Selva D, Newland HS. Prevalence of trachoma among a group of Aboriginal school children in remote South Australia. Clin Exp Ophthalmol. 2006;34:628–9.

762. Kain S, Morgan W, Riley D, Dorizzi K, Hogarth G, Yu D-Y. Prevalence of trachoma in school children of remote Western Australian communities between 1992 and 2003. Clin Exp Ophthalmol. 2007;35:119–23.

763. Van Buynder PG, Graham PJ. Trachoma in Australian Aboriginals in the Pilbara. Med J Aust. 1992;156:811.

764. Matters R, Wong I, Mak D. An outbreak of non-sexually transmitted gonococcal conjunctivitis in Central Australia and the Kimberly region. Comm Dis Intell. 1998;22:52–8.

765. Mak DB, Plant AJ. Trichiasis in Aboriginal people of the Kimberley region of Western Australia. Clin Exp Ophthalmol. 2001;29:7–11.

766. Landers J, Kleinschmidt A, Wu J, Burt B, Ewald D, Henderson T. Prevalence of cicatricial trachoma in an indigenous population of Central Australia: the Central Australian Trachomatous Trichiasis Study (CATTS). Clin Exp Ophthalmol. 2005;33:142–6.

767. Taylor V, Ewald D, Liddle H, Warchiver I. Review of the Implementation of the National Aboriginal and Torres Strait Islander Eye Health Program. Canberra: Commonwealth of Australia; 2004.

768. Laforest C, Durkin S, Selva D, Casson R, Newland H. Aboriginal versus non-Aboriginal ophthalmic disease: admission characteristics at the Royal Adelaide Hospital. Clin Exp Ophthalmol. 2006;34:324–32.

769. Wallace T. Trachoma treatment program in the Katherine region. The Northern Territory Communicable Diseases Bulletin 1996;3:13–15.

770. Johnson GH, Mak DB. An evaluation of a SAFE-style trachoma control program in central Australia. Med J Aust. 2003;179:116–17.

771. Lehmann D, Tennant MT, Silva DT, McAullay D, Lannigan F, Coates H, et al. Benefits of swimming pools in two remote Aboriginal communities in Western Australia: intervention study. Br Med J. 2003;327:415–19.

772. Anderson IPS. Mutual obligation, shared responsibility agreements & indigenous health strategy. Aust New Zealand Health Policy. 2006;3:10.

773. Australian Government. Response to the Review of the Implementation of the National Aboriginal and Torres Strait Islander Eye Health Program. Canberra: Commonwealth of Australia; 2004.

774. Bailie R. Housing. In: Carson B, Dunbar T, Chenhall RD, Bailie R, editors. Social Determinants of Indigenous Health. Crows Nest: Allen & Unwin; 2007:203–30.

775. Federal Race Discrimination Commissioner. Water: a report on the provision of water and sanitation in remote Aboriginal and Torres Strait Islander communities. Canberra: AGPS; 1994.

776. Communicable Diseases Network Australia. Guidelines for the public health management of trachoma in Australia. Canberra: Commonwealth of Australia; March 2006.

777. Thomas DP, Anderson IP. Getting the most from Indigenous health research. Med J Aust. 2006;184:500–1.

778. Si D, Bailie RS, Togni SJ, d'Abbs PHN, Robinson GW. Aboriginal health workers and diabetes care in remote community health centres: a mixed method analysis. Med J Aust. 2006;185:40–44.

779. Gruen RL, Bailie RS, Wang Z, Heard S, O'Rourke IC. Specialist outreach to isolated and disadvantaged communities: a population-based study. Lancet. 2006;368:130–38.

780. International Trachoma Initiative. 2006 Annual Report. New York: International Trachoma Initiative; 2006.

Index

Page numbers in **bold** refer to illustrations or tables.